Atlas of Human Cross-Sectional Anatomy

With CT and MR Images

Third Edition

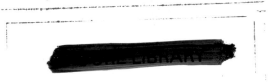
Atlas of Human Cross-Sectional Anatomy

With CT and MR Images

Third Edition

Donald R. Cahill, Ph.D.
Department of Anatomy
Mayo Medical School
Rochester, Minnesota

Matthew J. Orland, M.D.
Department of Medicine
Washington University
St. Louis, Missouri

Gary M. Miller, M.D.
Diagnostic Radiology
Mayo Clinic
Rochester, Minnesota

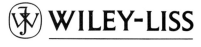 **WILEY-LISS**

A JOHN WILEY & SONS, INC., PUBLICATION
New York • Chichester • Brisbane • Toronto • Singapore

Address all Inquiries to the Publisher
Wiley-Liss, Inc., 605 Third Avenue, New York, NY 10158-0012

Printed in the United States of America.

Library of Congress Cataloging-in-Publication Data

Cahill, Donald R.
    Atlas of human cross-sectional anatomy : with CT and MR Images /
Donald R. Cahill, Matthew J. Orland, Gary M. Miller.—3rd ed.
        p.   cm.
    Includes bibliographical references and index.
    ISBN 0-471-59165-3 (alk. paper)
    1. Human anatomy—Atlases. 2. Tomography—Atlases. 3. Magnetic
resonance imaging—Atlases.   I. Orland, Matthew J. II. Miller,
Gary M. (Gary Michael), 1956–   . III. Title.
    [DNLM: 1. Anatomy, Regional—atlases. 2. Magnetic Resonance
Imaging—atlases. 3. Tomography, X-Ray Computed—atlases. QS 17
C132a 1955]
QM25.C24 1995
611′.0022′2—dc20
DNLM/DLC
for Library of Congress   94-42877
                                                                        CIP

The text of this book is printed on acid-free paper.
10 9 8 7 6 5 4 3 2

Dedicated to Susan, my wife.
Her pleasantness, encouragement, and continual
support have always helped in ways that
go beyond description.
DON

To Barbara, whose patience with this
project has been an inspiration.
MATT

To my wife, Joyce, and daughters,
Jaclyn and Natalie.
GARY

And to our colleagues and students
of anatomy, medicine, radiology, and surgery.
DRC, MJO, GMM

Contents

Preface

The *Atlas of Human Cross-Sectional Anatomy* is once again considerably revised and expanded in this, the third edition. Seven new chapters presenting anatomic drawings and magnetic resonance (MR) images of the shoulder, knee, and spine have been added. The chapters depicting the head and neck have been updated by Miller with newer, higher resolution MR images that show more anatomic detail and accommodate more labeling of identifiable soft tissue structures. Serial sections of the trunk, head and neck, and limbs are illustrated with the use of meticulously prepared pen and ink drawings by Cahill. Some of the computed tomography (CT) and MR images from the second edition presented by Carl C. Reading again appear in this edition.

All parts of the body are now displayed in the *Atlas* by CT and MR images of normal living subjects. The images were selected for correlation with the cadaver sections of the trunk, limbs, and head (including the new sections depicting the shoulder and the knee), except for the supplemental CT images of abdominal variations and the new MR images of the spine, which stand alone. The CT and MR images provide a clinical correlation with classical cross-sectional anatomy. The new axial images of the head were all presented from below, following the convention now developed among radiologists but not firmly established during the two previous publications of this atlas.

The anatomic sections were prepared by freezing and sectioning. Photographs were made of the frozen sections. The sections were then thawed and fixed, and dissection of the sections was performed to authenticate and complement the features shown on the surface photographs. The pen and ink drawings were made during dissection using the surface photographs as a guide. The drawings depict the basic histologic characteristics of the tissues and organs. Care has been taken not only to illustrate the surface image of a section, but also to demonstrate the important relationships occurring within a particular section not immediately apparent without the benefit of dissection. Such attention to detail complements radiographic correlations by demonstrating the thickness of a section rather than simply the surface features of the sections. Some of the original surface photographs of the trunk and head are still presented in this edition, but most have been replaced by CT and MR images as the work has evolved.

Orientation drawings were made from reassembled cadaver sections. These drawings were simplified to basic features to allow quick reference. New orientation drawings of the knee and shoulder defining sagittal and coronal planes were depicted from *above*, following classical anatomic conventions. In the spine, MR images were used for orientation. The axial images of the spine have been displayed from *below*.

Selection of CT or MR images was based on the current methods that best demonstrate anatomic detail. Regions of the body that are in involuntary motion, such as the trunk, are depicted primarily with CT images because the faster CT scanning time minimizes distortion of moving parts. On the other hand, MR imaging produces images of exquisite resolution of the head and limbs, which are regions that can be held motionless for the longer scanning times currently required. Because MR imaging can depict anatomy in any plane, it has fostered the inclusion of the sagittal and coronal views of the head, shoulder, knee, and spine in this *Atlas*. The zero degree axial images of the head and neck are now presented with MR images because they provide more detail and because this plane is more commonly imaged in the clinical setting using MR rather than CT. The technical note provides additional information on CT and MR imaging.

The *Atlas* is prepared in chapters, including (1) The Male Thorax (9 sections with drawings of both surfaces of the sections, photographs of the sections, and 8 matching CT scans), (2) The Male Abdomen (9 sections with drawings of both surfaces, photographs, and 9 matching CT scans), and an Upper Abdominal Supplement (4 drawings from a second cadaver, chosen to illustrate a common variation in upper abdominal anatomy, with 8 correlative CT scans including 4 scans that illustrate variations in liver morphology), (3) The Male Pelvis (8 sections with drawings of both surfaces, photographs, and 8 matching CT scans), (4) The Female Pelvis (14 sections, with drawings of both surfaces of the anatomic sections, photographs and 14 matching CT scans), (5) The Lower Limb (22 illustrated sections with 22 correlative MR images), (6) The Left Knee in Sagittal Planes (9 drawings with 9 correlative MR images), (7) The Left Knee in Coronal Planes (8 illustrated sections and 8 correlative MR images), (8) The Right Upper Limb (17 illustrated sections with 17 matching MR images), (9) The Right Shoulder in Sagittal Planes (9 illustrated sections and 9 matching MR images), (10) The Left Shoulder in Coronal Planes (6 illustrated sections with matching MR images), (11) The Head—20 Degrees from the Orbitomeatal Plane (7 sections with drawings of both surfaces and 14 matching CT scans), (12) The Head—0 Degrees from the Orbitomeatal Plane (14 sections with drawings of both surfaces and 28 matching MR images), (13) The Head in Sagittal Planes (6 sections with 15 drawings and 15 matching MR images), (14) The Head in Coronal Planes (6 sections with 12 illustrations and 12 matching MR images), (15) The Cervical Spine in Sagittal and Axial Planes (5 MR images), (16) The Thoracic Spine in Sagittal and Axial Planes (6 MR images), and (17) The Lumbar Spine in Sagittal, Axial, and Coronal Planes (10 MR images).

The anatomic drawings have been routinely presented with approximately 20–40 labels per drawing, typically shown above or beside a related CT or MR image which is less densely labeled. A nomenclature commonly used in American textbooks of anatomy, closely following the *Nomina Anatomica*, has been used in both the labeled drawings and images.

It is a pleasure to thank Associate Managing Editor, Rick Mumma, Head of Illustrations, Dean Gonzales, the senior staff members, Eric Swanson, Tom Mackey, Shawn Morton and Louise Page; and, indeed, the entire staff of Wiley-Liss, Inc., for their parts in bringing this book to fruition.

This *Atlas* is intended for use in the study of human cross-sectional anatomy and as a reference for the interpretation of CT and MR images obtained in clinical medicine. As such, this work is intended for a wide audience within the medical and paramedical fields including radiologists, anatomists, internists, surgeons, biomedical graduate students and radiologic technologists. As evidenced in the enclosed dedication, the authors hope that this new edition of the *Atlas of Human Cross-Sectional Anatomy* will continue to provide a valuable service to its readers.

Donald R. Cahill, PhD
Matthew J. Orland, MD
Gary M. Miller, MD

Technical Note: CT and MR Images in this Atlas

All MR Images were obtained using a 1.5 Tesla Superconducting Magnetic Resonance Imager (General Electric, Signa). The scans were obtained utilizing either a 512×512 matrix or 256×192 matrix (head, spine) or a 256×192 matrix (shoulder, knee), two signal acquisitions, and either a 3mm (head, shoulder, knee) or a 4mm (spine) slice thickness. Surface coils were used to obtain images of the spine while volume coils were used for the other body parts.

Because MR signal contrast is multiparametric and depends on proton density, T1 and T2 relaxation times, and blood flow, different pulse sequences were chosen to highlight specific anatomic aspects of the different regions of the body. Short repetition times (TR) and echo times (TE) were used to emphasize T1 relaxation time characteristics, whereas long repetition and echo times were used to highlight T2 relaxation time characteristics. Structures with a large number of mobile hydrogen protons, such as adipose tissue, generate a strong signal and appear bright on T1 and somewhat less bright on T2-weighted images. Other structures such as cortical bone and tendons, which have few mobile hydrogen protons, generate a weak signal and appear dark on both T1 and T2-weighted images. Fluids such as cerebrospinal fluid, bile, and urine have T1 and T2 characteristics which cause the fluid to appear dark on T1-weighted images but bright on T2-weighted images Blood vessels are unique structures in that they contain a rapidly flowing liquid which has the potential to generate a very strong signal. In this atlas imaging techniques were used to suppress this signal and therefore, generally, blood vessels appear as dark structures. There are many additional factors which contribute to the MR image which are beyond the scope of this brief introduction to the subject. The interested reader is referred to the bibliography at the end of this section.

The CT images were obtained using fourth generation CT scanners (GE 9800 and Picker 1200). Scans of ten mm slice thickness were obtained of the head and neck after the administration of iodinated intravenous contrast material. Similarly, scans of ten mm slice thickness were obtained of the abdomen and pelvis following the administration of both iodinated intravenous and oral contrast material. Window settings were adjusted to demonstrate the soft tissue components of the sections, except in the base of the skull where the window settings were chosen to highlight the bony structures. The appearance of the anatomic structures in the CT images depends upon the differential degree of attenuation of the x-ray beam by the different tissue types. Adipose, for example, causes very little attenuation of x-rays and therefore appears dark on CT scans. Bone, which is very dense, on the other hand, attenuates a considerable portion of the x-ray beam and appears white on the CT scans. Iodinated contrast material in the intestine and blood vessels also attenuates the beam to cause these structures to appear whiter than would be seen without contrast material.

Considerable effort went into acquiring the best possible CT and MR images for this atlas at the time it was sent to press. Already, however, new advances in both CT and MR imaging are on the horizon which promise to provide even better anatomic detail than is presently available. We look forward to these new advances in technology as a means to improve our understanding and to provide a greater insight into the cross-sectional anatomy of the human body.

References

Berquist TH, Ehman RL, Richardson ML: Magnetic resonance of the musculoskeletal system. New York, New York, Raven Press, 1987.

Brant-Zawadzki M, Norman D: Magnetic resonance imaging of the central nervous system. New York, New York, Raven Press, 1987.

Stark DD, Bradley W: Magnetic resonance imaging. St. Louis, Missouri, CV Mosby Company, 1988.

Young, SW: Magnetic resonance imaging–basic principles. New York, New York, Raven Press, 1988.

Gary M. Miller

The Male Thorax

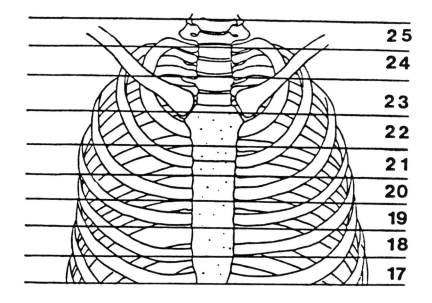

25
24
23
22
21
20
19
18
17

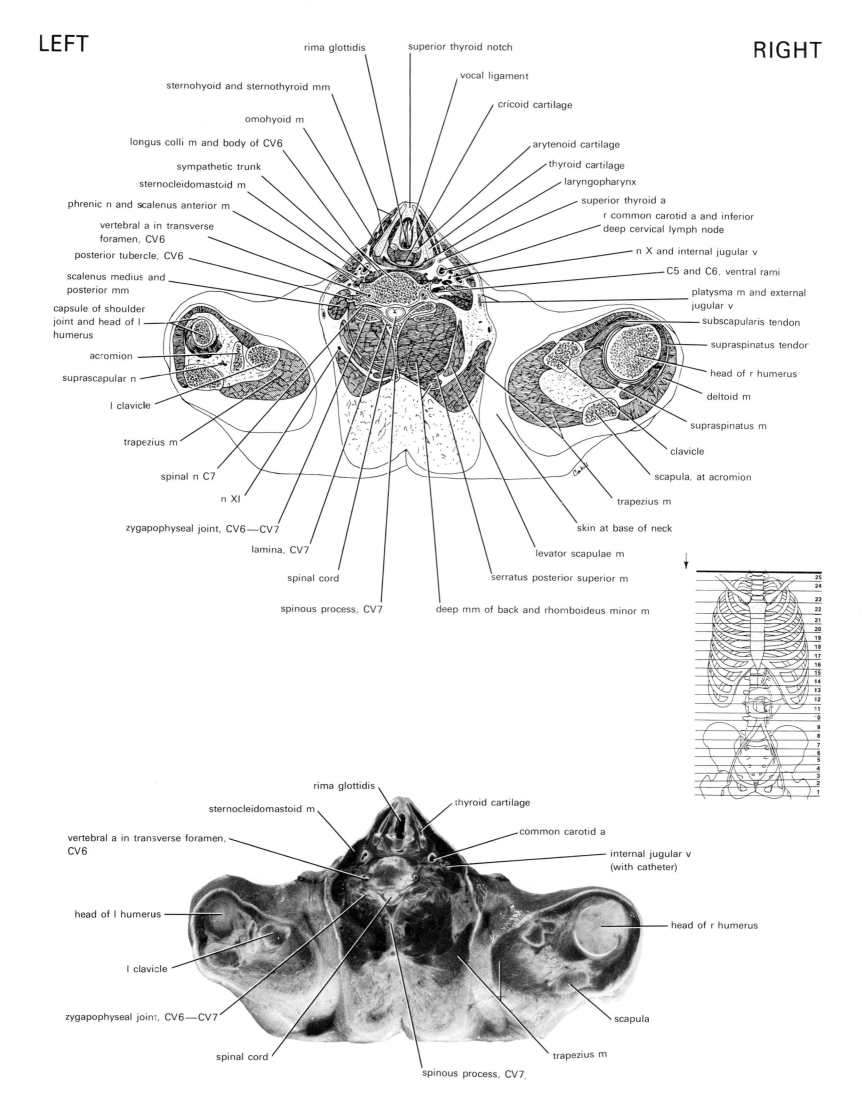

rima glottidis
superior thyroid notch
vocal ligament
sternohyoid and sternothyroid mm
cricoid cartilage
omohyoid m
longus colli m and body of CV6
arytenoid cartilage
sympathetic trunk
thyroid cartilage
sternocleidomastoid m
laryngopharynx
phrenic n and scalenus anterior m
superior thyroid a
vertebral a in transverse foramen, CV6
r common carotid a and inferior deep cervical lymph node
posterior tubercle, CV6
n X and internal jugular v
scalenus medius and posterior mm
C5 and C6, ventral rami
capsule of shoulder joint and head of l humerus
platysma m and external jugular v
subscapularis tendon
acromion
suprascapular n
supraspinatus tendon
l clavicle
head of r humerus
trapezius m
deltoid m
spinal n C7
supraspinatus m
n XI
clavicle
zygapophyseal joint, CV6—CV7
scapula, at acromion
lamina, CV7
trapezius m
spinal cord
skin at base of neck
spinous process, CV7
levator scapulae m
serratus posterior superior m
deep mm of back and rhomboideus minor m

rima glottidis
thyroid cartilage
sternocleidomastoid m
common carotid a
vertebral a in transverse foramen, CV6
internal jugular v (with catheter)
head of l humerus
head of r humerus
l clavicle
zygapophyseal joint, CV6—CV7
scapula
spinal cord
trapezius m
spinous process, CV7

Section 25 from above.

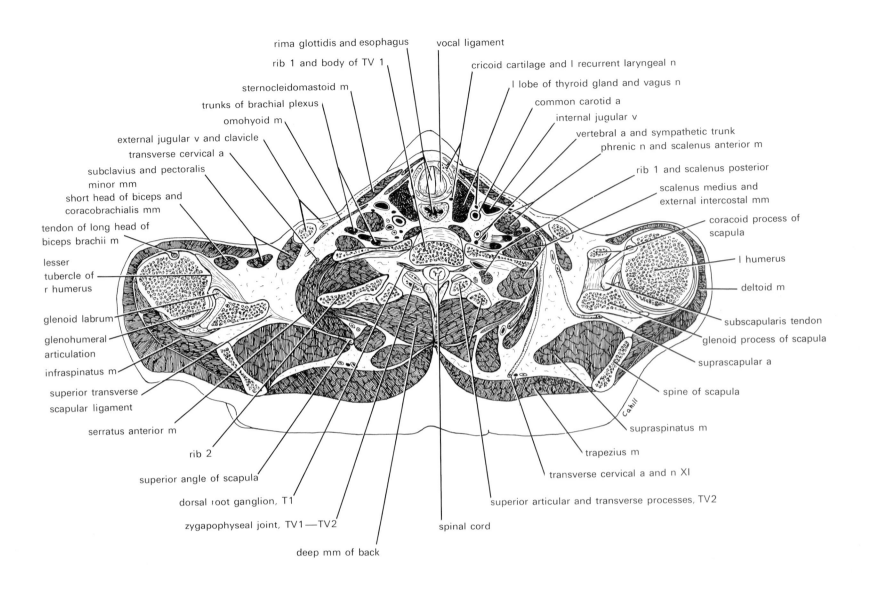

rima glottidis and esophagus
rib 1 and body of TV 1
sternocleidomastoid m
trunks of brachial plexus
omohyoid m
external jugular v and clavicle
transverse cervical a
subclavius and pectoralis minor mm
short head of biceps and coracobrachialis mm
tendon of long head of biceps brachii m
lesser tubercle of r humerus
glenoid labrum
glenohumeral articulation
infraspinatus m
superior transverse scapular ligament
serratus anterior m
rib 2
superior angle of scapula
dorsal root ganglion, T1
zygapophyseal joint, TV1—TV2
deep mm of back
spinal cord

vocal ligament
cricoid cartilage and l recurrent laryngeal n
l lobe of thyroid gland and vagus n
common carotid a
internal jugular v
vertebral a and sympathetic trunk
phrenic n and scalenus anterior m
rib 1 and scalenus posterior
scalenus medius and external intercostal mm
coracoid process of scapula
l humerus
deltoid m
subscapularis tendon
glenoid process of scapula
suprascapular a
spine of scapula
supraspinatus m
trapezius m
transverse cervical a and n XI
superior articular and transverse processes, TV2

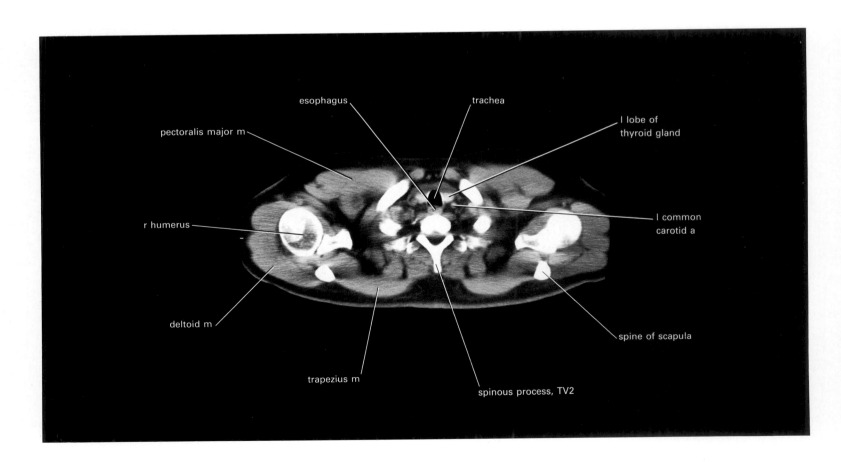

esophagus
trachea
pectoralis major m
l lobe of thyroid gland
r humerus
l common carotid a
deltoid m
spine of scapula
trapezius m
spinous process, TV2

Section 25 from below.

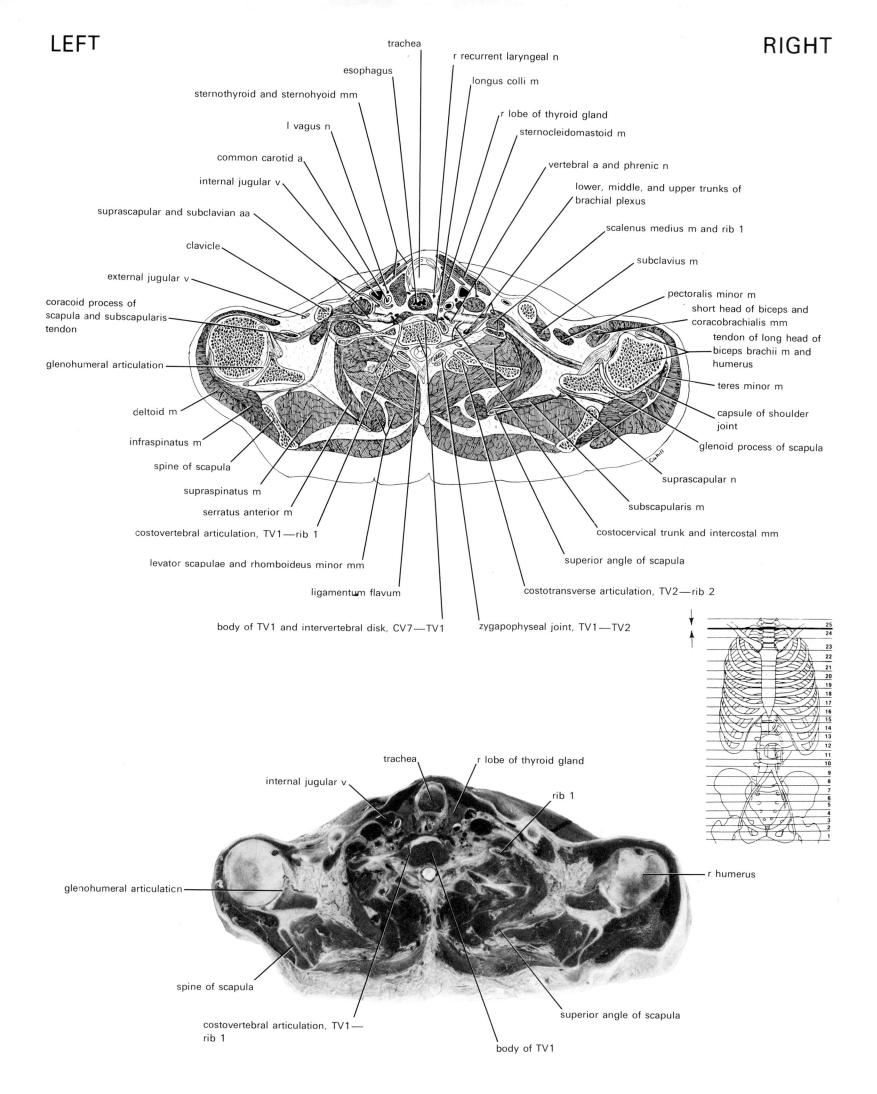

trachea
r recurrent laryngeal n
esophagus
longus colli m
sternothyroid and sternohyoid mm
l vagus n
r lobe of thyroid gland
sternocleidomastoid m
common carotid a
internal jugular v
vertebral a and phrenic n
lower, middle, and upper trunks of brachial plexus
suprascapular and subclavian aa
scalenus medius m and rib 1
clavicle
subclavius m
external jugular v
pectoralis minor m
short head of biceps and coracobrachialis mm
coracoid process of scapula and subscapularis tendon
tendon of long head of biceps brachii m and humerus
glenohumeral articulation
teres minor m
deltoid m
capsule of shoulder joint
infraspinatus m
glenoid process of scapula
spine of scapula
suprascapular n
supraspinatus m
subscapularis m
serratus anterior m
costocervical trunk and intercostal mm
costovertebral articulation, TV1—rib 1
superior angle of scapula
levator scapulae and rhomboideus minor mm
costotransverse articulation, TV2—rib 2
ligamentum flavum
body of TV1 and intervertebral disk, CV7—TV1
zygapophyseal joint, TV1—TV2

trachea
r lobe of thyroid gland
internal jugular v
rib 1
r humerus
glenohumeral articulation
spine of scapula
superior angle of scapula
costovertebral articulation, TV1—rib 1
body of TV1

Section 24 from above.

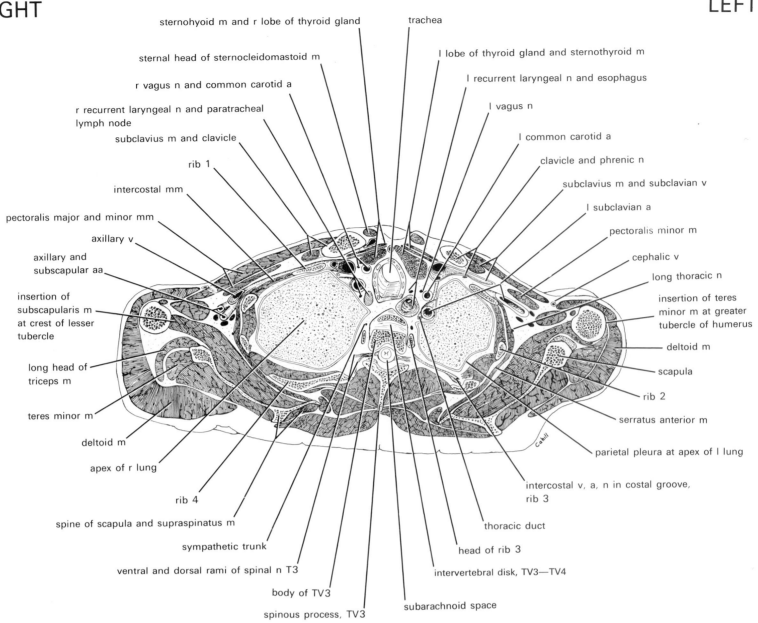

sternohyoid m and r lobe of thyroid gland

trachea

sternal head of sternocleidomastoid m

l lobe of thyroid gland and sternothyroid m

r vagus n and common carotid a

l recurrent laryngeal n and esophagus

r recurrent laryngeal n and paratracheal
lymph node

l vagus n

subclavius m and clavicle

l common carotid a

rib 1

clavicle and phrenic n

intercostal mm

subclavius m and subclavian v

pectoralis major and minor mm

l subclavian a

axillary v

pectoralis minor m

axillary and
subscapular aa

cephalic v

long thoracic n

insertion of
subscapularis m
at crest of lesser
tubercle

insertion of teres
minor m at greater
tubercle of humerus

deltoid m

long head of
triceps m

scapula

teres minor m

rib 2

deltoid m

serratus anterior m

apex of r lung

parietal pleura at apex of l lung

rib 4

intercostal v, a, n in costal groove,
rib 3

spine of scapula and supraspinatus m

thoracic duct

sympathetic trunk

head of rib 3

ventral and dorsal rami of spinal n T3

intervertebral disk, TV3—TV4

body of TV3

subarachnoid space

spinous process, TV3

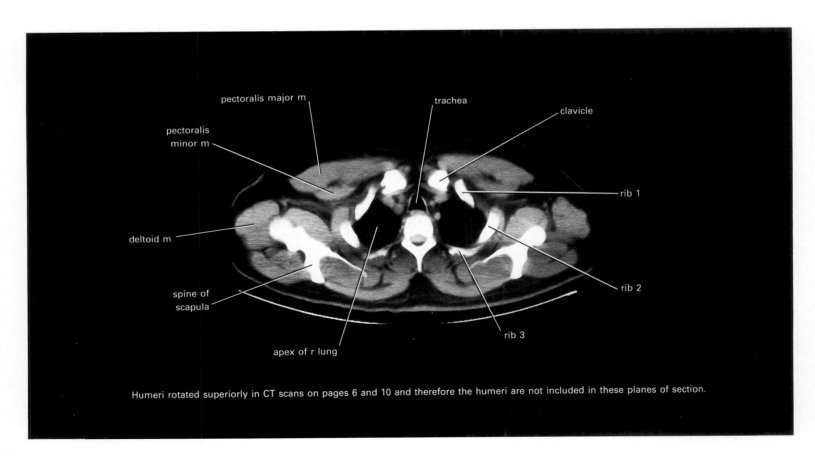

pectoralis major m

trachea

clavicle

pectoralis
minor m

rib 1

deltoid m

rib 2

spine of
scapula

rib 3

apex of r lung

Humeri rotated superiorly in CT scans on pages 6 and 10 and therefore the humeri are not included in these planes of section.

Section 24 from below.

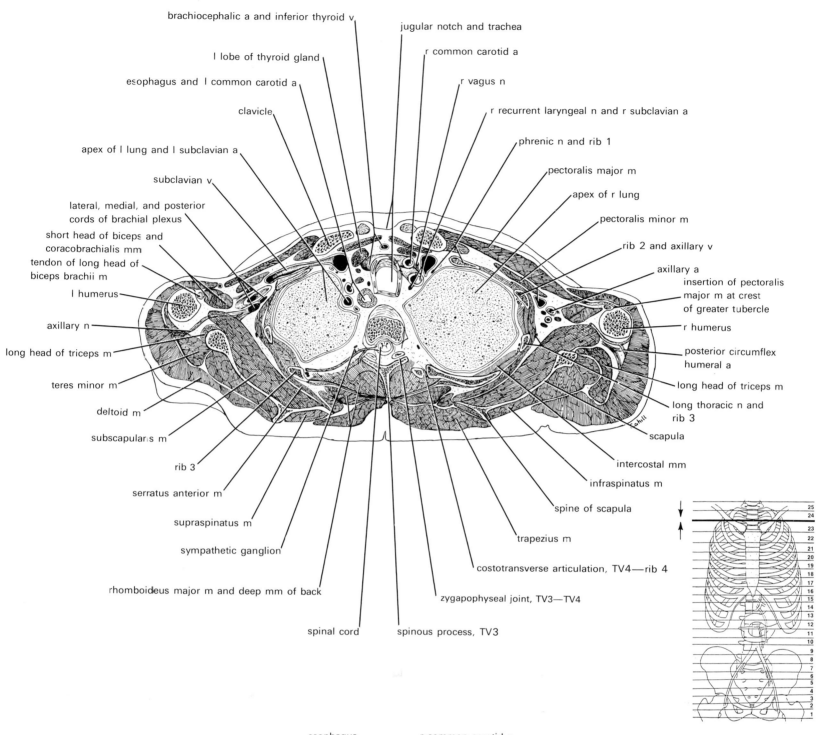

brachiocephalic a and inferior thyroid v

jugular notch and trachea

r common carotid a

l lobe of thyroid gland

r vagus n

esophagus and l common carotid a

r recurrent laryngeal n and r subclavian a

clavicle

phrenic n and rib 1

apex of l lung and l subclavian a

pectoralis major m

subclavian v

apex of r lung

lateral, medial, and posterior
cords of brachial plexus

pectoralis minor m

short head of biceps and
coracobrachialis mm

rib 2 and axillary v

tendon of long head of
biceps brachii m

axillary a

l humerus

insertion of pectoralis
major m at crest
of greater tubercle

axillary n

r humerus

long head of triceps m

posterior circumflex
humeral a

teres minor m

long head of triceps m

deltoid m

long thoracic n and
rib 3

subscapularis m

scapula

rib 3

intercostal mm

serratus anterior m

infraspinatus m

supraspinatus m

spine of scapula

sympathetic ganglion

trapezius m

rhomboideus major m and deep mm of back

costotransverse articulation, TV4—rib 4

zygapophyseal joint, TV3—TV4

spinal cord

spinous process, TV3

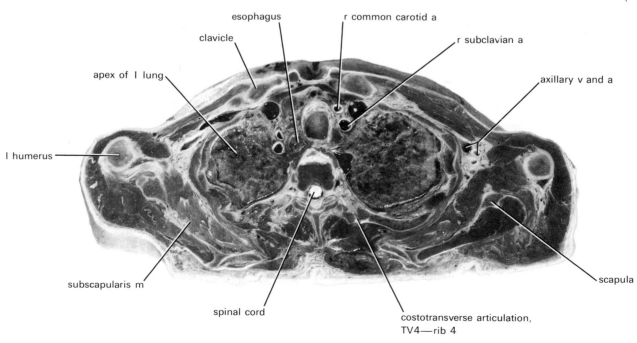

esophagus

r common carotid a

clavicle

r subclavian a

apex of l lung

axillary v and a

l humerus

subscapularis m

spinal cord

scapula

costotransverse articulation,
TV4—rib 4

Section 23 from above.

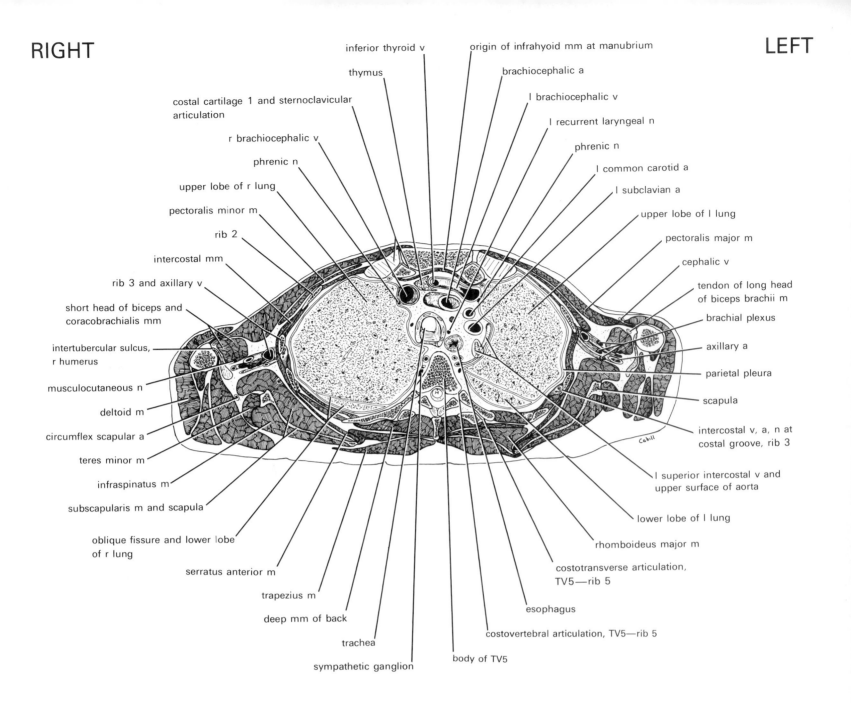

inferior thyroid v

origin of infrahyoid mm at manubrium

thymus

brachiocephalic a

costal cartilage 1 and sternoclavicular
articulation

l brachiocephalic v

r brachiocephalic v

l recurrent laryngeal n

phrenic n

phrenic n

upper lobe of r lung

l common carotid a

pectoralis minor m

l subclavian a

rib 2

upper lobe of l lung

intercostal mm

pectoralis major m

rib 3 and axillary v

cephalic v

short head of biceps and
coracobrachialis mm

tendon of long head
of biceps brachii m

brachial plexus

intertubercular sulcus,
r humerus

axillary a

musculocutaneous n

parietal pleura

deltoid m

scapula

circumflex scapular a

intercostal v, a, n at
costal groove, rib 3

teres minor m

infraspinatus m

l superior intercostal v and
upper surface of aorta

subscapularis m and scapula

lower lobe of l lung

oblique fissure and lower lobe
of r lung

rhomboideus major m

serratus anterior m

costotransverse articulation,
TV5—rib 5

trapezius m

esophagus

deep mm of back

costovertebral articulation, TV5—rib 5

trachea

body of TV5

sympathetic ganglion

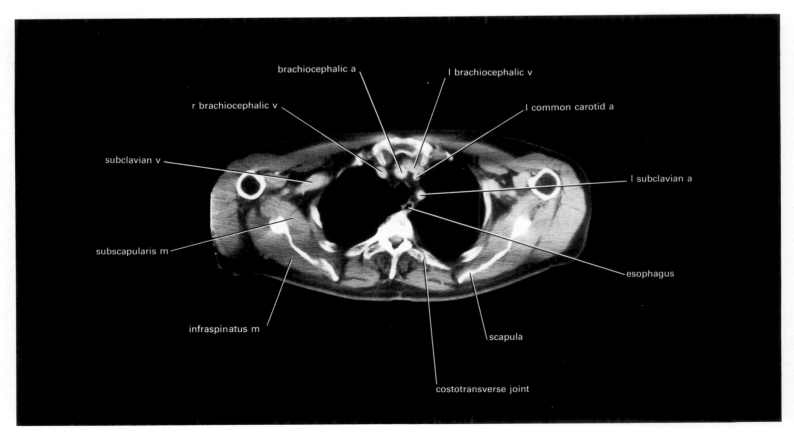

brachiocephalic a

l brachiocephalic v

r brachiocephalic v

l common carotid a

subclavian v

l subclavian a

subscapularis m

esophagus

infraspinatus m

scapula

costotransverse joint

Section 23 from below.

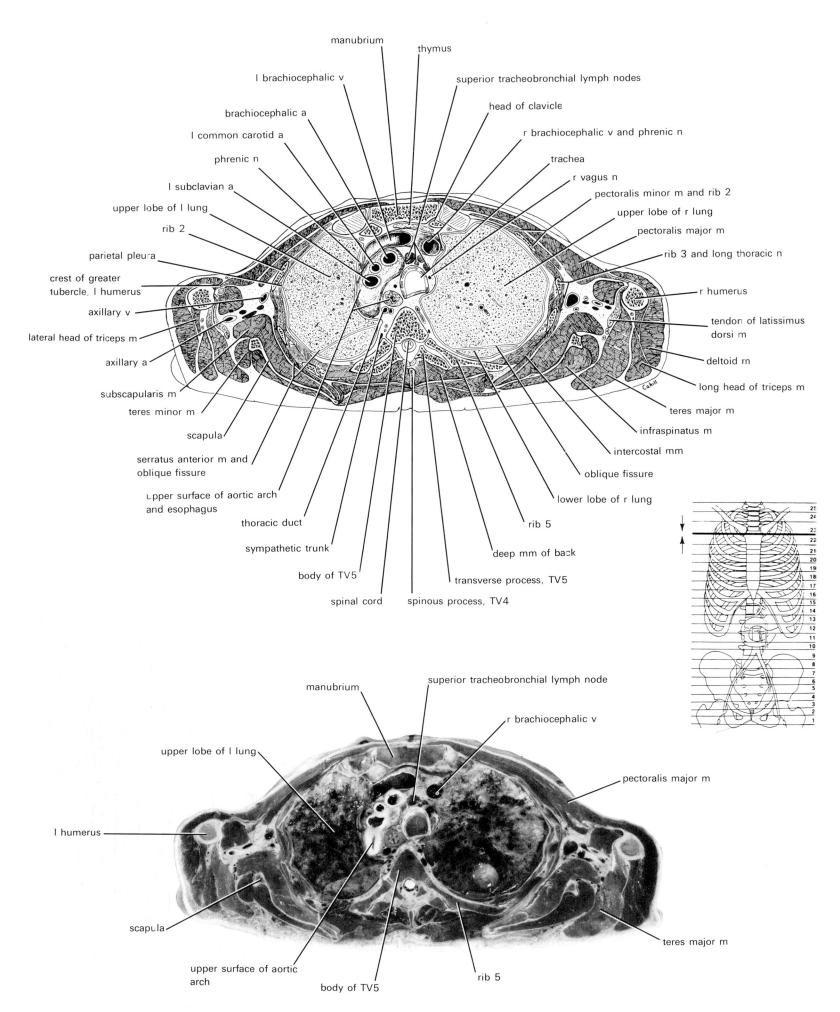

manubrium
thymus
l brachiocephalic v
superior tracheobronchial lymph nodes
brachiocephalic a
head of clavicle
l common carotid a
r brachiocephalic v and phrenic n
phrenic n
trachea
l subclavian a
r vagus n
upper lobe of l lung
pectoralis minor m and rib 2
rib 2
upper lobe of r lung
parietal pleura
pectoralis major m
crest of greater
tubercle, l humerus
rib 3 and long thoracic n
axillary v
r humerus
lateral head of triceps m
tendon of latissimus
dorsi m
axillary a
deltoid m
subscapularis m
long head of triceps m
teres minor m
teres major m
scapula
infraspinatus m
serratus anterior m and
oblique fissure
intercostal mm
upper surface of aortic arch
and esophagus
oblique fissure
thoracic duct
lower lobe of r lung
sympathetic trunk
rib 5
body of TV5
deep mm of back
spinal cord
transverse process, TV5
spinous process, TV4

manubrium
superior tracheobronchial lymph node
upper lobe of l lung
r brachiocephalic v
l humerus
pectoralis major m
scapula
teres major m
upper surface of aortic
arch
rib 5
body of TV5

Section 22 from above.

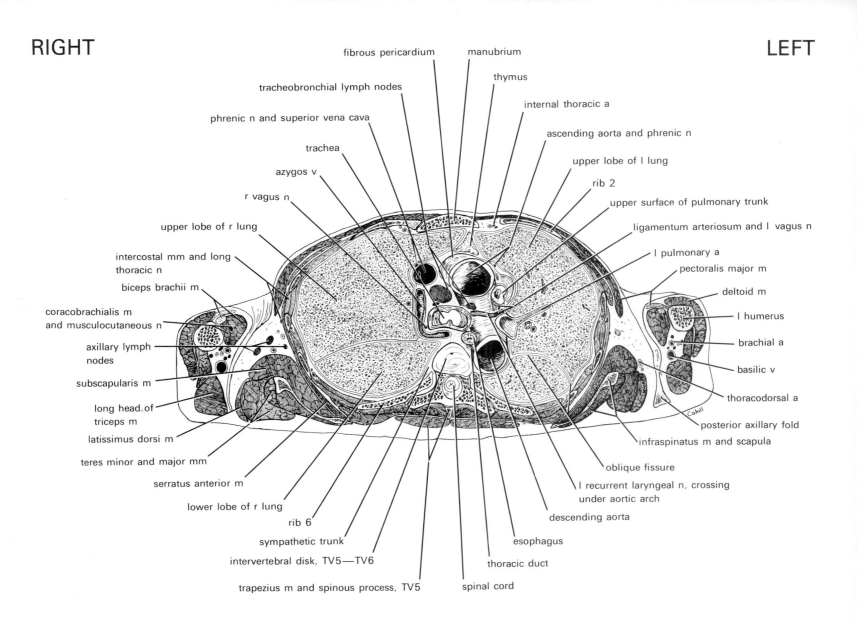

fibrous pericardium
manubrium
tracheobronchial lymph nodes
thymus
internal thoracic a
phrenic n and superior vena cava
ascending aorta and phrenic n
trachea
upper lobe of l lung
azygos v
rib 2
r vagus n
upper surface of pulmonary trunk
upper lobe of r lung
ligamentum arteriosum and l vagus n
intercostal mm and long
thoracic n
l pulmonary a
biceps brachii m
pectoralis major m
coracobrachialis m
and musculocutaneous n
deltoid m
l humerus
axillary lymph
nodes
brachial a
subscapularis m
basilic v
long head of
triceps m
thoracodorsal a
latissimus dorsi m
posterior axillary fold
teres minor and major mm
infraspinatus m and scapula
serratus anterior m
oblique fissure
lower lobe of r lung
l recurrent laryngeal n, crossing
under aortic arch
rib 6
descending aorta
sympathetic trunk
intervertebral disk, TV5—TV6
esophagus
trapezius m and spinous process, TV5
thoracic duct
spinal cord

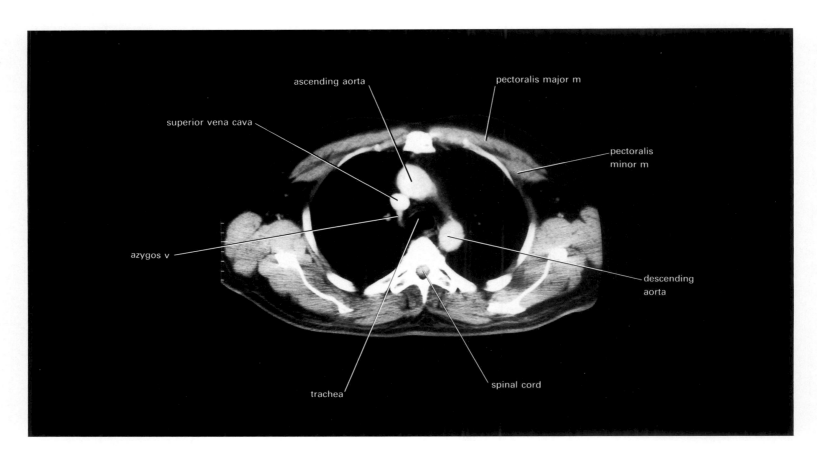

ascending aorta
pectoralis major m
superior vena cava
pectoralis
minor m
azygos v
descending
aorta
trachea
spinal cord

Section 22 from below.

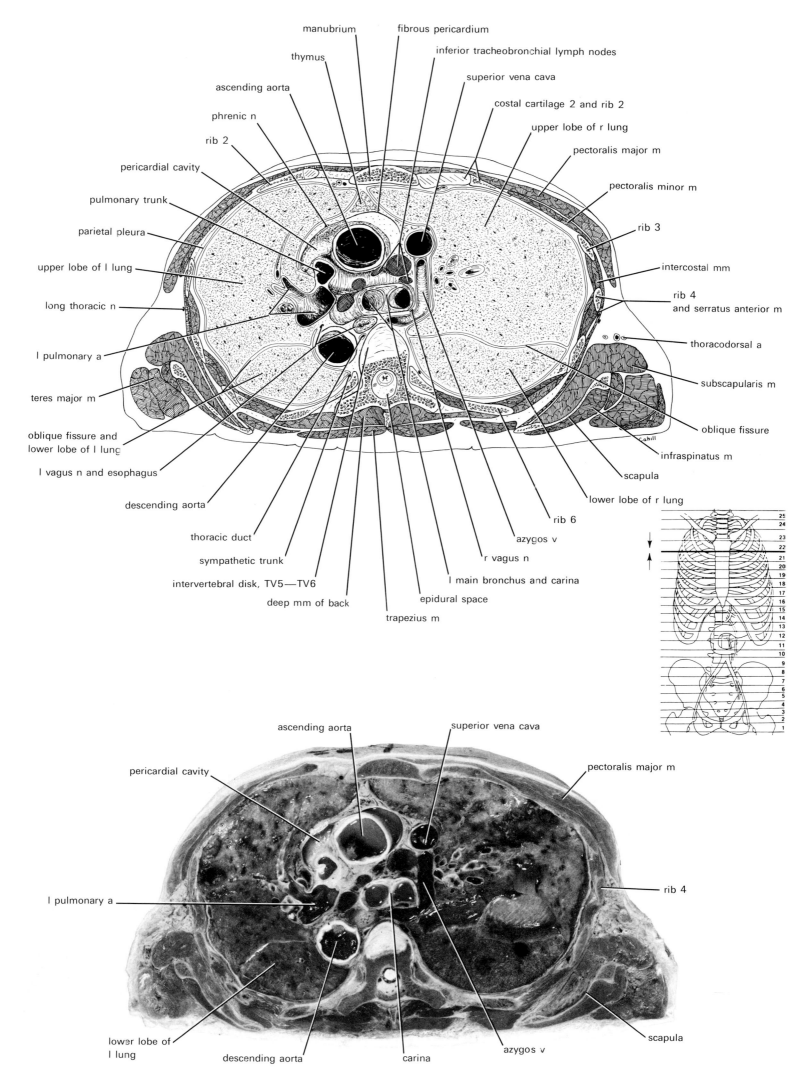

manubrium

fibrous pericardium

thymus

inferior tracheobronchial lymph nodes

ascending aorta

superior vena cava

phrenic n

costal cartilage 2 and rib 2

rib 2

upper lobe of r lung

pericardial cavity

pectoralis major m

pulmonary trunk

pectoralis minor m

parietal pleura

rib 3

upper lobe of l lung

intercostal mm

long thoracic n

rib 4
and serratus anterior m

l pulmonary a

thoracodorsal a

teres major m

subscapularis m

oblique fissure and
lower lobe of l lung

oblique fissure

l vagus n and esophagus

infraspinatus m

descending aorta

scapula

thoracic duct

lower lobe of r lung

sympathetic trunk

rib 6

intervertebral disk, TV5—TV6

azygos v

deep mm of back

r vagus n

trapezius m

l main bronchus and carina

epidural space

ascending aorta

superior vena cava

pericardial cavity

pectoralis major m

l pulmonary a

rib 4

lower lobe of
l lung

scapula

descending aorta

carina

azygos v

Section 21 from above.

RIGHT   LEFT

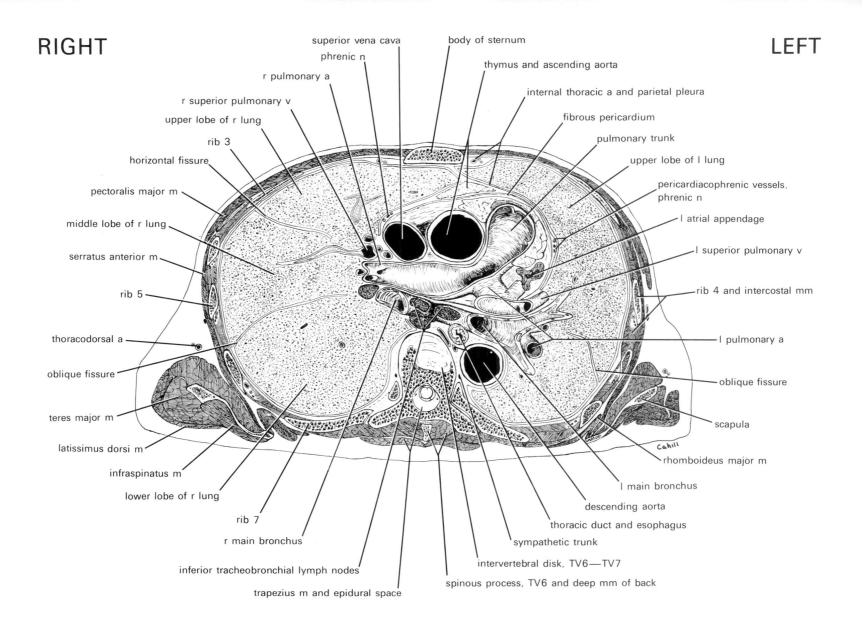

superior vena cava — body of sternum
phrenic n — thymus and ascending aorta
r pulmonary a — internal thoracic a and parietal pleura
r superior pulmonary v — fibrous pericardium
upper lobe of r lung — pulmonary trunk
rib 3 — upper lobe of l lung
horizontal fissure — pericardiacophrenic vessels, phrenic n
pectoralis major m — l atrial appendage
middle lobe of r lung — l superior pulmonary v
serratus anterior m — rib 4 and intercostal mm
rib 5 — l pulmonary a
thoracodorsal a — oblique fissure
oblique fissure — scapula
teres major m — rhomboideus major m
latissimus dorsi m — l main bronchus
infraspinatus m — descending aorta
lower lobe of r lung — thoracic duct and esophagus
rib 7 — sympathetic trunk
r main bronchus — intervertebral disk, TV6—TV7
inferior tracheobronchial lymph nodes — spinous process, TV6 and deep mm of back
trapezius m and epidural space

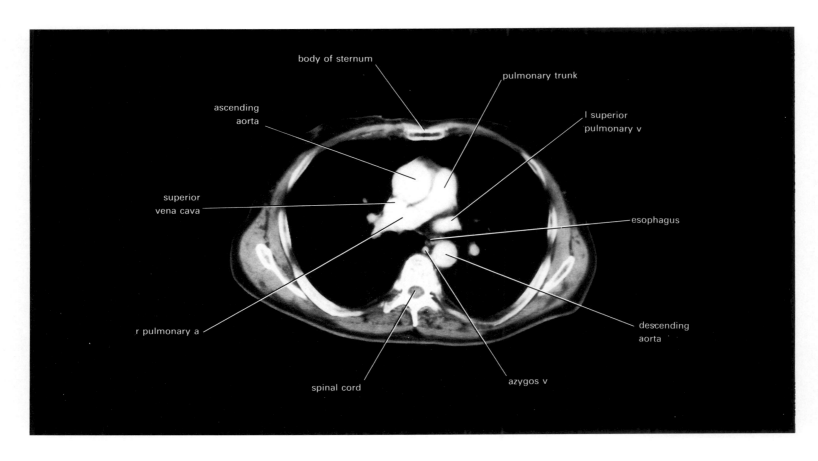

body of sternum
pulmonary trunk
ascending aorta
l superior pulmonary v
superior vena cava
esophagus
r pulmonary a
descending aorta
spinal cord
azygos v

Section 21 from below.

LEFT   RIGHT

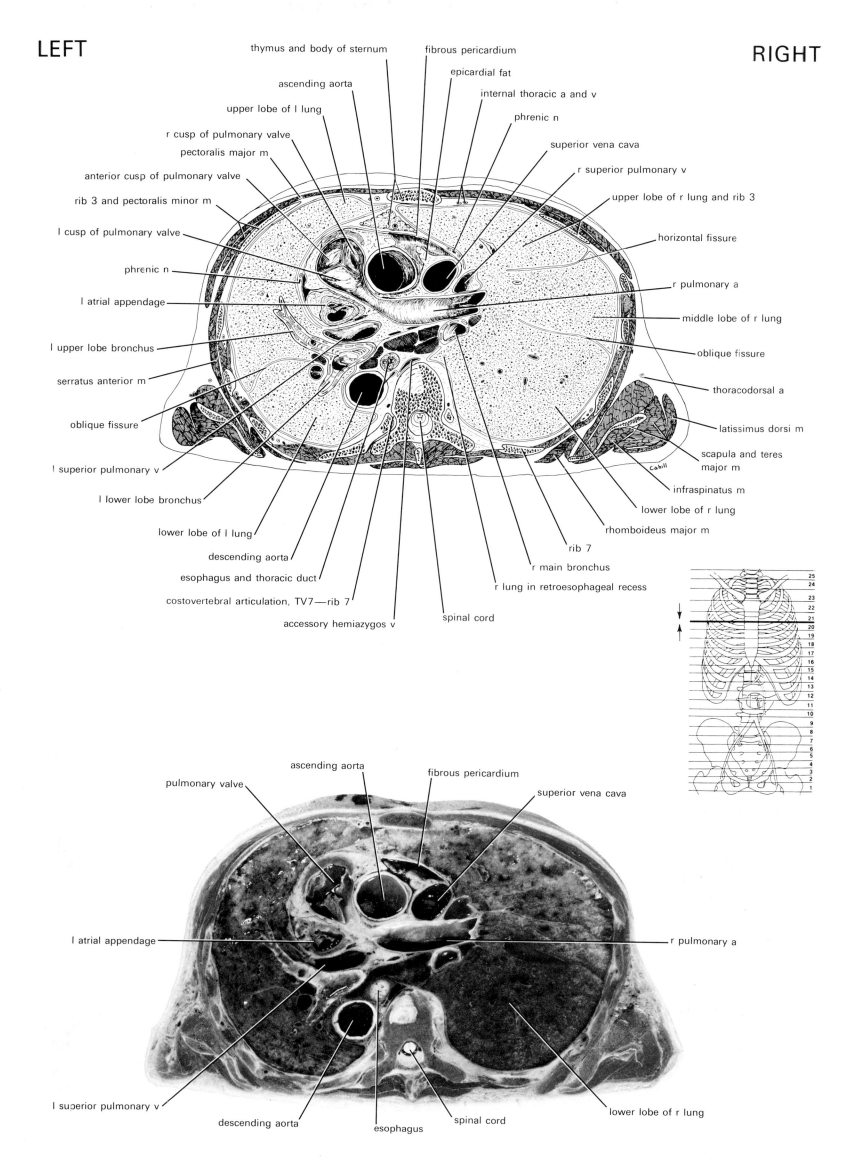

thymus and body of sternum — fibrous pericardium
ascending aorta — epicardial fat
upper lobe of l lung — internal thoracic a and v
r cusp of pulmonary valve — phrenic n
pectoralis major m — superior vena cava
anterior cusp of pulmonary valve — r superior pulmonary v
rib 3 and pectoralis minor m — upper lobe of r lung and rib 3
l cusp of pulmonary valve — horizontal fissure
phrenic n — r pulmonary a
l atrial appendage — middle lobe of r lung
l upper lobe bronchus — oblique fissure
serratus anterior m — thoracodorsal a
oblique fissure — latissimus dorsi m
l superior pulmonary v — scapula and teres major m
l lower lobe bronchus — infraspinatus m
lower lobe of l lung — lower lobe of r lung
descending aorta — rhomboideus major m
esophagus and thoracic duct — rib 7
costovertebral articulation, TV7—rib 7 — r main bronchus
accessory hemiazygos v — r lung in retroesophageal recess
spinal cord

pulmonary valve — ascending aorta — fibrous pericardium — superior vena cava
l atrial appendage — r pulmonary a
l superior pulmonary v — lower lobe of r lung
descending aorta — esophagus — spinal cord

Section 20 from above.

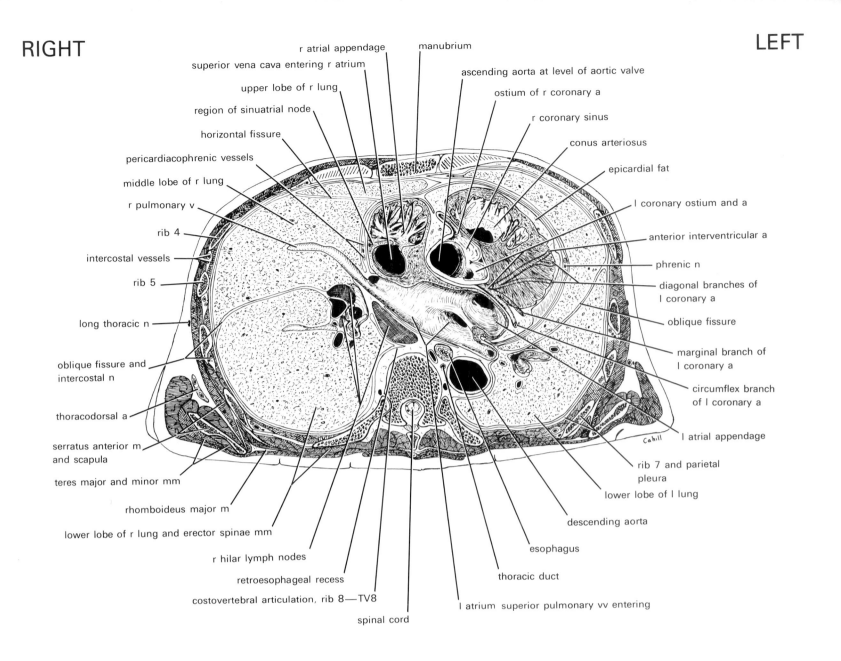

r atrial appendage
superior vena cava entering r atrium
upper lobe of r lung
region of sinuatrial node
horizontal fissure
pericardiacophrenic vessels
middle lobe of r lung
r pulmonary v
rib 4
intercostal vessels
rib 5
long thoracic n
oblique fissure and intercostal n
thoracodorsal a
serratus anterior m and scapula
teres major and minor mm
rhomboideus major m
lower lobe of r lung and erector spinae mm
r hilar lymph nodes
retroesophageal recess
costovertebral articulation, rib 8—TV8
spinal cord

manubrium
ascending aorta at level of aortic valve
ostium of r coronary a
r coronary sinus
conus arteriosus
epicardial fat
l coronary ostium and a
anterior interventricular a
phrenic n
diagonal branches of l coronary a
oblique fissure
marginal branch of l coronary a
circumflex branch of l coronary a
l atrial appendage
rib 7 and parietal pleura
lower lobe of l lung
descending aorta
esophagus
thoracic duct
l atrium superior pulmonary vv entering

Cahill

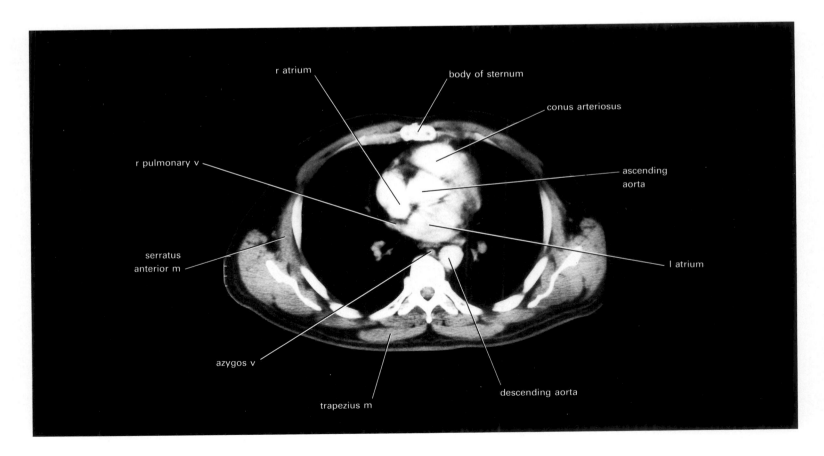

r atrium
body of sternum
conus arteriosus
r pulmonary v
ascending aorta
serratus anterior m
l atrium
azygos v
trapezius m
descending aorta

Section 20 from below.

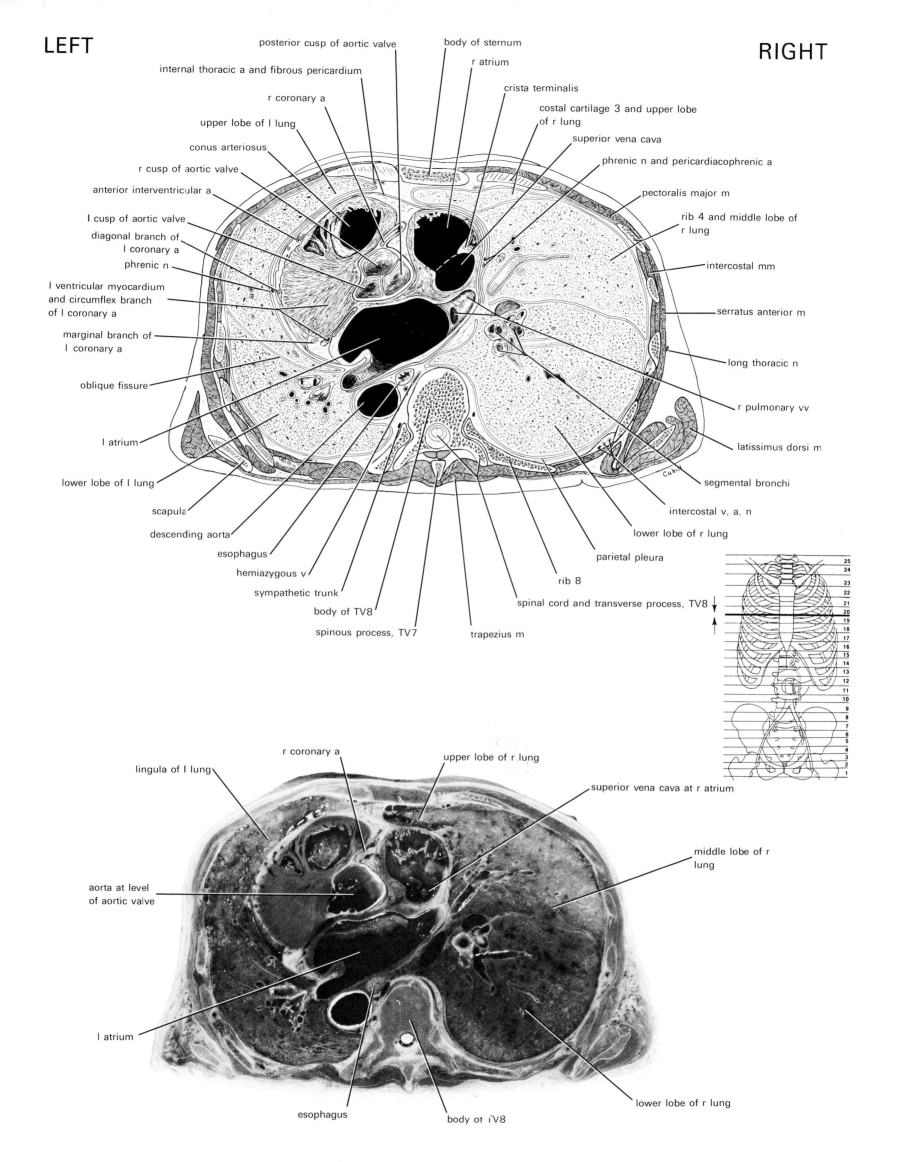

LEFT   RIGHT

posterior cusp of aortic valve
body of sternum
r atrium
internal thoracic a and fibrous pericardium
crista terminalis
r coronary a
costal cartilage 3 and upper lobe of r lung
upper lobe of l lung
superior vena cava
conus arteriosus
phrenic n and pericardiacophrenic a
r cusp of aortic valve
pectoralis major m
anterior interventricular a
rib 4 and middle lobe of r lung
l cusp of aortic valve
diagonal branch of l coronary a
intercostal mm
phrenic n
l ventricular myocardium and circumflex branch of l coronary a
serratus anterior m
marginal branch of l coronary a
long thoracic n
oblique fissure
r pulmonary vv
l atrium
latissimus dorsi m
lower lobe of l lung
segmental bronchi
scapula
intercostal v, a, n
descending aorta
lower lobe of r lung
esophagus
parietal pleura
hemiazygous v
rib 8
sympathetic trunk
spinal cord and transverse process, TV8
body of TV8
spinous process, TV7
trapezius m

Section 19 from above.

lingula of l lung
r coronary a
upper lobe of r lung
superior vena cava at r atrium
aorta at level of aortic valve
middle lobe of r lung
l atrium
esophagus
body of TV8
lower lobe of r lung

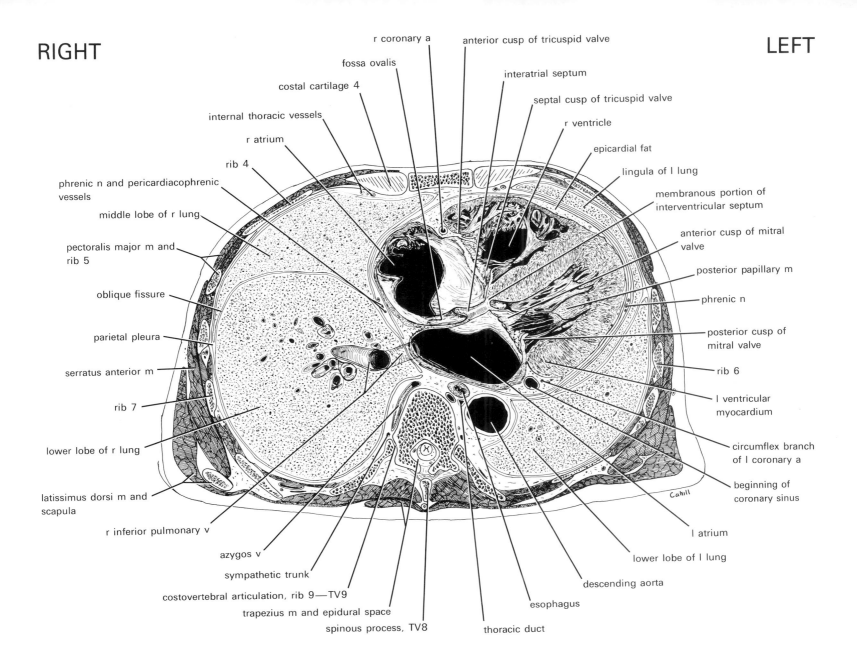

r coronary a
anterior cusp of tricuspid valve
fossa ovalis
interatrial septum
costal cartilage 4
septal cusp of tricuspid valve
internal thoracic vessels
r ventricle
r atrium
epicardial fat
rib 4
lingula of l lung
phrenic n and pericardiacophrenic
vessels
membranous portion of
interventricular septum
middle lobe of r lung
anterior cusp of mitral
valve
pectoralis major m and
rib 5
posterior papillary m
oblique fissure
phrenic n
parietal pleura
posterior cusp of
mitral valve
serratus anterior m
rib 6
rib 7
l ventricular
myocardium
lower lobe of r lung
circumflex branch
of l coronary a
beginning of
coronary sinus
latissimus dorsi m and
scapula
l atrium
r inferior pulmonary v
lower lobe of l lung
azygos v
descending aorta
sympathetic trunk
costovertebral articulation, rib 9—TV9
esophagus
trapezius m and epidural space
spinous process, TV8
thoracic duct

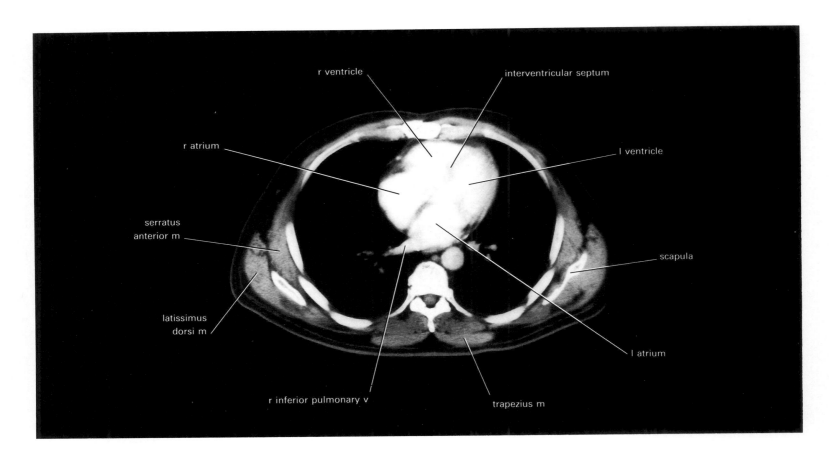

r ventricle
interventricular septum
r atrium
l ventricle
serratus
anterior m
scapula
latissimus
dorsi m
l atrium
r inferior pulmonary v
trapezius m

Section 19 from below.

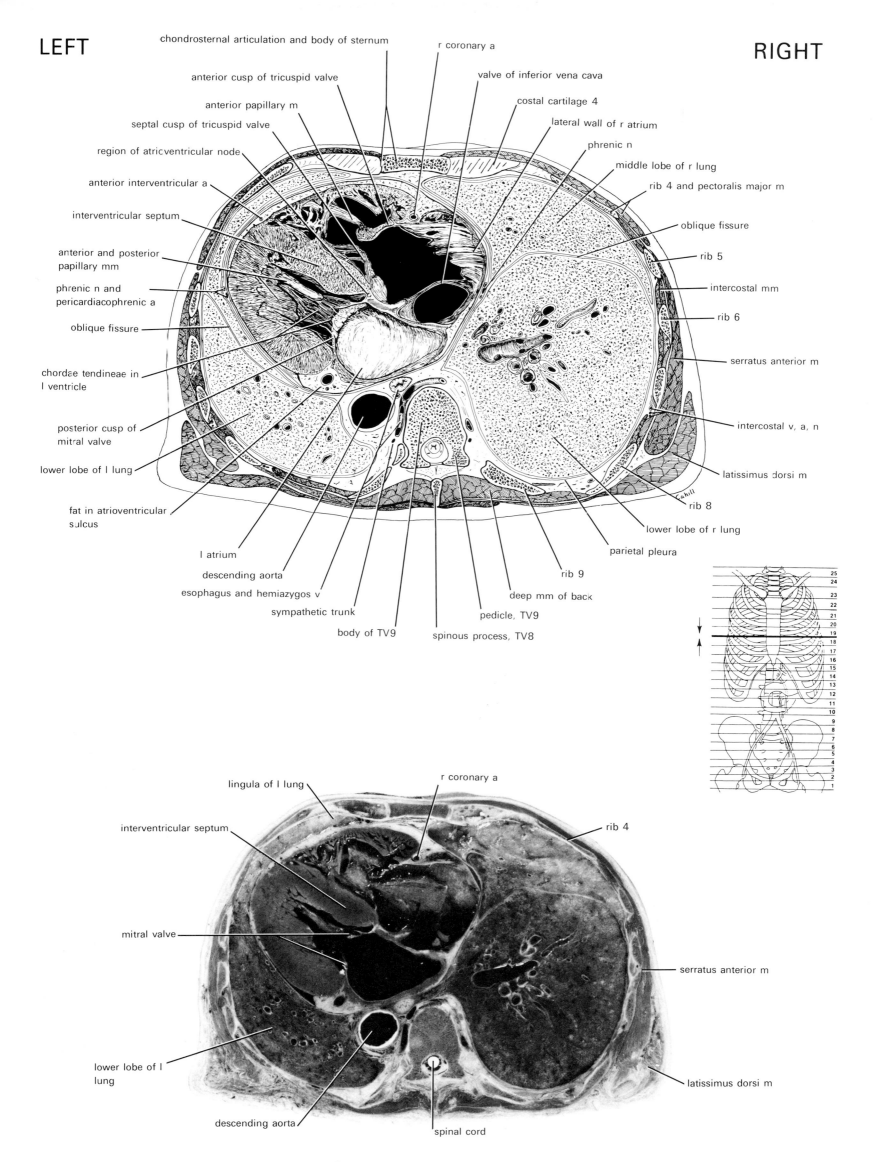

chondrosternal articulation and body of sternum
anterior cusp of tricuspid valve
anterior papillary m
septal cusp of tricuspid valve
region of atricventricular node
anterior interventricular a
interventricular septum
anterior and posterior papillary mm
phrenic n and pericardiacophrenic a
oblique fissure
chordae tendineae in l ventricle
posterior cusp of mitral valve
lower lobe of l lung
fat in atrioventricular sulcus

r coronary a
valve of inferior vena cava
costal cartilage 4
lateral wall of r atrium
phrenic n
middle lobe of r lung
rib 4 and pectoralis major m
oblique fissure
rib 5
intercostal mm
rib 6
serratus anterior m
intercostal v, a, n
latissimus dorsi m
rib 8
lower lobe of r lung
parietal pleura
rib 9
deep mm of back
pedicle, TV9
spinous process, TV8

l atrium
descending aorta
esophagus and hemiazygos v
sympathetic trunk
body of TV9

lingula of l lung
r coronary a
interventricular septum
rib 4
mitral valve
serratus anterior m
lower lobe of l lung
descending aorta
spinal cord
latissimus dorsi m

Section 18 from above.

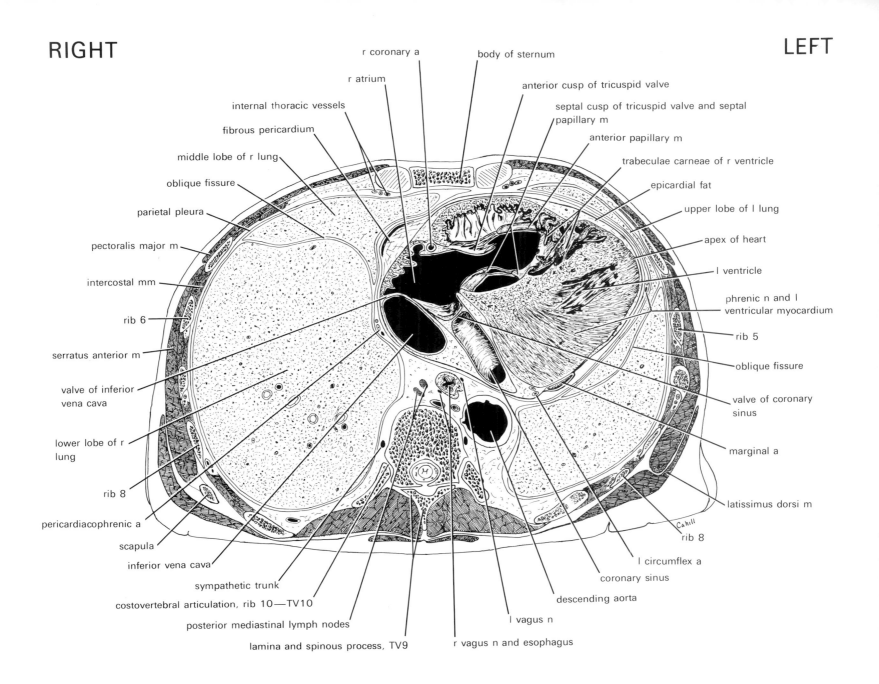

r coronary a
body of sternum
r atrium
anterior cusp of tricuspid valve
internal thoracic vessels
septal cusp of tricuspid valve and septal papillary m
fibrous pericardium
anterior papillary m
middle lobe of r lung
trabeculae carneae of r ventricle
oblique fissure
epicardial fat
parietal pleura
upper lobe of l lung
pectoralis major m
apex of heart
intercostal mm
l ventricle
rib 6
phrenic n and l ventricular myocardium
serratus anterior m
rib 5
valve of inferior vena cava
oblique fissure
valve of coronary sinus
lower lobe of r lung
marginal a
rib 8
latissimus dorsi m
pericardiacophrenic a
rib 8
scapula
l circumflex a
inferior vena cava
coronary sinus
sympathetic trunk
descending aorta
costovertebral articulation, rib 10—TV10
l vagus n
posterior mediastinal lymph nodes
r vagus n and esophagus
lamina and spinous process, TV9

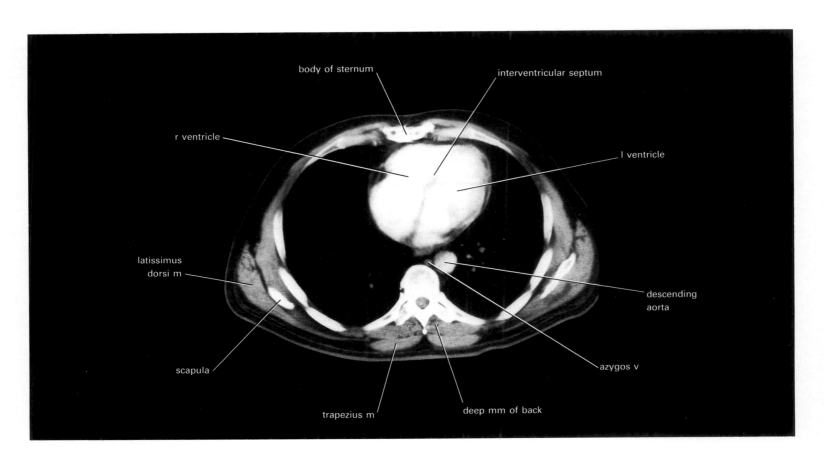

body of sternum
interventricular septum
r ventricle
l ventricle
latissimus dorsi m
descending aorta
scapula
azygos v
trapezius m
deep mm of back

Section 18 from below.

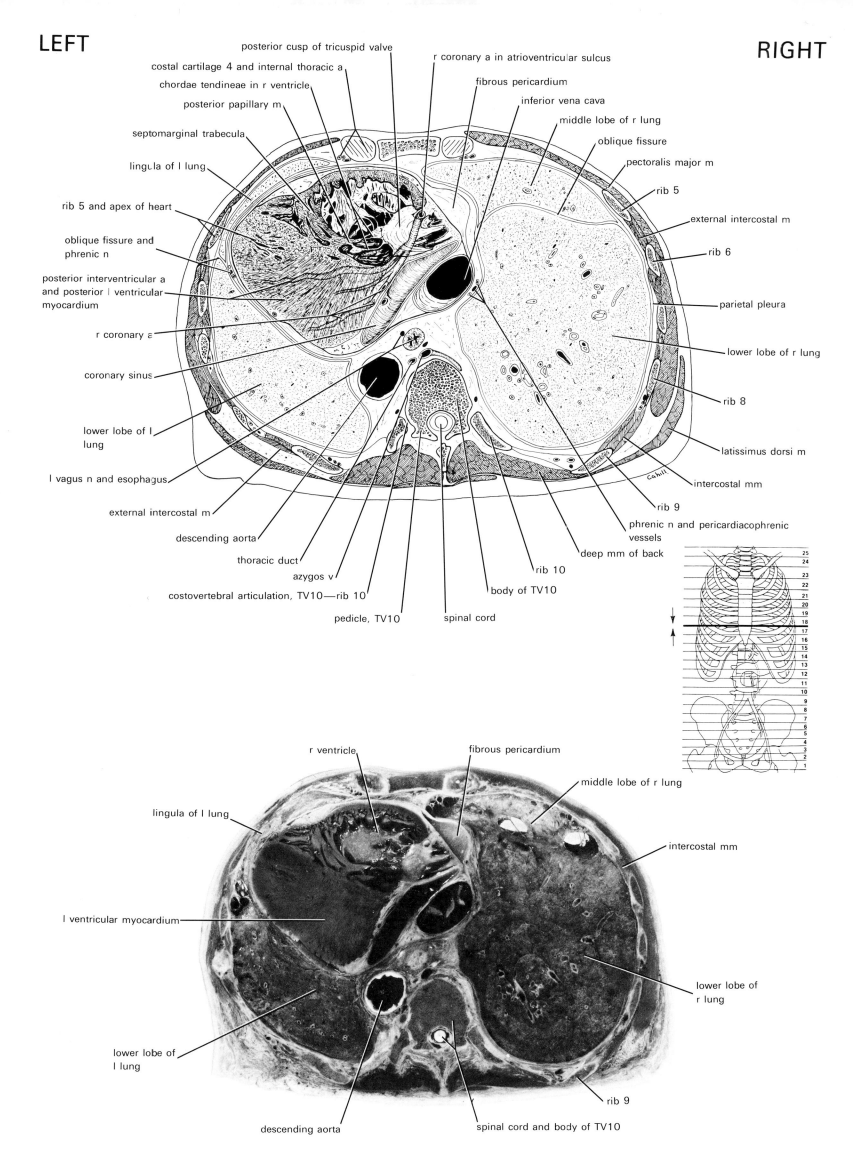

posterior cusp of tricuspid valve
r coronary a in atrioventricular sulcus
costal cartilage 4 and internal thoracic a
fibrous pericardium
chordae tendineae in r ventricle
inferior vena cava
posterior papillary m
middle lobe of r lung
septomarginal trabecula
oblique fissure
lingula of l lung
pectoralis major m
rib 5
rib 5 and apex of heart
external intercostal m
oblique fissure and
phrenic n
rib 6
posterior interventricular a
and posterior l ventricular
myocardium
parietal pleura
r coronary a
lower lobe of r lung
coronary sinus
rib 8
lower lobe of l
lung
latissimus dorsi m
l vagus n and esophagus
intercostal mm
external intercostal m
rib 9
descending aorta
phrenic n and pericardiacophrenic
vessels
thoracic duct
deep mm of back
azygos v
rib 10
costovertebral articulation, TV10—rib 10
body of TV10
pedicle, TV10
spinal cord

r ventricle
fibrous pericardium
lingula of l lung
middle lobe of r lung
intercostal mm
l ventricular myocardium
lower lobe of
r lung
lower lobe of
l lung
rib 9
descending aorta
spinal cord and body of TV10

Section 17 from above.

The Male Abdomen

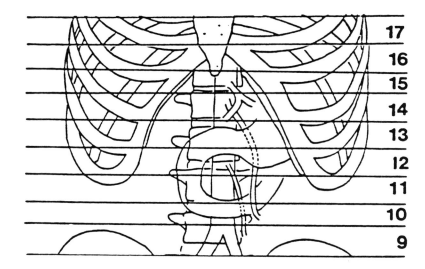

17
16
15
14
13
12
11
10
9

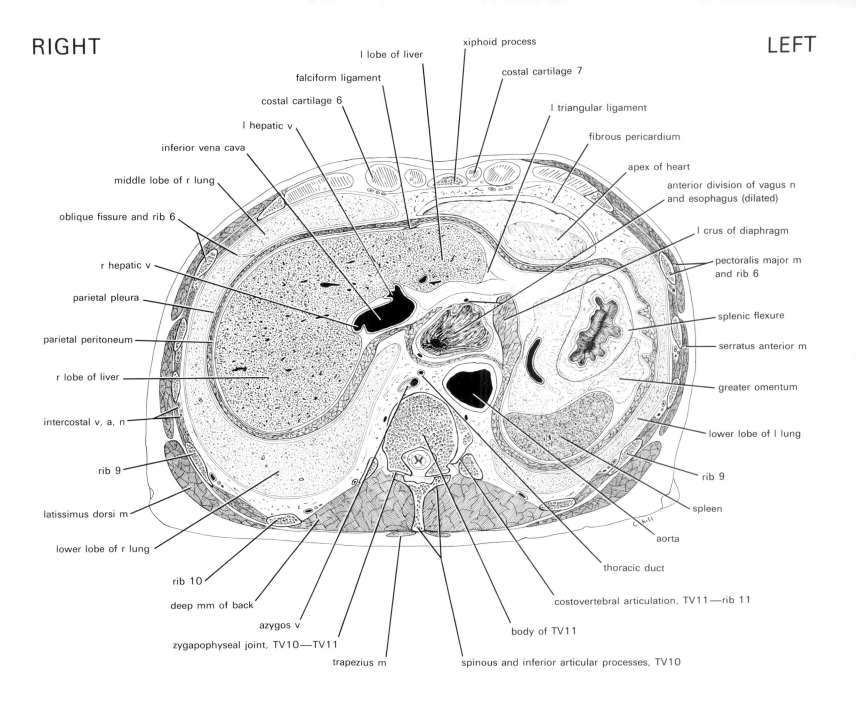

- l lobe of liver
- xiphoid process
- falciform ligament
- costal cartilage 7
- costal cartilage 6
- l triangular ligament
- l hepatic v
- fibrous pericardium
- inferior vena cava
- apex of heart
- middle lobe of r lung
- anterior division of vagus n and esophagus (dilated)
- oblique fissure and rib 6
- l crus of diaphragm
- r hepatic v
- pectoralis major m and rib 6
- parietal pleura
- splenic flexure
- parietal peritoneum
- serratus anterior m
- r lobe of liver
- greater omentum
- intercostal v, a, n
- lower lobe of l lung
- rib 9
- rib 9
- latissimus dorsi m
- spleen
- lower lobe of r lung
- aorta
- rib 10
- thoracic duct
- deep mm of back
- costovertebral articulation, TV11—rib 11
- azygos v
- body of TV11
- zygapophyseal joint, TV10—TV11
- trapezius m
- spinous and inferior articular processes, TV10

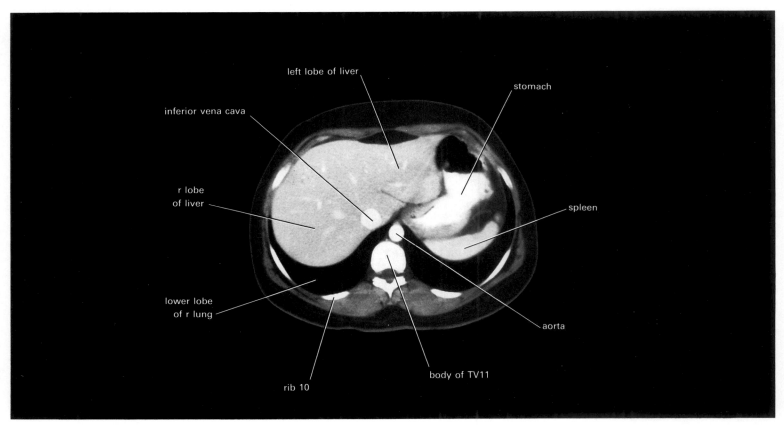

- left lobe of liver
- stomach
- inferior vena cava
- r lobe of liver
- spleen
- lower lobe of r lung
- aorta
- rib 10
- body of TV11

Section 17 from below.

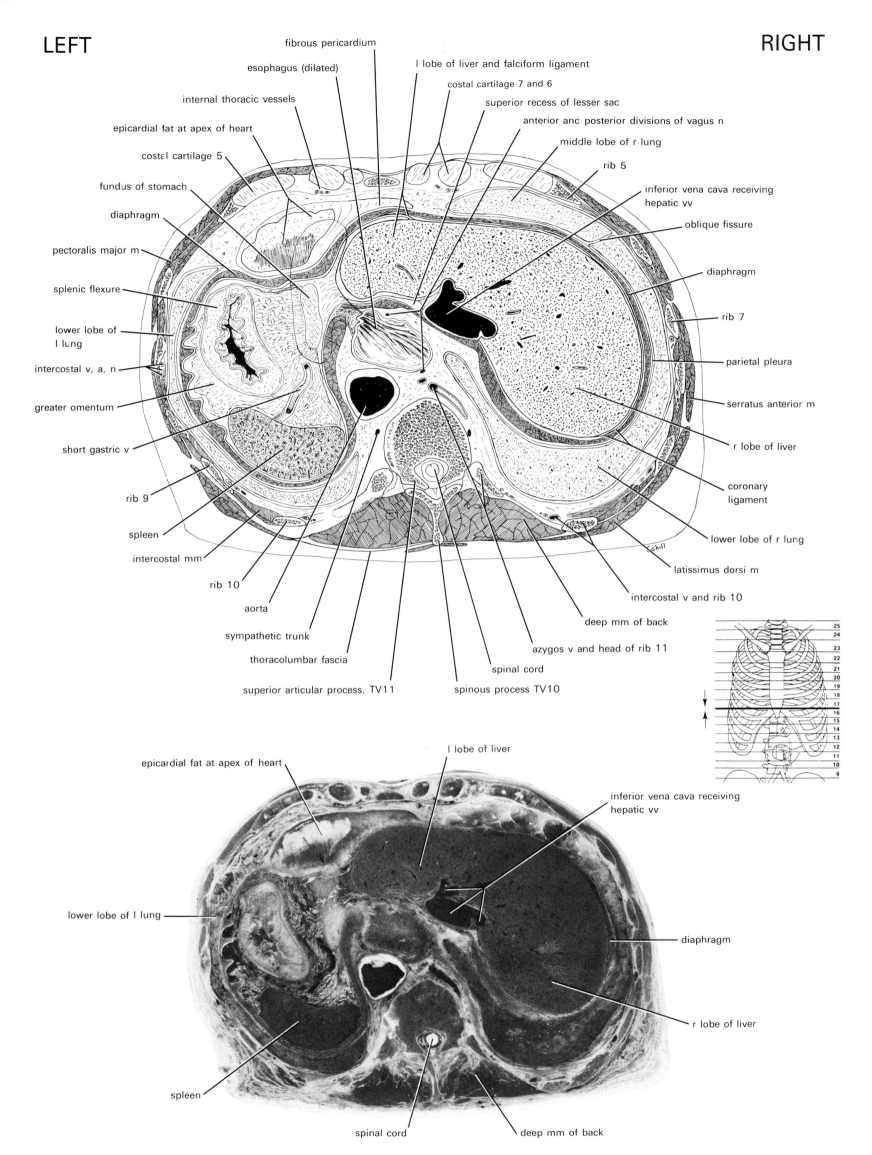

fibrous pericardium

esophagus (dilated)

internal thoracic vessels

epicardial fat at apex of heart

costal cartilage 5

fundus of stomach

diaphragm

pectoralis major m

splenic flexure

lower lobe of l lung

intercostal v, a, n

greater omentum

short gastric v

rib 9

spleen

intercostal mm

rib 10

aorta

sympathetic trunk

thoracolumbar fascia

superior articular process, TV11

l lobe of liver and falciform ligament

costal cartilage 7 and 6

superior recess of lesser sac

anterior and posterior divisions of vagus n

middle lobe of r lung

rib 5

inferior vena cava receiving hepatic vv

oblique fissure

diaphragm

rib 7

parietal pleura

serratus anterior m

r lobe of liver

coronary ligament

lower lobe of r lung

latissimus dorsi m

intercostal v and rib 10

deep mm of back

azygos v and head of rib 11

spinal cord

spinous process TV10

Cahill

epicardial fat at apex of heart

l lobe of liver

inferior vena cava receiving hepatic vv

lower lobe of l lung

diaphragm

r lobe of liver

spleen

spinal cord

deep mm of back

Section 16 from above.

25 24 23 22 21 20 19 18 17 16 15 14 13 12 11 10 9

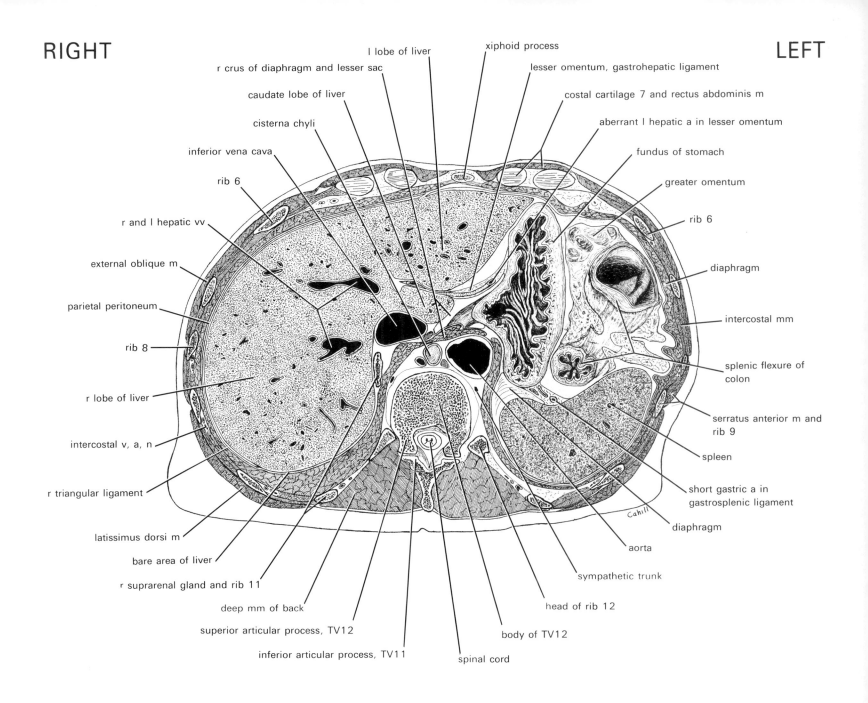

l lobe of liver

r crus of diaphragm and lesser sac

caudate lobe of liver

cisterna chyli

inferior vena cava

rib 6

r and l hepatic vv

external oblique m

parietal peritoneum

rib 8

r lobe of liver

intercostal v, a, n

r triangular ligament

latissimus dorsi m

bare area of liver

r suprarenal gland and rib 11

deep mm of back

superior articular process, TV12

inferior articular process, TV11

xiphoid process

lesser omentum, gastrohepatic ligament

costal cartilage 7 and rectus abdominis m

aberrant l hepatic a in lesser omentum

fundus of stomach

greater omentum

rib 6

diaphragm

intercostal mm

splenic flexure of colon

serratus anterior m and rib 9

spleen

short gastric a in gastrosplenic ligament

diaphragm

aorta

sympathetic trunk

head of rib 12

body of TV12

spinal cord

Cahill

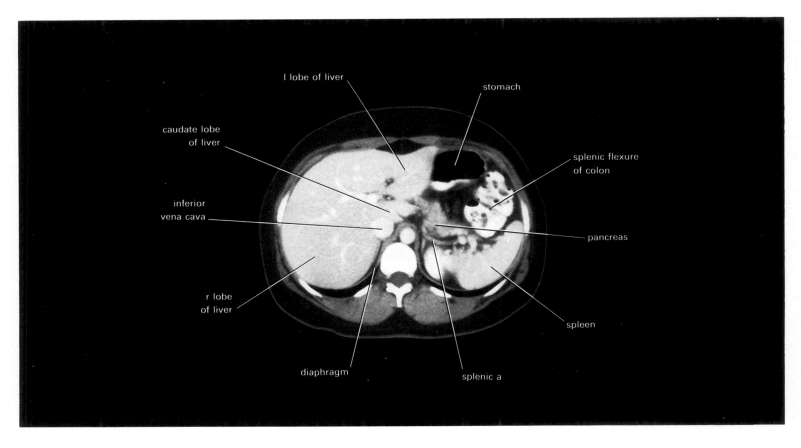

l lobe of liver

caudate lobe of liver

inferior vena cava

r lobe of liver

diaphragm

stomach

splenic flexure of colon

pancreas

spleen

splenic a

Section 16 from below.

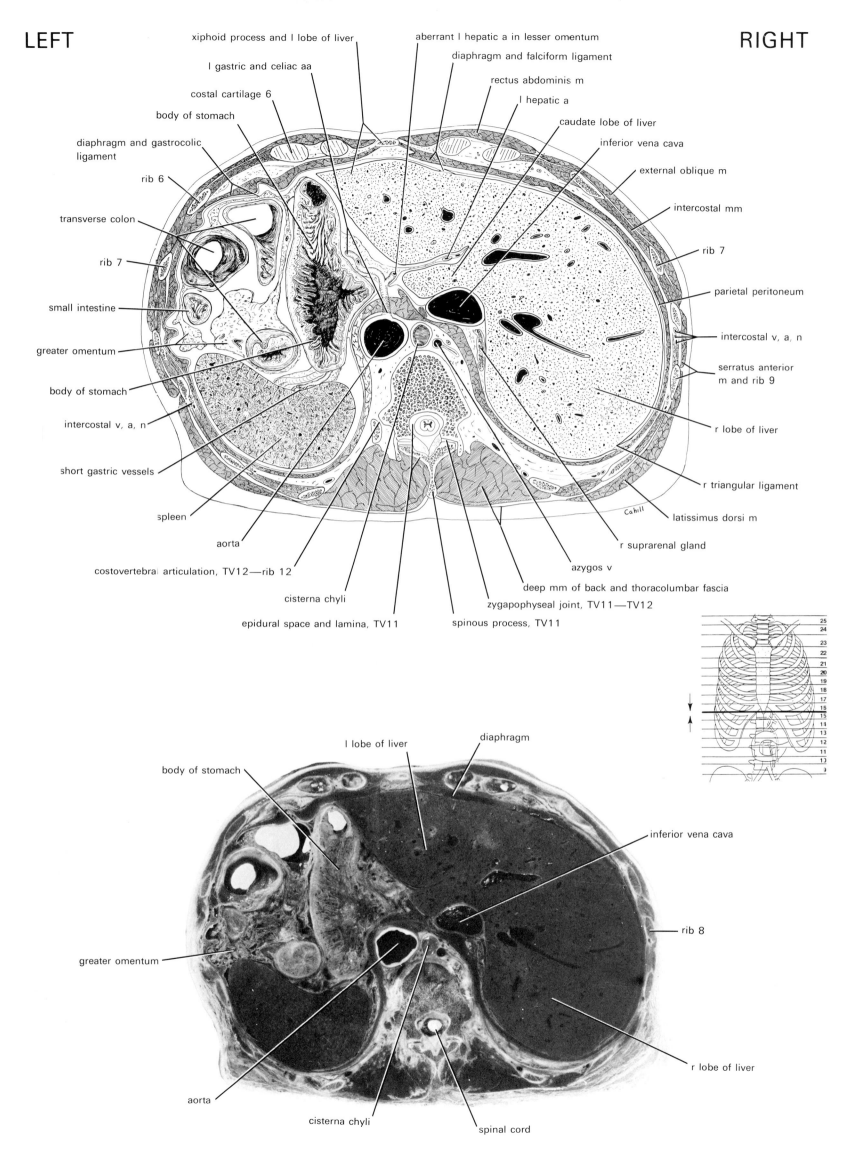

xiphoid process and l lobe of liver

l gastric and celiac aa

costal cartilage 6

body of stomach

diaphragm and gastrocolic
ligament

rib 6

transverse colon

rib 7

small intestine

greater omentum

body of stomach

intercostal v, a, n

short gastric vessels

spleen

aorta

costovertebral articulation, TV12—rib 12

cisterna chyli

epidural space and lamina, TV11

aberrant l hepatic a in lesser omentum

diaphragm and falciform ligament

rectus abdominis m

l hepatic a

caudate lobe of liver

inferior vena cava

external oblique m

intercostal mm

rib 7

parietal peritoneum

intercostal v, a, n

serratus anterior
m and rib 9

r lobe of liver

r triangular ligament

latissimus dorsi m

r suprarenal gland

azygos v

deep mm of back and thoracolumbar fascia

zygapophyseal joint, TV11—TV12

spinous process, TV11

Cahill

l lobe of liver

diaphragm

body of stomach

inferior vena cava

rib 8

greater omentum

r lobe of liver

aorta

cisterna chyli

spinal cord

Section 15 from above.

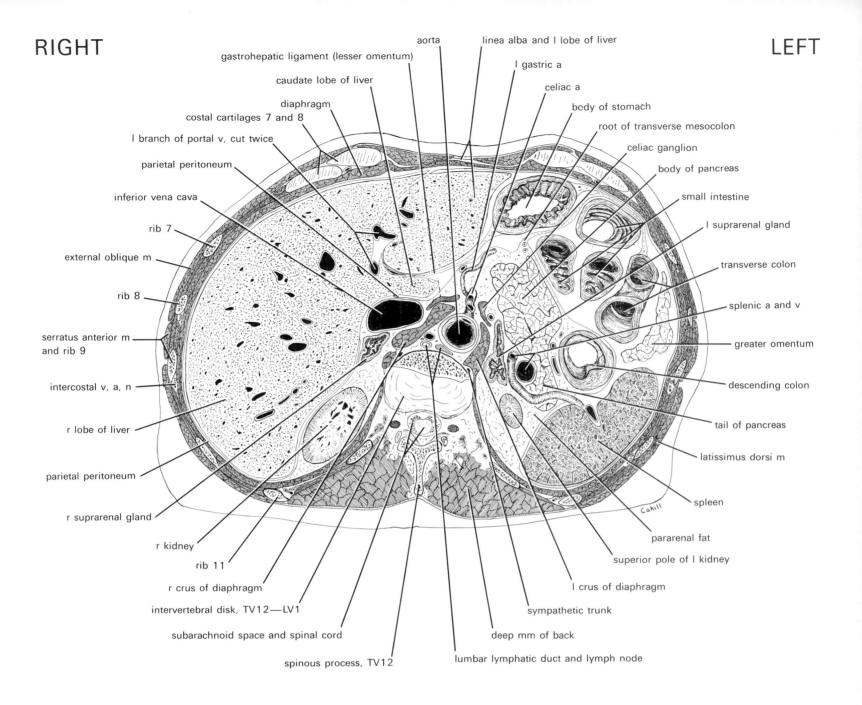

aorta

linea alba and l lobe of liver

gastrohepatic ligament (lesser omentum)

l gastric a

caudate lobe of liver

celiac a

diaphragm

body of stomach

costal cartilages 7 and 8

root of transverse mesocolon

l branch of portal v, cut twice

celiac ganglion

parietal peritoneum

body of pancreas

inferior vena cava

small intestine

rib 7

l suprarenal gland

external oblique m

transverse colon

rib 8

splenic a and v

serratus anterior m
and rib 9

greater omentum

intercostal v, a, n

descending colon

r lobe of liver

tail of pancreas

parietal peritoneum

latissimus dorsi m

r suprarenal gland

spleen

r kidney

pararenal fat

rib 11

superior pole of l kidney

r crus of diaphragm

l crus of diaphragm

intervertebral disk, TV12—LV1

sympathetic trunk

subarachnoid space and spinal cord

deep mm of back

spinous process, TV12

lumbar lymphatic duct and lymph node

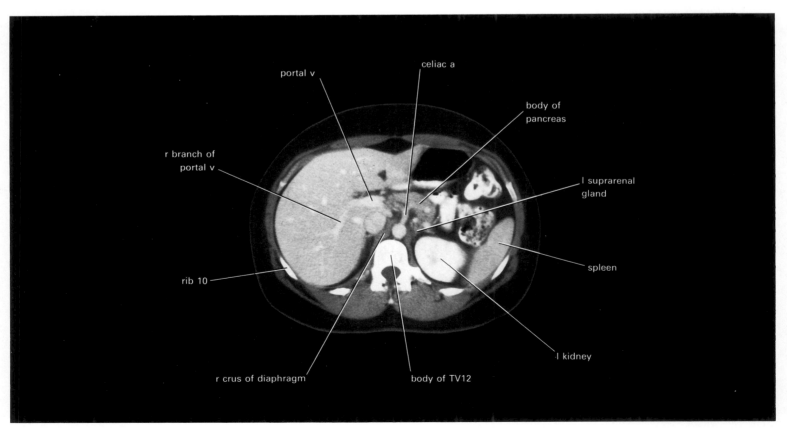

portal v

celiac a

body of
pancreas

r branch of
portal v

l suprarenal
gland

spleen

rib 10

l kidney

r crus of diaphragm

body of TV12

Section 15 from below.

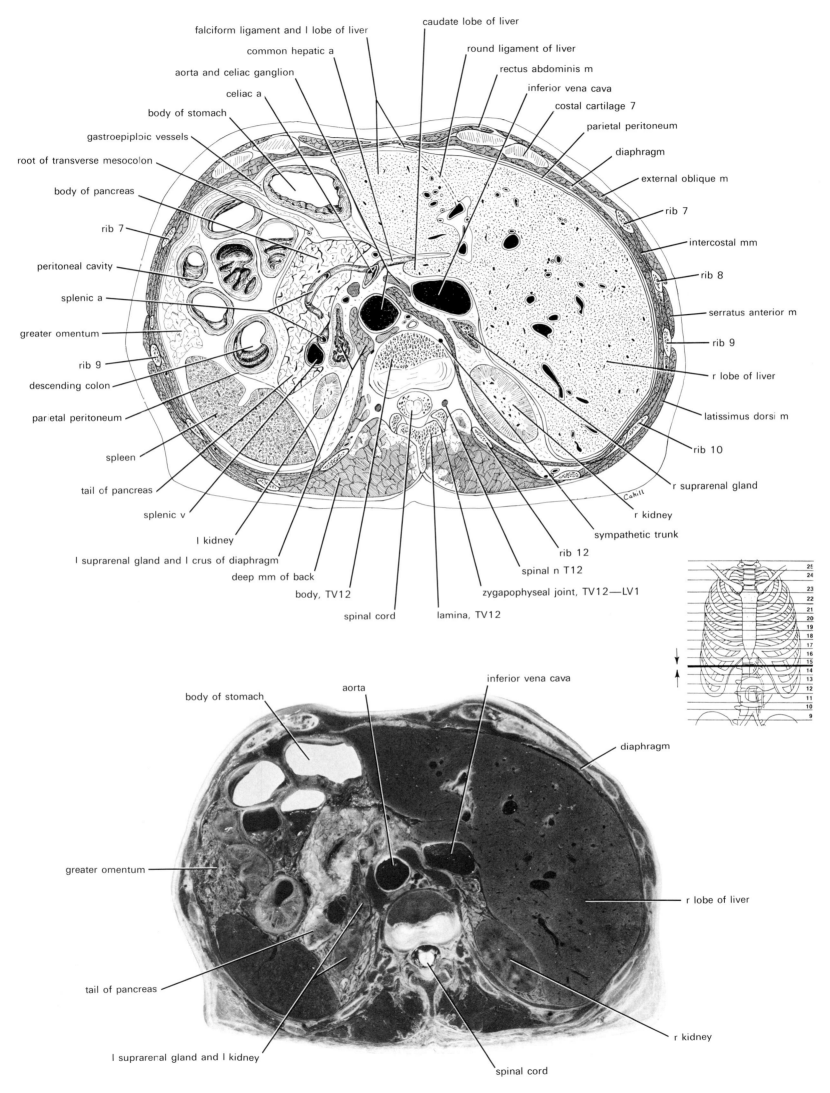

falciform ligament and l lobe of liver
caudate lobe of liver
common hepatic a
round ligament of liver
aorta and celiac ganglion
rectus abdominis m
celiac a
inferior vena cava
body of stomach
costal cartilage 7
gastroepiploic vessels
parietal peritoneum
root of transverse mesocolon
diaphragm
body of pancreas
external oblique m
rib 7
rib 7
peritoneal cavity
intercostal mm
splenic a
rib 8
greater omentum
serratus anterior m
rib 9
rib 9
descending colon
r lobe of liver
parietal peritoneum
latissimus dorsi m
spleen
rib 10
tail of pancreas
r suprarenal gland
splenic v
r kidney
l kidney
sympathetic trunk
l suprarenal gland and l crus of diaphragm
rib 12
deep mm of back
spinal n T12
body, TV12
zygapophyseal joint, TV12—LV1
spinal cord
lamina, TV12

body of stomach
aorta
inferior vena cava
diaphragm
greater omentum
r lobe of liver
tail of pancreas
r kidney
l suprarenal gland and l kidney
spinal cord

Section 14 from above.

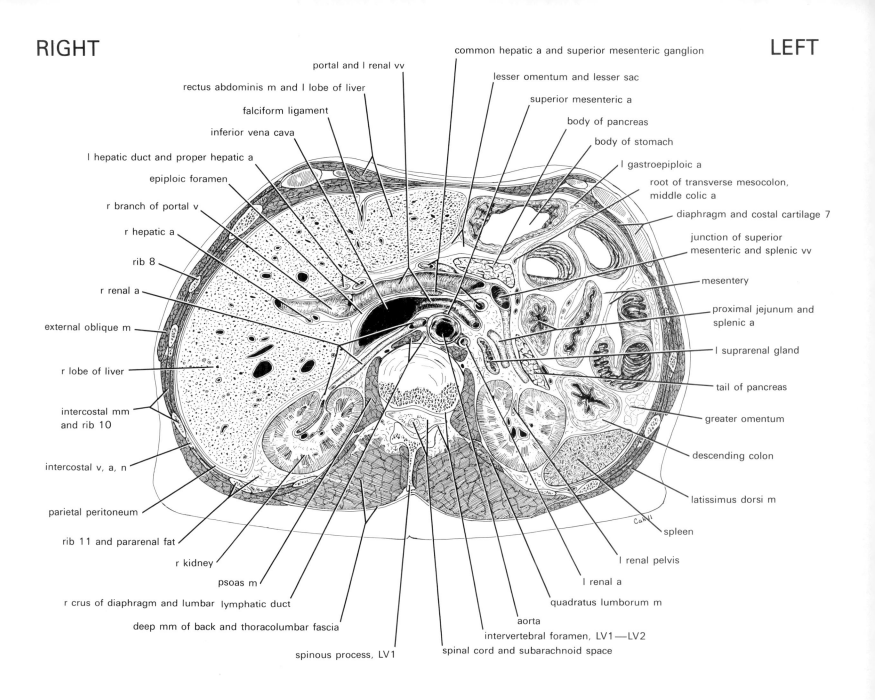

portal and l renal vv
common hepatic a and superior mesenteric ganglion
rectus abdominis m and l lobe of liver
lesser omentum and lesser sac
falciform ligament
superior mesenteric a
inferior vena cava
body of pancreas
l hepatic duct and proper hepatic a
body of stomach
epiploic foramen
l gastroepiploic a
r branch of portal v
root of transverse mesocolon, middle colic a
r hepatic a
diaphragm and costal cartilage 7
rib 8
junction of superior mesenteric and splenic vv
r renal a
mesentery
external oblique m
proximal jejunum and splenic a
r lobe of liver
l suprarenal gland
intercostal mm and rib 10
tail of pancreas
intercostal v, a, n
greater omentum
parietal peritoneum
descending colon
rib 11 and pararenal fat
latissimus dorsi m
r kidney
spleen
psoas m
l renal pelvis
r crus of diaphragm and lumbar   lymphatic duct
l renal a
deep mm of back and thoracolumbar fascia
quadratus lumborum m
spinous process, LV1
aorta
spinal cord and subarachnoid space
intervertebral foramen, LV1—LV2

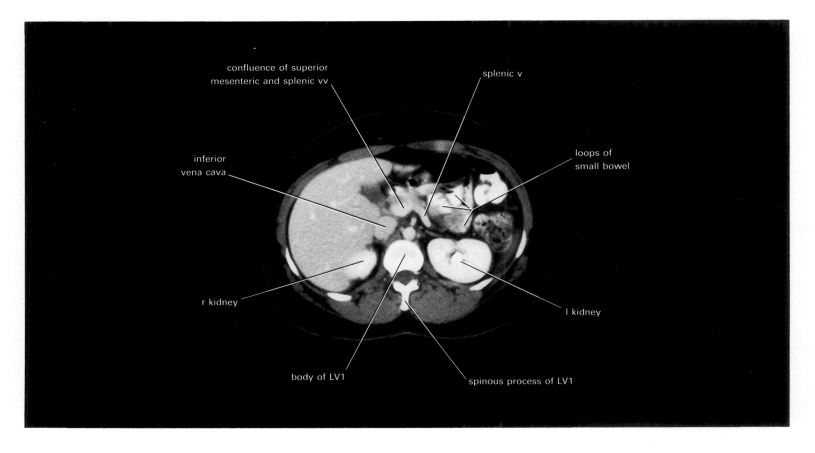

confluence of superior mesenteric and splenic vv
splenic v
inferior vena cava
loops of small bowel
r kidney
l kidney
body of LV1
spinous process of LV1

Section 14 from below.

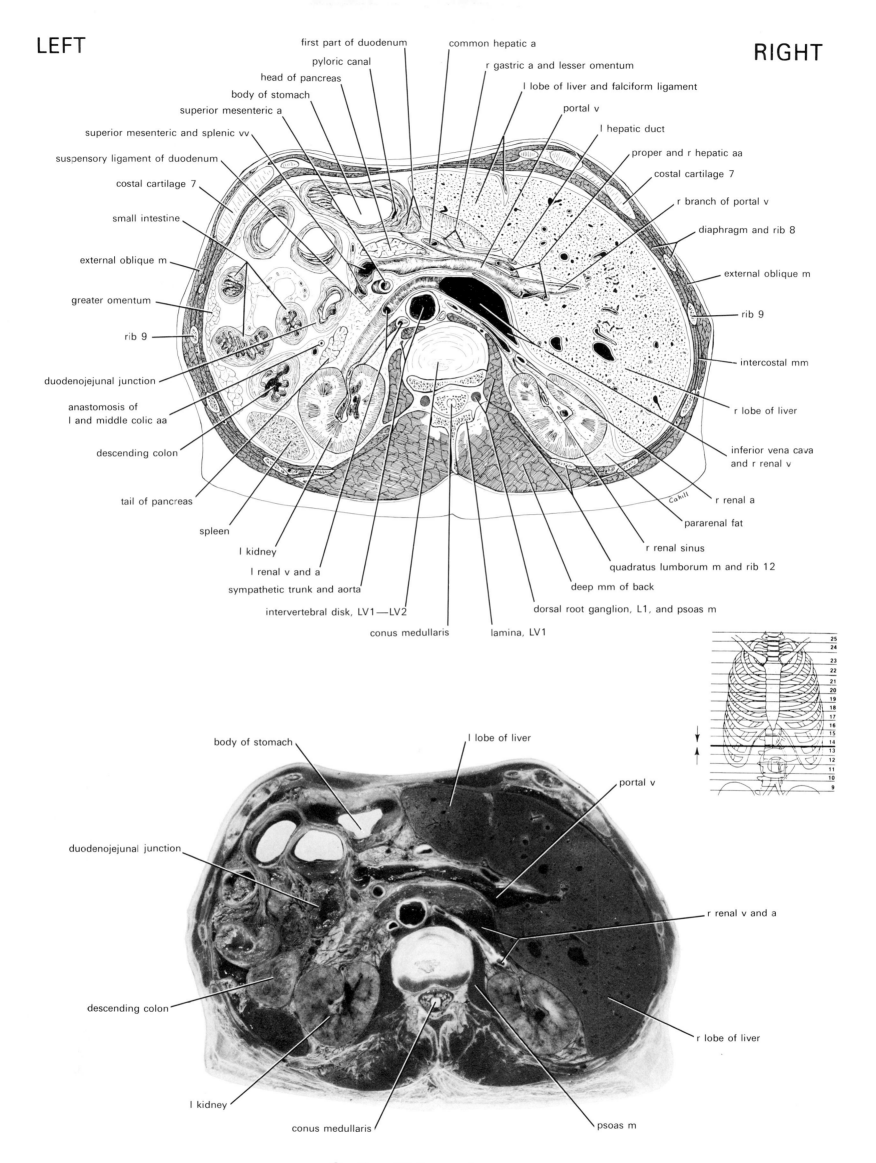

first part of duodenum
pyloric canal
head of pancreas
body of stomach
superior mesenteric a
superior mesenteric and splenic vv
suspensory ligament of duodenum
costal cartilage 7
small intestine
external oblique m
greater omentum
rib 9
duodenojejunal junction
anastomosis of
l and middle colic aa
descending colon
tail of pancreas
spleen
l kidney
l renal v and a
sympathetic trunk and aorta
intervertebral disk, LV1—LV2
conus medullaris

common hepatic a
r gastric a and lesser omentum
l lobe of liver and falciform ligament
portal v
l hepatic duct
proper and r hepatic aa
costal cartilage 7
r branch of portal v
diaphragm and rib 8
external oblique m
rib 9
intercostal mm
r lobe of liver
inferior vena cava
and r renal v
r renal a
pararenal fat
r renal sinus
quadratus lumborum m and rib 12
deep mm of back
dorsal root ganglion, L1, and psoas m
lamina, LV1

Cahill

body of stomach
duodenojejunal junction
descending colon
l kidney
conus medullaris

l lobe of liver
portal v
r renal v and a
r lobe of liver
psoas m

Section 13 from above.

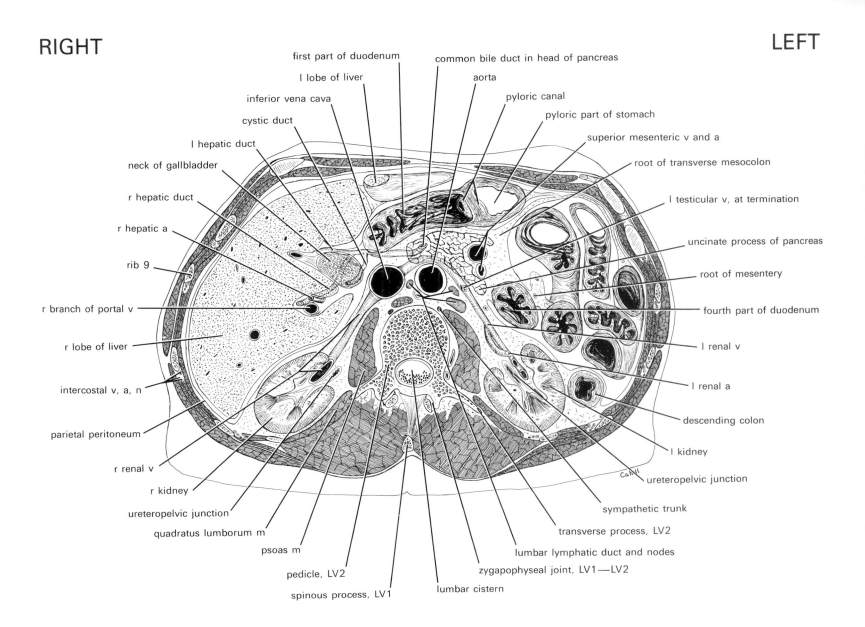

first part of duodenum
l lobe of liver
inferior vena cava
cystic duct
l hepatic duct
neck of gallbladder
r hepatic duct
r hepatic a
rib 9
r branch of portal v
r lobe of liver
intercostal v, a, n
parietal peritoneum
r renal v
r kidney
ureteropelvic junction
quadratus lumborum m
psoas m
pedicle, LV2
spinous process, LV1

common bile duct in head of pancreas
aorta
pyloric canal
pyloric part of stomach
superior mesenteric v and a
root of transverse mesocolon
l testicular v, at termination
uncinate process of pancreas
root of mesentery
fourth part of duodenum
l renal v
l renal a
descending colon
l kidney
ureteropelvic junction
sympathetic trunk
transverse process, LV2
lumbar lymphatic duct and nodes
zygapophyseal joint, LV1—LV2
lumbar cistern

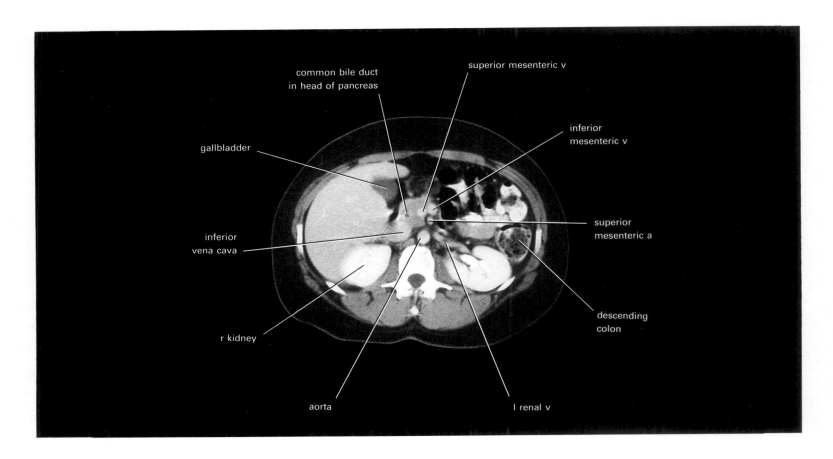

common bile duct
in head of pancreas
gallbladder
inferior
vena cava
r kidney
aorta

superior mesenteric v
inferior
mesenteric v
superior
mesenteric a
descending
colon
l renal v

Section 13 from below.

LEFT   RIGHT

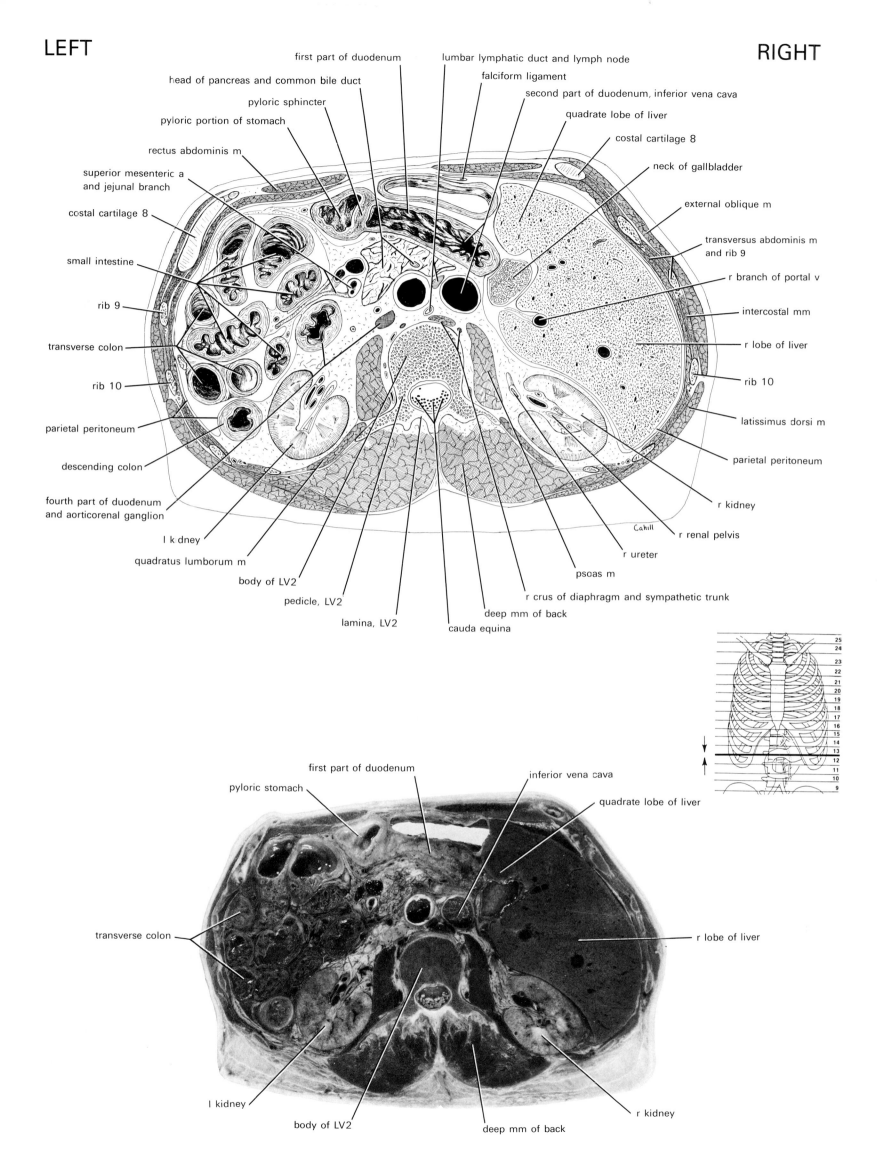

first part of duodenum
head of pancreas and common bile duct
lumbar lymphatic duct and lymph node
pyloric sphincter
falciform ligament
pyloric portion of stomach
second part of duodenum, inferior vena cava
rectus abdominis m
quadrate lobe of liver
superior mesenteric a
and jejunal branch
costal cartilage 8
neck of gallbladder
costal cartilage 8
external oblique m
small intestine
transversus abdominis m
and rib 9
rib 9
r branch of portal v
transverse colon
intercostal mm
rib 10
r lobe of liver
parietal peritoneum
rib 10
descending colon
latissimus dorsi m
fourth part of duodenum
and aorticorenal ganglion
parietal peritoneum
l k dney
r kidney
quadratus lumborum m
r renal pelvis
body of LV2
r ureter
pedicle, LV2
psoas m
lamina, LV2
r crus of diaphragm and sympathetic trunk
cauda equina
deep mm of back

first part of duodenum
pyloric stomach
inferior vena cava
quadrate lobe of liver

transverse colon
r lobe of liver

l kidney
r kidney
body of LV2
deep mm of back

Section 12 from above.

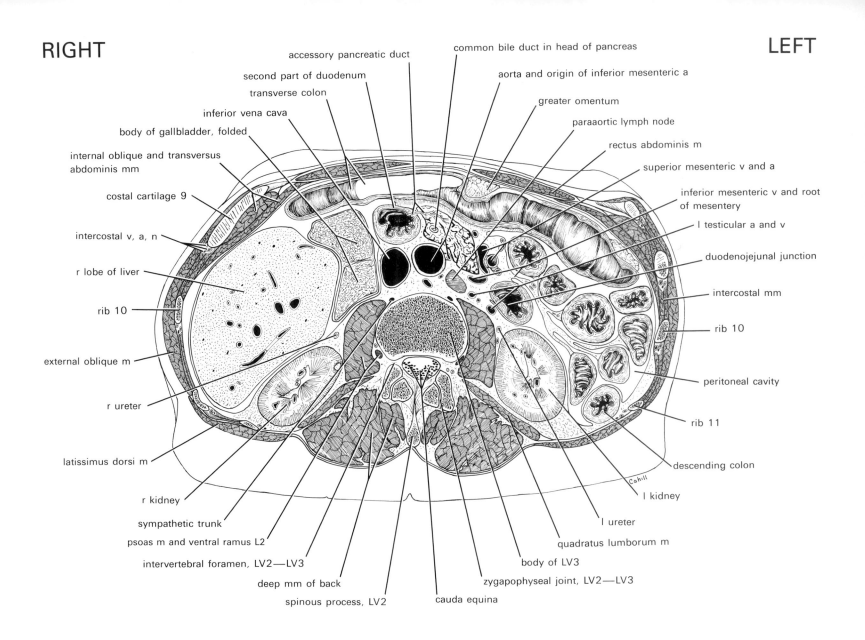

accessory pancreatic duct

common bile duct in head of pancreas

second part of duodenum

aorta and origin of inferior mesenteric a

transverse colon

greater omentum

inferior vena cava

paraaortic lymph node

body of gallbladder, folded

rectus abdominis m

internal oblique and transversus abdominis mm

superior mesenteric v and a

costal cartilage 9

inferior mesenteric v and root of mesentery

intercostal v, a, n

l testicular a and v

r lobe of liver

duodenojejunal junction

rib 10

intercostal mm

external oblique m

rib 10

r ureter

peritoneal cavity

latissimus dorsi m

rib 11

r kidney

descending colon

sympathetic trunk

l kidney

psoas m and ventral ramus L2

l ureter

intervertebral foramen, LV2—LV3

quadratus lumborum m

deep mm of back

body of LV3

spinous process, LV2

zygapophyseal joint, LV2—LV3

cauda equina

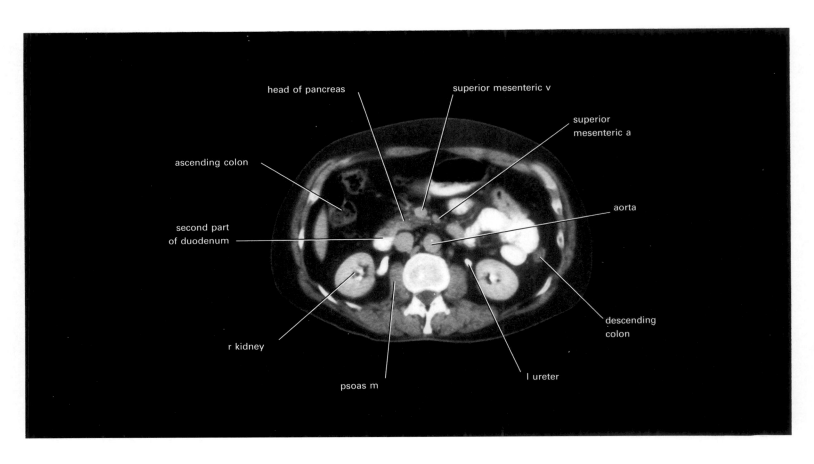

head of pancreas

superior mesenteric v

superior mesenteric a

ascending colon

second part of duodenum

aorta

r kidney

descending colon

psoas m

l ureter

Section 12 from below.

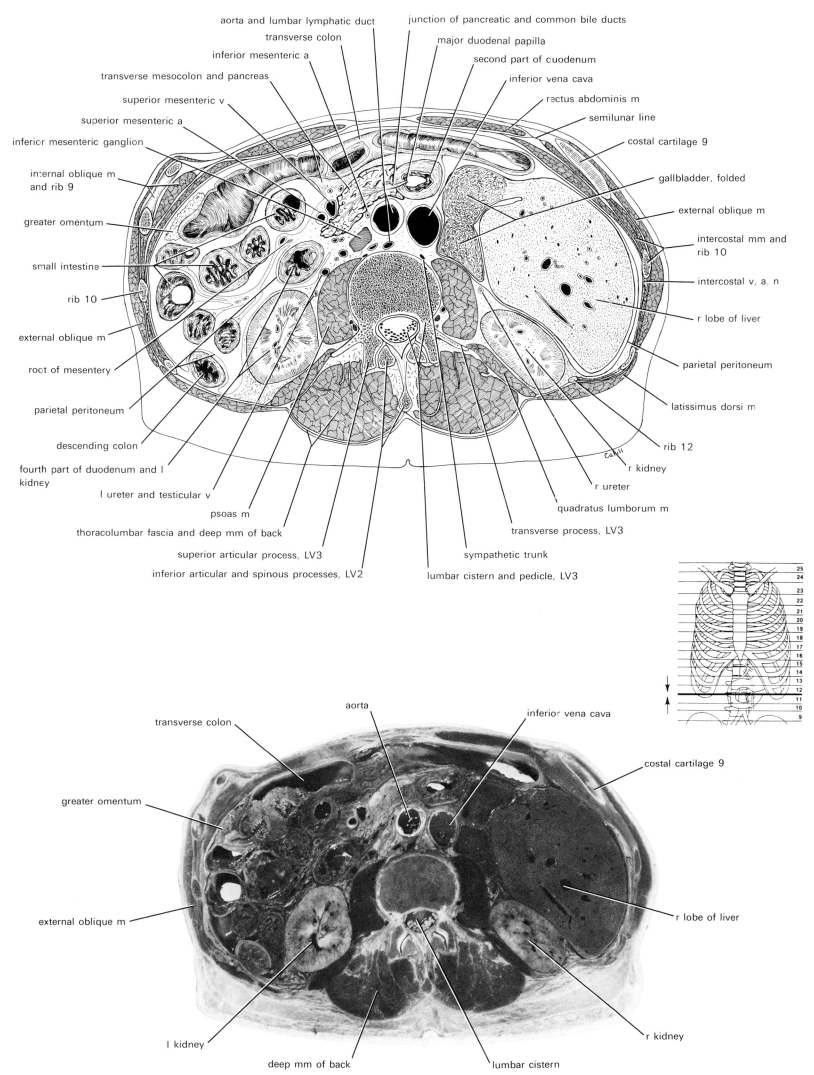

aorta and lumbar lymphatic duct
transverse colon
inferior mesenteric a
transverse mesocolon and pancreas
superior mesenteric v
superior mesenteric a
inferior mesenteric ganglion
internal oblique m and rib 9
greater omentum
small intestine
rib 10
external oblique m
root of mesentery
parietal peritoneum
descending colon
fourth part of duodenum and l kidney
l ureter and testicular v
psoas m
thoracolumbar fascia and deep mm of back
superior articular process, LV3
inferior articular and spinous processes, LV2

junction of pancreatic and common bile ducts
major duodenal papilla
second part of duodenum
inferior vena cava
rectus abdominis m
semilunar line
costal cartilage 9
gallbladder, folded
external oblique m
intercostal mm and rib 10
intercostal v, a, n
r lobe of liver
parietal peritoneum
latissimus dorsi m
rib 12
r kidney
r ureter
quadratus lumborum m
transverse process, LV3
sympathetic trunk
lumbar cistern and pedicle, LV3

transverse colon
greater omentum
external oblique m
l kidney
deep mm of back

aorta
inferior vena cava
costal cartilage 9
r lobe of liver
r kidney
lumbar cistern

Section 11 from above.

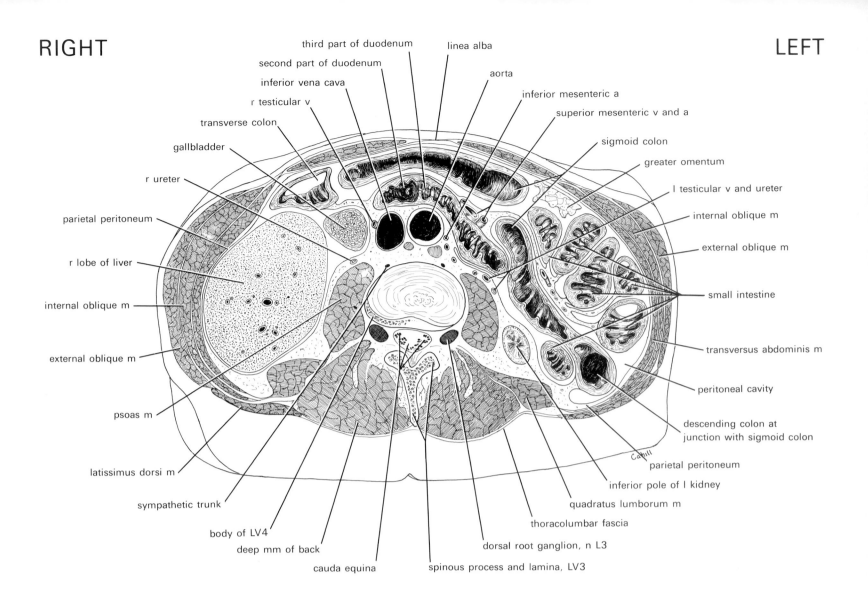

third part of duodenum
second part of duodenum
inferior vena cava
r testicular v
transverse colon
gallbladder
r ureter
parietal peritoneum
r lobe of liver
internal oblique m
external oblique m
psoas m
latissimus dorsi m
sympathetic trunk
body of LV4
deep mm of back
cauda equina

linea alba
aorta
inferior mesenteric a
superior mesenteric v and a
sigmoid colon
greater omentum
l testicular v and ureter
internal oblique m
external oblique m
small intestine
transversus abdominis m
peritoneal cavity
descending colon at junction with sigmoid colon
parietal peritoneum
inferior pole of l kidney
quadratus lumborum m
thoracolumbar fascia
dorsal root ganglion, n L3
spinous process and lamina, LV3

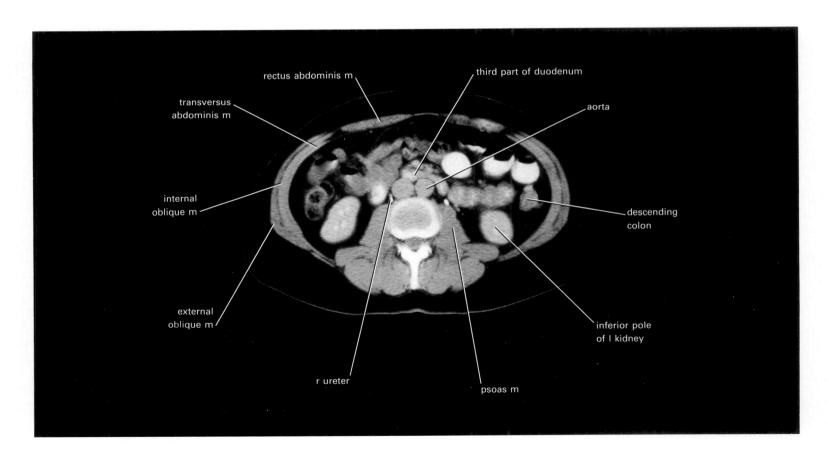

rectus abdominis m
transversus abdominis m
internal oblique m
external oblique m
r ureter
third part of duodenum
aorta
descending colon
inferior pole of l kidney
psoas m

Section 11 from below.

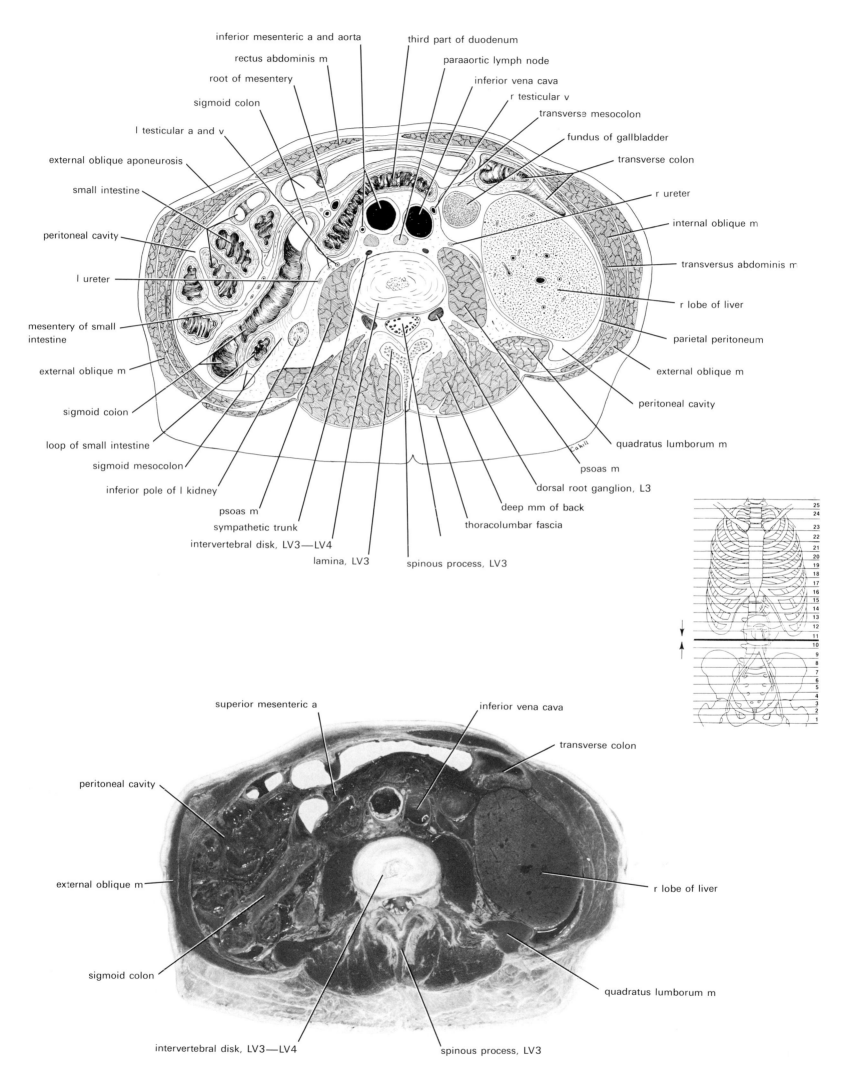

inferior mesenteric a and aorta

rectus abdominis m

root of mesentery

sigmoid colon

l testicular a and v

external oblique aponeurosis

small intestine

peritoneal cavity

l ureter

mesentery of small intestine

external oblique m

sigmoid colon

loop of small intestine

sigmoid mesocolon

inferior pole of l kidney

psoas m

sympathetic trunk

intervertebral disk, LV3—LV4

lamina, LV3

third part of duodenum

paraaortic lymph node

inferior vena cava

r testicular v

transverse mesocolon

fundus of gallbladder

transverse colon

r ureter

internal oblique m

transversus abdominis m

r lobe of liver

parietal peritoneum

external oblique m

peritoneal cavity

quadratus lumborum m

psoas m

dorsal root ganglion, L3

deep mm of back

thoracolumbar fascia

spinous process, LV3

superior mesenteric a

peritoneal cavity

external oblique m

sigmoid colon

intervertebral disk, LV3—LV4

inferior vena cava

transverse colon

r lobe of liver

quadratus lumborum m

spinous process, LV3

Section 10 from above.

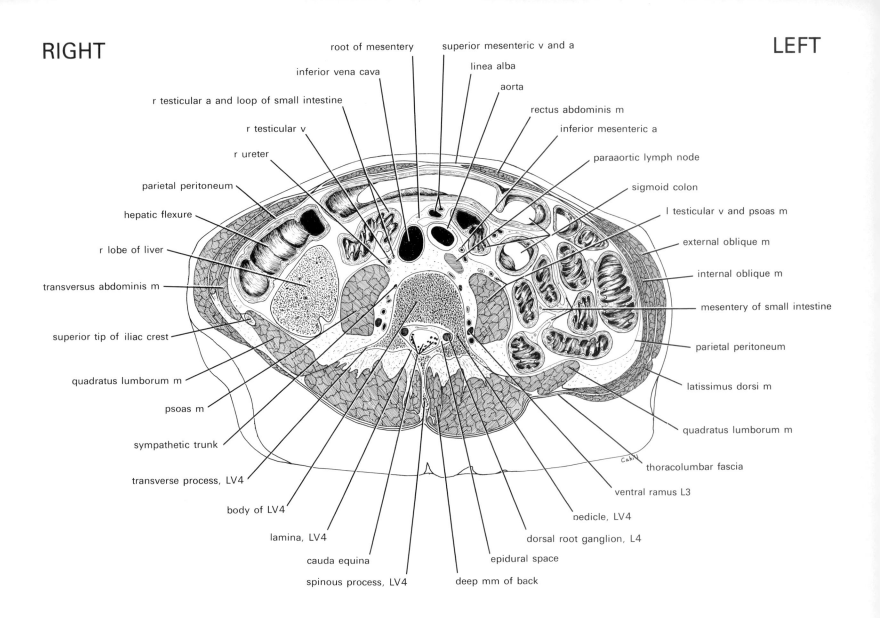

root of mesentery
superior mesenteric v and a
inferior vena cava
linea alba
aorta
r testicular a and loop of small intestine
rectus abdominis m
inferior mesenteric a
r testicular v
r ureter
paraaortic lymph node
parietal peritoneum
sigmoid colon
hepatic flexure
l testicular v and psoas m
r lobe of liver
external oblique m
internal oblique m
transversus abdominis m
mesentery of small intestine
superior tip of iliac crest
parietal peritoneum
latissimus dorsi m
quadratus lumborum m
psoas m
quadratus lumborum m
sympathetic trunk
thoracolumbar fascia
transverse process, LV4
ventral ramus L3
body of LV4
pedicle, LV4
lamina, LV4
dorsal root ganglion, L4
cauda equina
epidural space
spinous process, LV4
deep mm of back

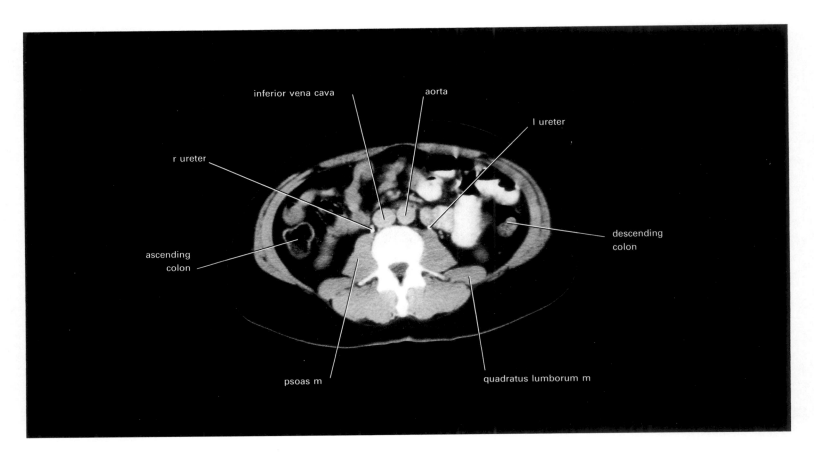

inferior vena cava
aorta
l ureter
r ureter
ascending colon
descending colon
psoas m
quadratus lumborum m

Section 10 from below.

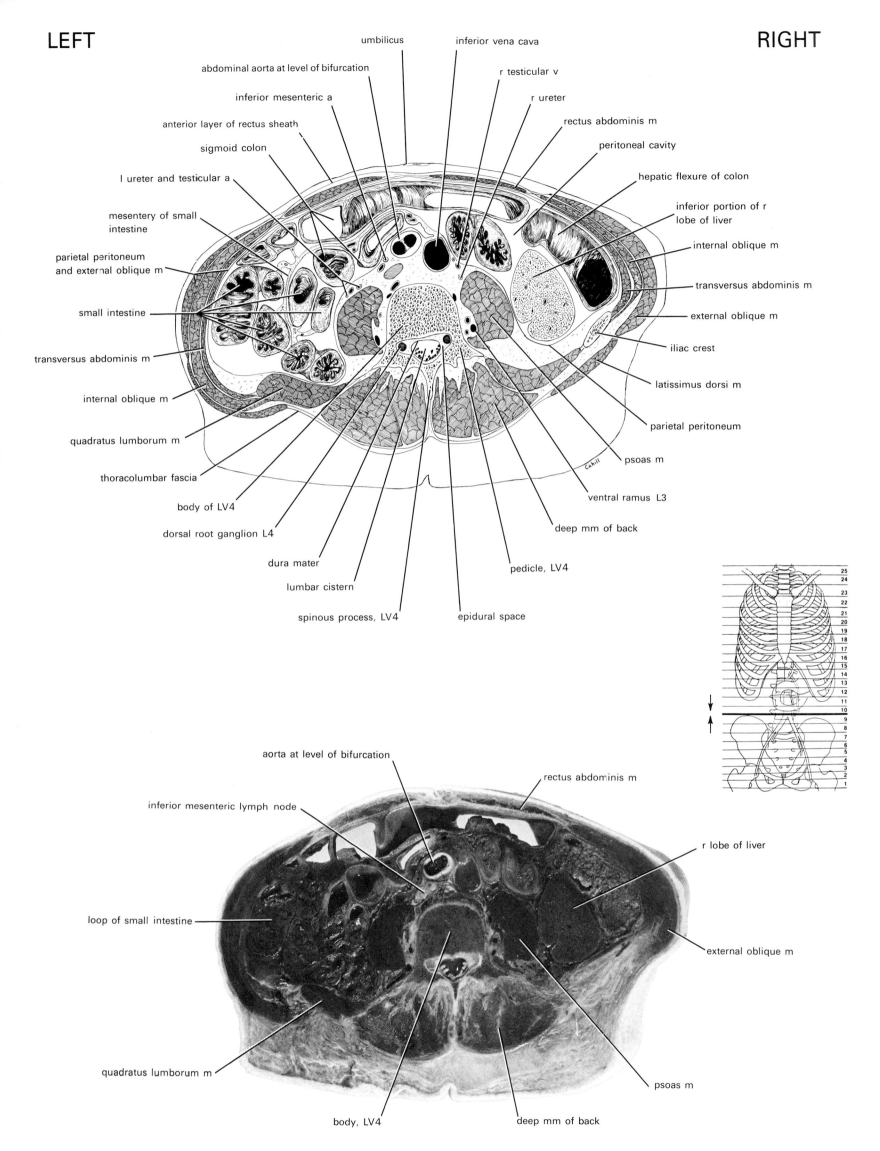

umbilicus

inferior vena cava

abdominal aorta at level of bifurcation

r testicular v

inferior mesenteric a

r ureter

anterior layer of rectus sheath

rectus abdominis m

sigmoid colon

peritoneal cavity

l ureter and testicular a

hepatic flexure of colon

mesentery of small intestine

inferior portion of r lobe of liver

parietal peritoneum and external oblique m

internal oblique m

small intestine

transversus abdominis m

external oblique m

transversus abdominis m

iliac crest

internal oblique m

latissimus dorsi m

quadratus lumborum m

parietal peritoneum

thoracolumbar fascia

psoas m

body of LV4

ventral ramus L3

dorsal root ganglion L4

deep mm of back

dura mater

pedicle, LV4

lumbar cistern

spinous process, LV4

epidural space

Cahill

aorta at level of bifurcation

rectus abdominis m

inferior mesenteric lymph node

r lobe of liver

loop of small intestine

external oblique m

quadratus lumborum m

psoas m

body, LV4

deep mm of back

Section 9 from above.

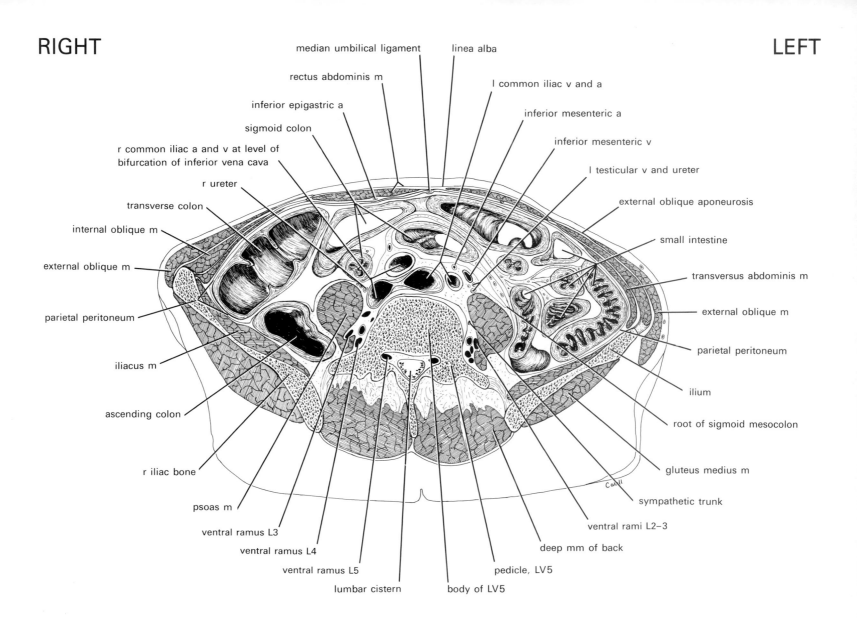

median umbilical ligament
linea alba
rectus abdominis m
l common iliac v and a
inferior epigastric a
inferior mesenteric a
sigmoid colon
inferior mesenteric v
r common iliac a and v at level of
bifurcation of inferior vena cava
l testicular v and ureter
r ureter
external oblique aponeurosis
transverse colon
small intestine
internal oblique m
transversus abdominis m
external oblique m
external oblique m
parietal peritoneum
parietal peritoneum
ilium
iliacus m
root of sigmoid mesocolon
ascending colon
gluteus medius m
r iliac bone
sympathetic trunk
psoas m
ventral rami L2-3
ventral ramus L3
deep mm of back
ventral ramus L4
pedicle, LV5
ventral ramus L5
body of LV5
lumbar cistern

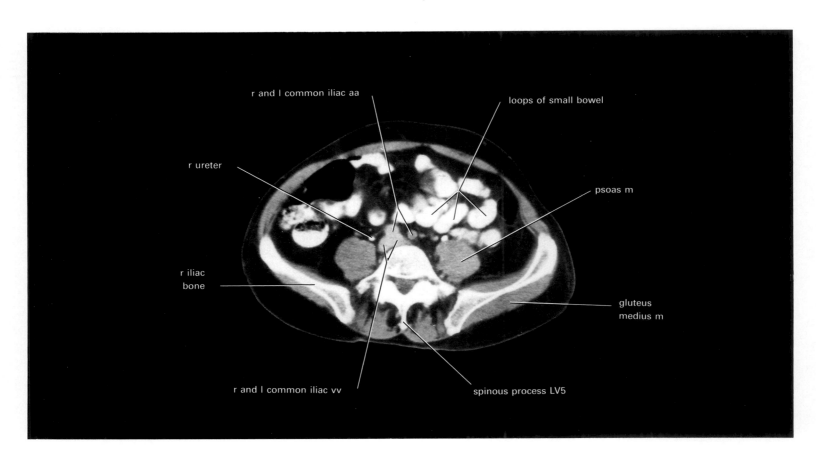

r and l common iliac aa
loops of small bowel
r ureter
psoas m
r iliac
bone
gluteus
medius m
r and l common iliac vv
spinous process LV5

Section 9 from below.

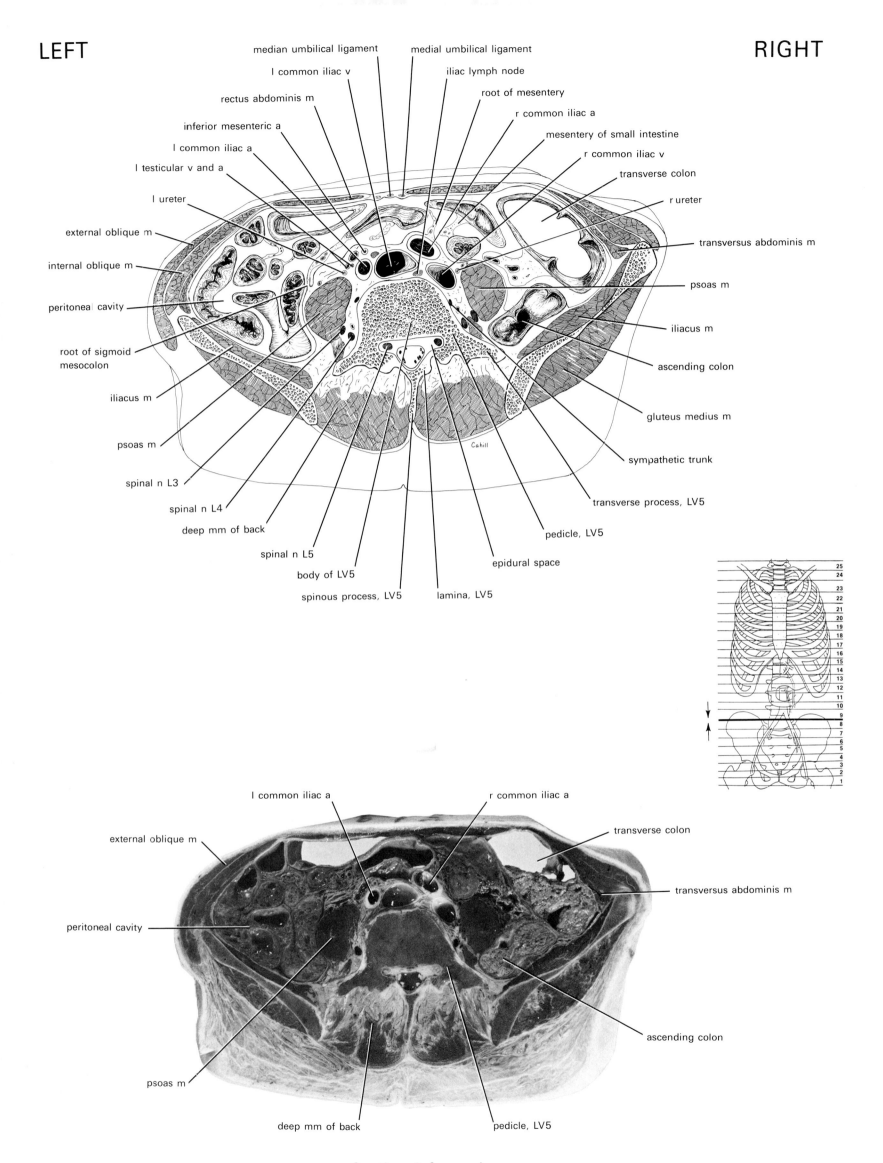

median umbilical ligament
l common iliac v
rectus abdominis m
inferior mesenteric a
l common iliac a
l testicular v and a
l ureter
external oblique m
internal oblique m
peritoneal cavity
root of sigmoid mesocolon
iliacus m
psoas m
spinal n L3
spinal n L4
deep mm of back
spinal n L5
body of LV5
spinous process, LV5
lamina, LV5
epidural space
pedicle, LV5
transverse process, LV5
sympathetic trunk
gluteus medius m
ascending colon
iliacus m
psoas m
transversus abdominis m
r ureter
transverse colon
r common iliac v
mesentery of small intestine
r common iliac a
root of mesentery
iliac lymph node
medial umbilical ligament

Cahill

l common iliac a
external oblique m
peritoneal cavity
psoas m
deep mm of back
pedicle, LV5
ascending colon
transversus abdominis m
transverse colon
r common iliac a

Section 8 from above.

Upper Abdomen Supplement

The next four sections, drawn from a second cadaver, illustrate a common variation of upper abdominal anatomy referenced by levels 16–13.

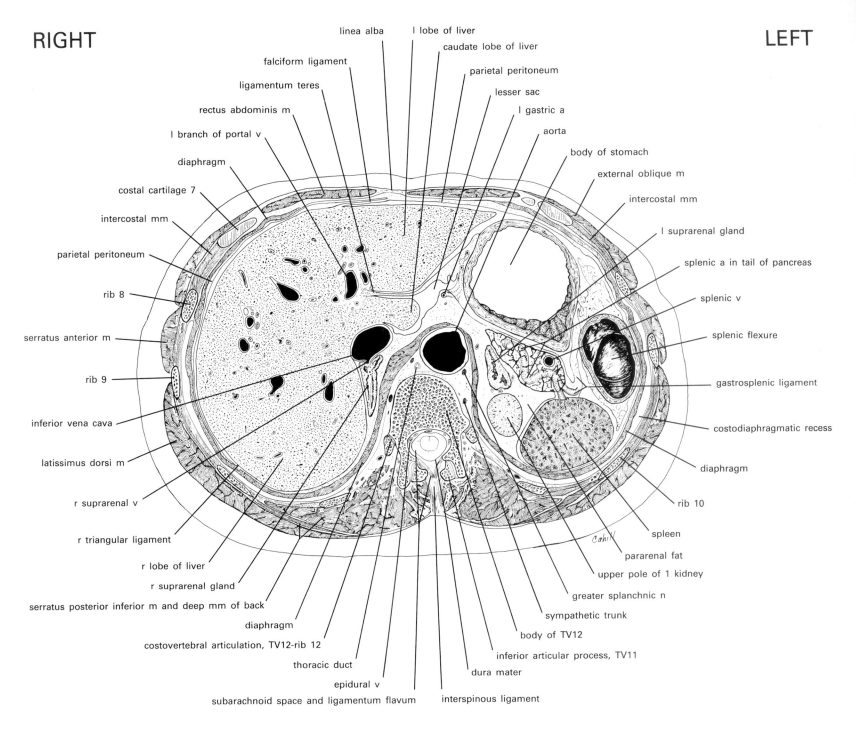

linea alba
falciform ligament
ligamentum teres
rectus abdominis m
l branch of portal v
diaphragm
costal cartilage 7
intercostal mm
parietal peritoneum
rib 8
serratus anterior m
rib 9
inferior vena cava
latissimus dorsi m
r suprarenal v
r triangular ligament
r lobe of liver
r suprarenal gland
serratus posterior inferior m and deep mm of back
diaphragm
costovertebral articulation, TV12-rib 12
thoracic duct
epidural v
subarachnoid space and ligamentum flavum

l lobe of liver
caudate lobe of liver
parietal peritoneum
lesser sac
l gastric a
aorta
body of stomach
external oblique m
intercostal mm
l suprarenal gland
splenic a in tail of pancreas
splenic v
splenic flexure
gastrosplenic ligament
costodiaphragmatic recess
diaphragm
rib 10
spleen
pararenal fat
upper pole of 1 kidney
greater splanchnic n
sympathetic trunk
body of TV12
inferior articular process, TV11
dura mater
interspinous ligament

Cahil

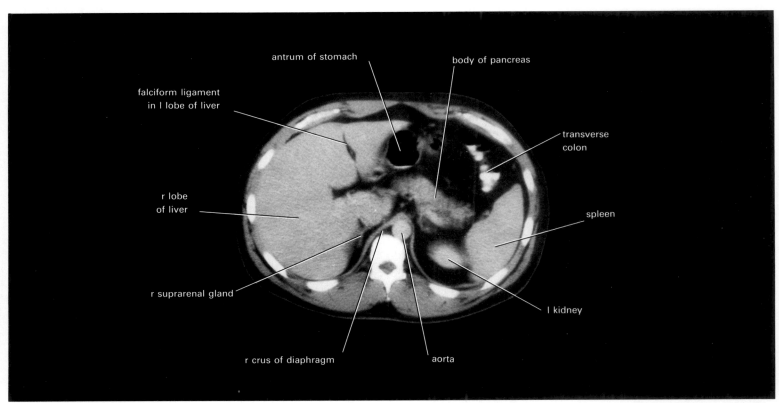

antrum of stomach
falciform ligament
in l lobe of liver
r lobe
of liver
r suprarenal gland
r crus of diaphragm

body of pancreas
transverse
colon
spleen
l kidney
aorta

Supplemental level 16.

RIGHT   LEFT

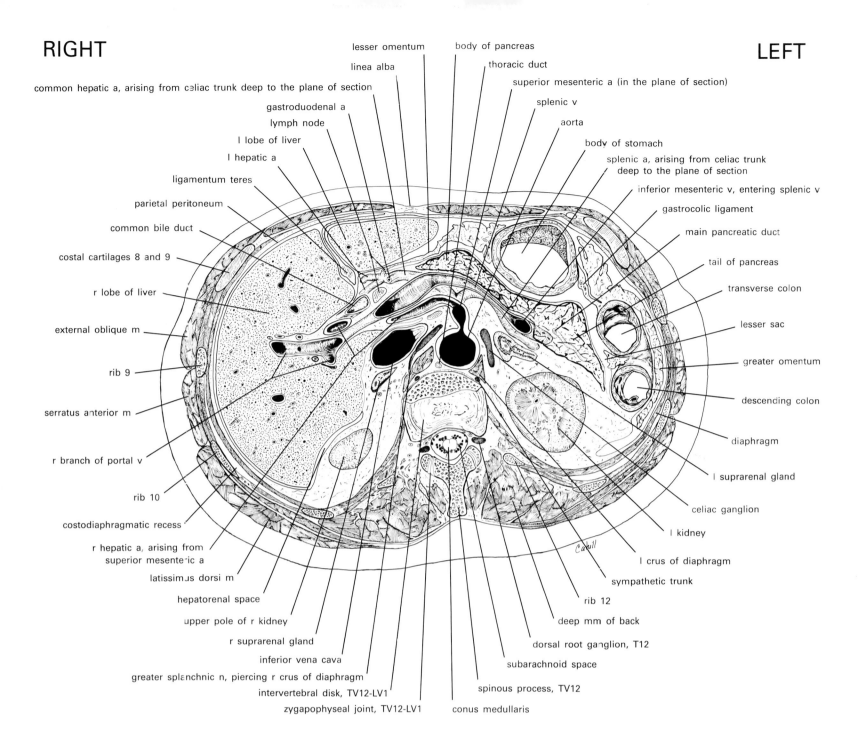

lesser omentum
linea alba
body of pancreas
thoracic duct
common hepatic a, arising from celiac trunk deep to the plane of section
superior mesenteric a (in the plane of section)
gastroduodenal a
splenic v
lymph node
aorta
l lobe of liver
body of stomach
l hepatic a
splenic a, arising from celiac trunk
deep to the plane of section
ligamentum teres
inferior mesenteric v, entering splenic v
parietal peritoneum
gastrocolic ligament
common bile duct
main pancreatic duct
costal cartilages 8 and 9
tail of pancreas
r lobe of liver
transverse colon
external oblique m
lesser sac
rib 9
greater omentum
serratus anterior m
descending colon
r branch of portal v
diaphragm
rib 10
l suprarenal gland
costodiaphragmatic recess
celiac ganglion
r hepatic a, arising from
superior mesenteric a
l kidney
latissimus dorsi m
l crus of diaphragm
hepatorenal space
sympathetic trunk
upper pole of r kidney
rib 12
r suprarenal gland
deep mm of back
inferior vena cava
dorsal root ganglion, T12
greater splanchnic n, piercing r crus of diaphragm
subarachnoid space
intervertebral disk, TV12-LV1
spinous process, TV12
zygapophyseal joint, TV12-LV1
conus medullaris

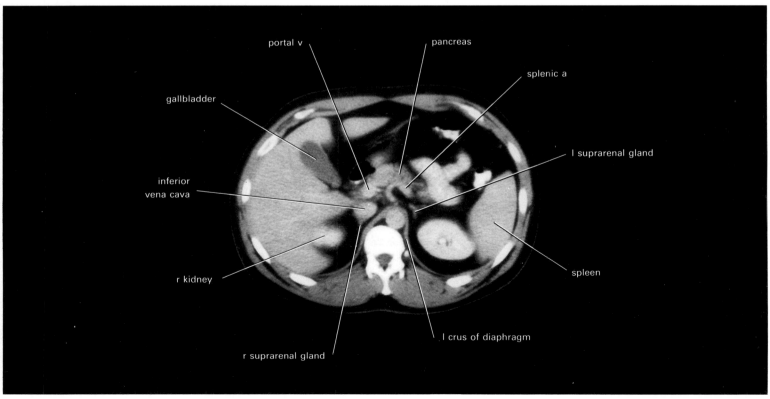

portal v
pancreas
splenic a
gallbladder
l suprarenal gland
inferior
vena cava
spleen
r kidney
r suprarenal gland
l crus of diaphragm

Supplemental level 15.

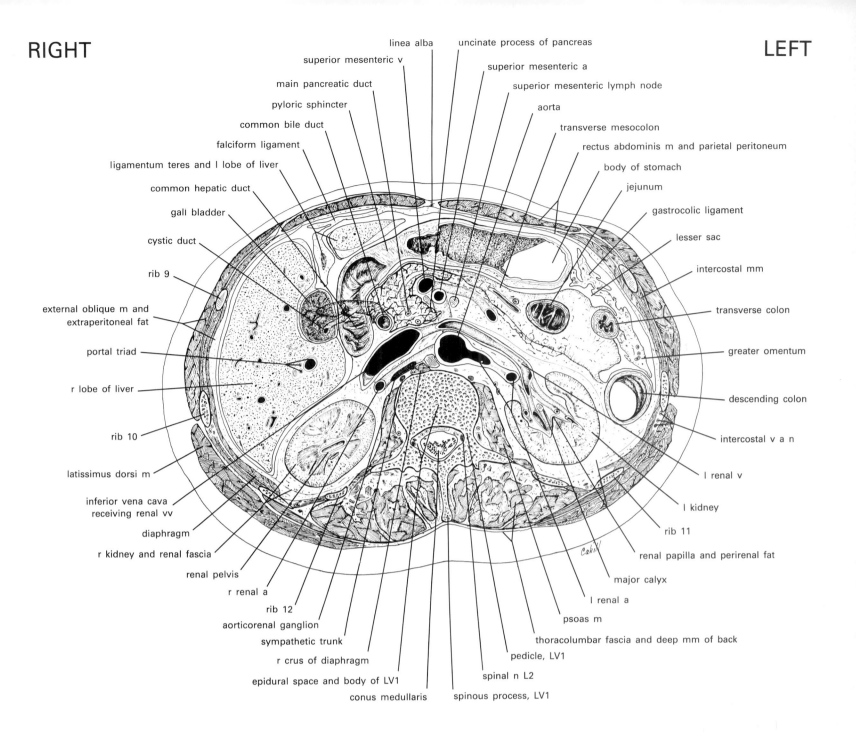

linea alba
uncinate process of pancreas
superior mesenteric v
superior mesenteric a
main pancreatic duct
superior mesenteric lymph node
pyloric sphincter
aorta
common bile duct
transverse mesocolon
falciform ligament
rectus abdominis m and parietal peritoneum
ligamentum teres and l lobe of liver
body of stomach
common hepatic duct
jejunum
gall bladder
gastrocolic ligament
cystic duct
lesser sac
rib 9
intercostal mm
external oblique m and
extraperitoneal fat
transverse colon
portal triad
greater omentum
r lobe of liver
descending colon
rib 10
intercostal v a n
latissimus dorsi m
l renal v
inferior vena cava
receiving renal vv
l kidney
diaphragm
rib 11
r kidney and renal fascia
renal papilla and perirenal fat
renal pelvis
major calyx
r renal a
l renal a
rib 12
psoas m
aorticorenal ganglion
thoracolumbar fascia and deep mm of back
sympathetic trunk
pedicle, LV1
r crus of diaphragm
spinal n L2
epidural space and body of LV1
conus medullaris
spinous process, LV1

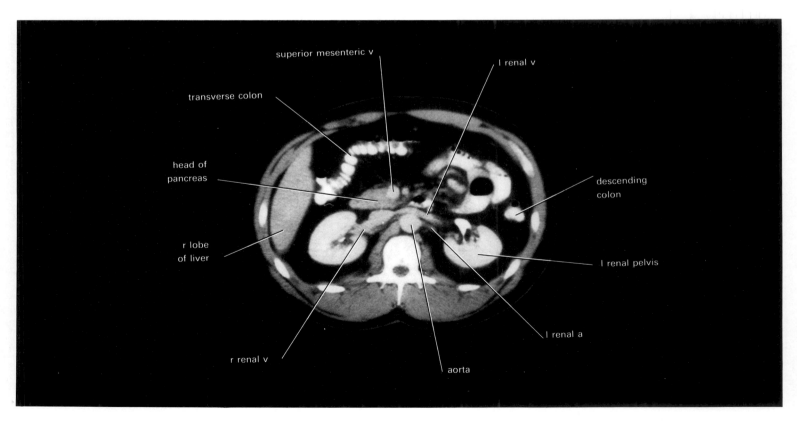

superior mesenteric v
l renal v
transverse colon
head of
pancreas
descending
colon
r lobe
of liver
l renal pelvis
r renal v
l renal a
aorta

Supplemental level 14.

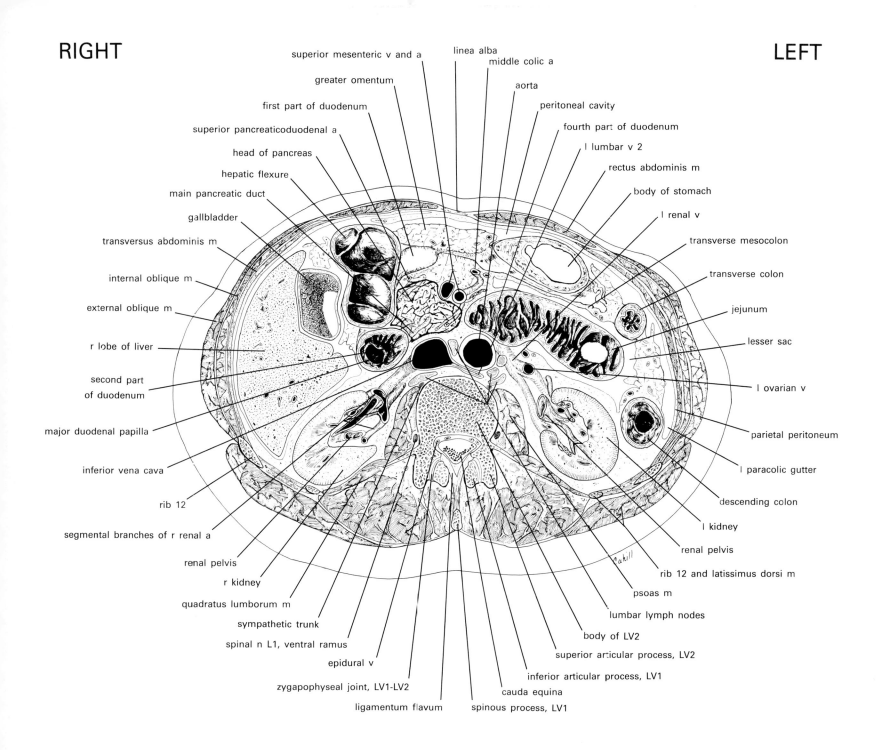

superior mesenteric v and a
linea alba
middle colic a
aorta
greater omentum
peritoneal cavity
first part of duodenum
fourth part of duodenum
superior pancreaticoduodenal a
l lumbar v 2
head of pancreas
rectus abdominis m
hepatic flexure
body of stomach
main pancreatic duct
l renal v
gallbladder
transverse mesocolon
transversus abdominis m
transverse colon
internal oblique m
jejunum
external oblique m
lesser sac
r lobe of liver
l ovarian v
second part
of duodenum
parietal peritoneum
major duodenal papilla
l paracolic gutter
inferior vena cava
descending colon
rib 12
l kidney
segmental branches of r renal a
renal pelvis
renal pelvis
rib 12 and latissimus dorsi m
r kidney
psoas m
quadratus lumborum m
lumbar lymph nodes
sympathetic trunk
body of LV2
spinal n L1, ventral ramus
superior articular process, LV2
epidural v
inferior articular process, LV1
zygapophyseal joint, LV1-LV2
cauda equina
ligamentum flavum
spinous process, LV1

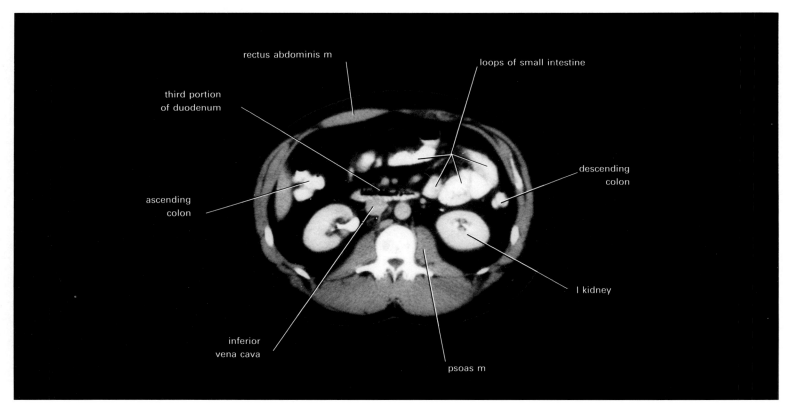

rectus abdominis m
loops of small intestine
third portion
of duodenum
descending
colon
ascending
colon
l kidney
inferior
vena cava
psoas m

Supplemental level 13.

Upper Abdominal Variations, CT

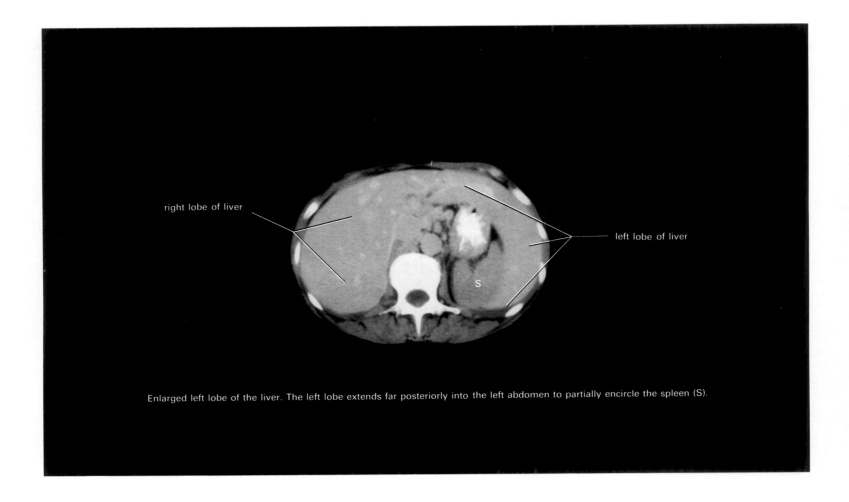

Enlarged left lobe of the liver. The left lobe extends far posteriorly into the left abdomen to partially encircle the spleen (S).

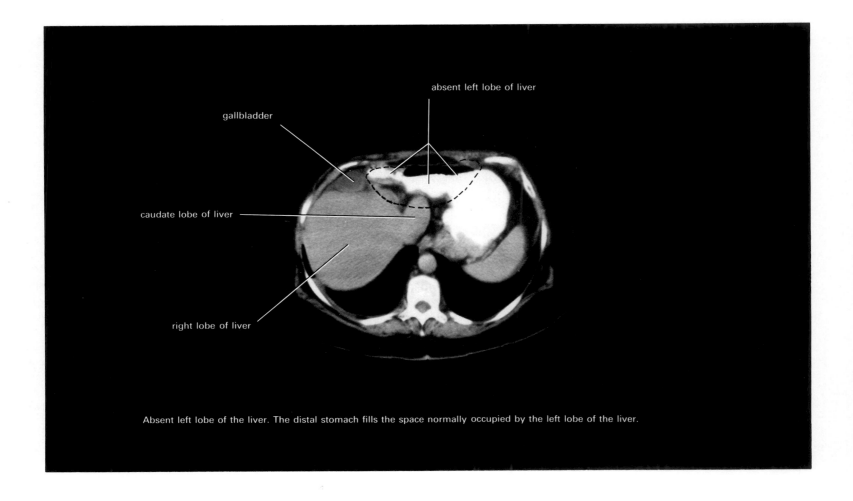

Absent left lobe of the liver. The distal stomach fills the space normally occupied by the left lobe of the liver.

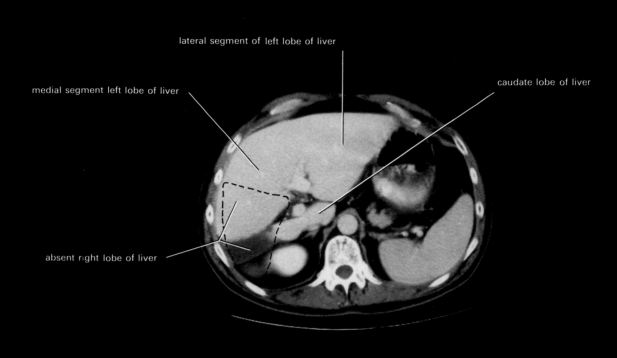

lateral segment of left lobe of liver

medial segment left lobe of liver

caudate lobe of liver

absent right lobe of liver

Absent right lobe of the liver. Compensatory hypertrophy of the remaining left and caudate lobes which partially fill the space normally occupied by the right lobe of the liver.

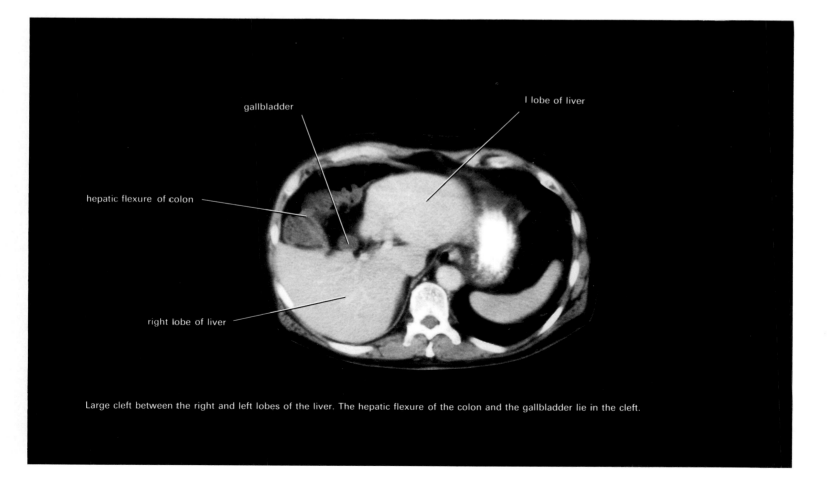

gallbladder

l lobe of liver

hepatic flexure of colon

right lobe of liver

Large cleft between the right and left lobes of the liver. The hepatic flexure of the colon and the gallbladder lie in the cleft.

The Male Pelvis

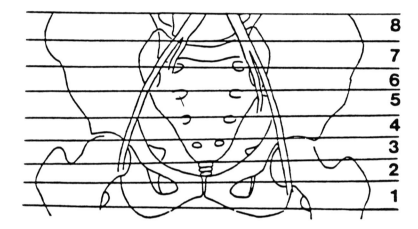

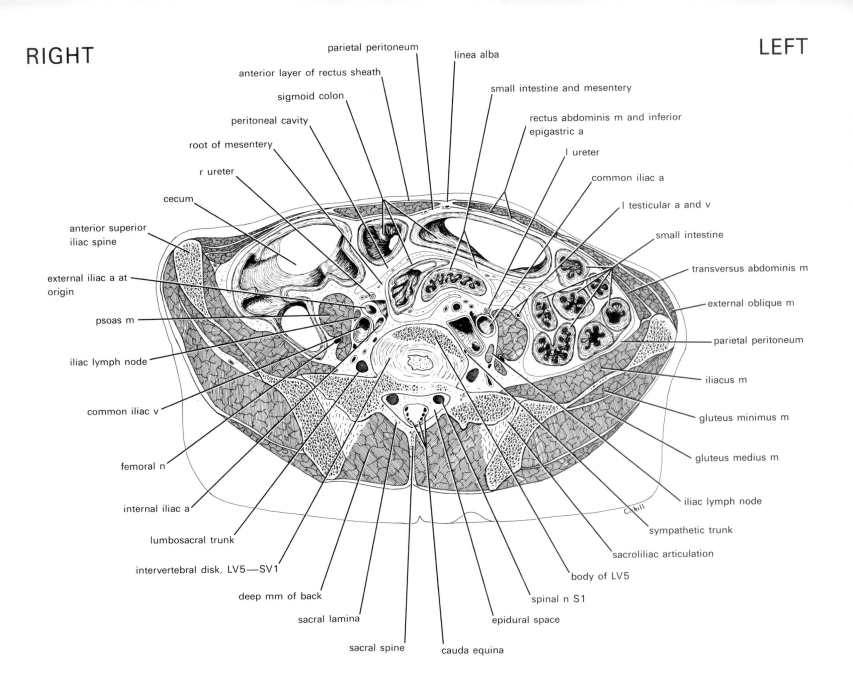

parietal peritoneum

linea alba

anterior layer of rectus sheath

small intestine and mesentery

sigmoid colon

rectus abdominis m and inferior epigastric a

peritoneal cavity

l ureter

root of mesentery

common iliac a

r ureter

l testicular a and v

cecum

small intestine

anterior superior iliac spine

transversus abdominis m

external iliac a at origin

external oblique m

psoas m

parietal peritoneum

iliac lymph node

iliacus m

gluteus minimus m

common iliac v

gluteus medius m

femoral n

iliac lymph node

internal iliac a

sympathetic trunk

lumbosacral trunk

sacroiliac articulation

intervertebral disk, LV5—SV1

body of LV5

deep mm of back

spinal n S1

sacral lamina

epidural space

sacral spine

cauda equina

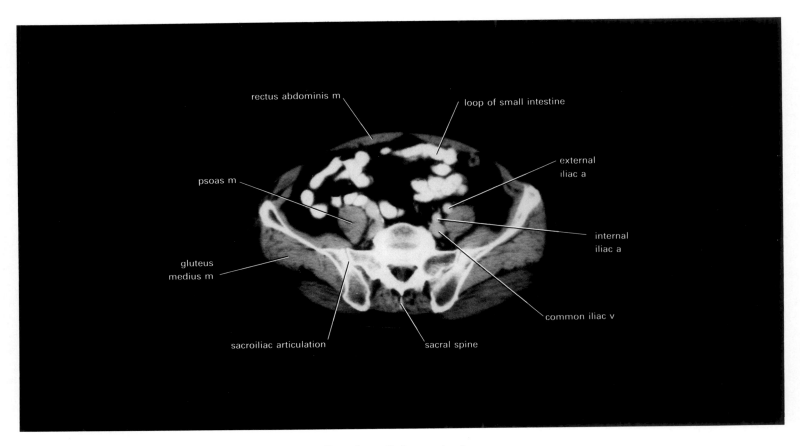

rectus abdominis m

loop of small intestine

psoas m

external iliac a

gluteus medius m

internal iliac a

common iliac v

sacroiliac articulation

sacral spine

Section 8 from below.

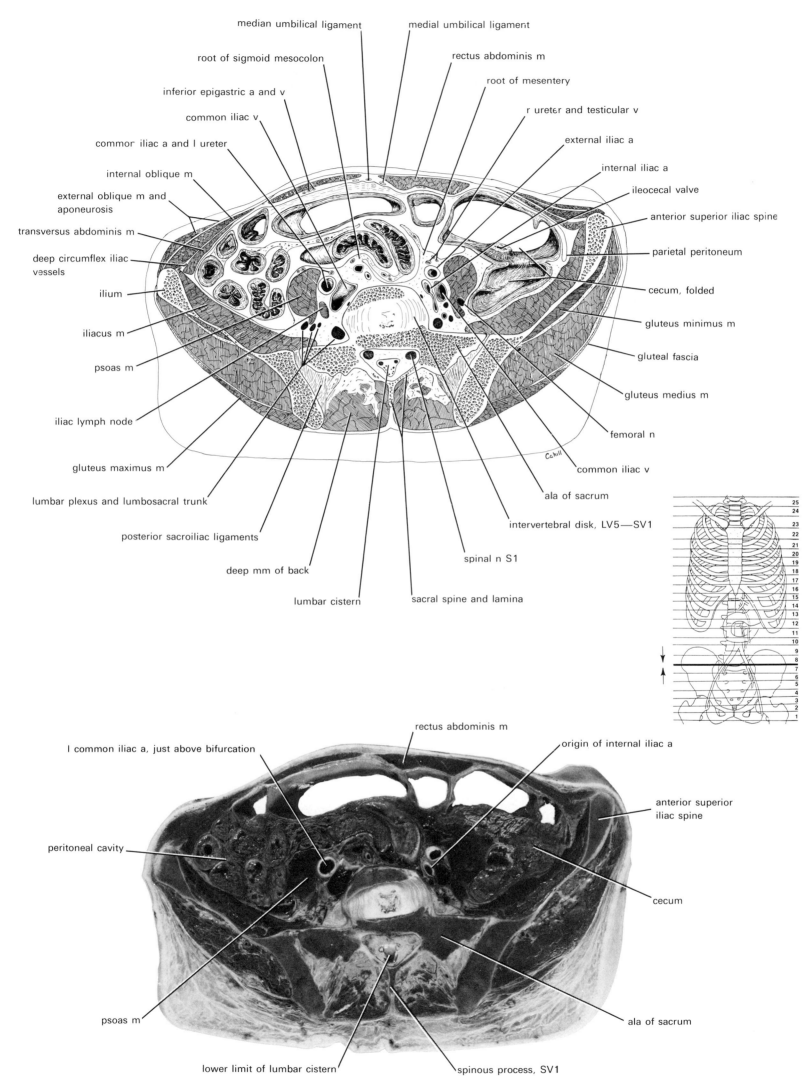

median umbilical ligament

medial umbilical ligament

root of sigmoid mesocolon

rectus abdominis m

inferior epigastric a and v

root of mesentery

common iliac v

r ureter and testicular v

common iliac a and l ureter

external iliac a

internal oblique m

internal iliac a

external oblique m and aponeurosis

ileocecal valve

transversus abdominis m

anterior superior iliac spine

deep circumflex iliac vessels

parietal peritoneum

ilium

cecum, folded

iliacus m

gluteus minimus m

psoas m

gluteal fascia

iliac lymph node

gluteus medius m

gluteus maximus m

femoral n

lumbar plexus and lumbosacral trunk

common iliac v

posterior sacroiliac ligaments

ala of sacrum

deep mm of back

intervertebral disk, LV5—SV1

lumbar cistern

spinal n S1

sacral spine and lamina

Section 7 from above.

l common iliac a, just above bifurcation

rectus abdominis m

origin of internal iliac a

peritoneal cavity

anterior superior iliac spine

psoas m

cecum

lower limit of lumbar cistern

ala of sacrum

spinous process, SV1

25
24
23
22
21
20
19
18
17
16
15
14
13
12
11
10
9
8
7
6
5
4
3
2
1

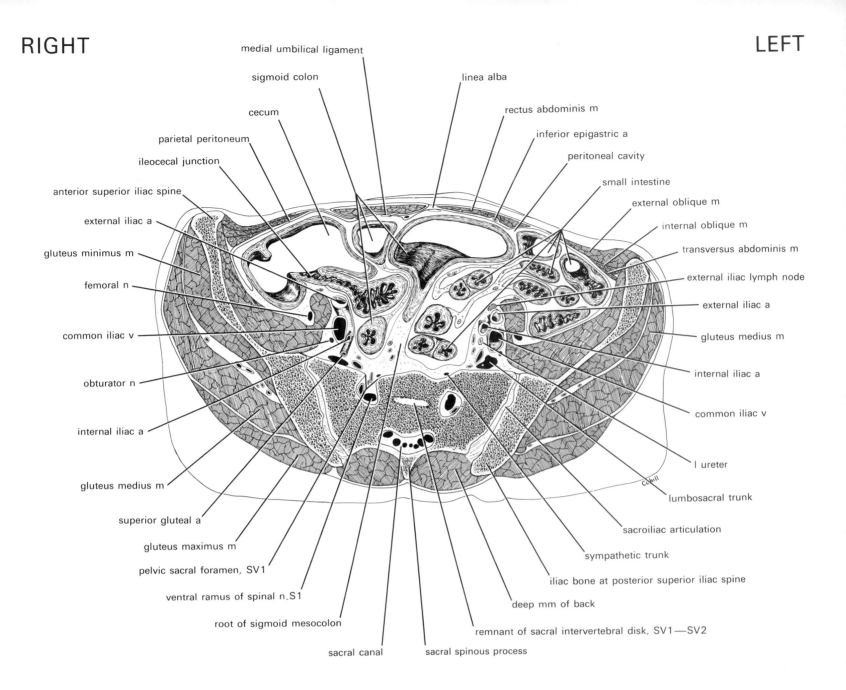

medial umbilical ligament
sigmoid colon
cecum
parietal peritoneum
ileocecal junction
anterior superior iliac spine
external iliac a
gluteus minimus m
femoral n
common iliac v
obturator n
internal iliac a
gluteus medius m
superior gluteal a
gluteus maximus m
pelvic sacral foramen, SV1
ventral ramus of spinal n. S1
root of sigmoid mesocolon
sacral canal
sacral spinous process

linea alba
rectus abdominis m
inferior epigastric a
peritoneal cavity
small intestine
external oblique m
internal oblique m
transversus abdominis m
external iliac lymph node
external iliac a
gluteus medius m
internal iliac a
common iliac v
l ureter
lumbosacral trunk
sacroiliac articulation
sympathetic trunk
iliac bone at posterior superior iliac spine
deep mm of back
remnant of sacral intervertebral disk, SV1—SV2

Cahill

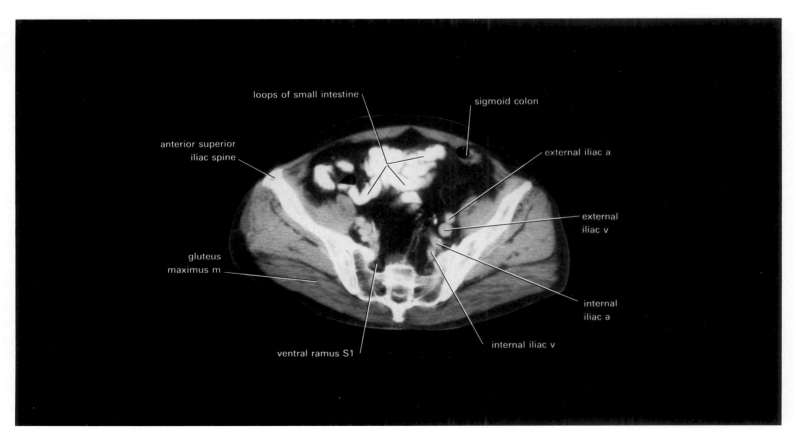

loops of small intestine
sigmoid colon
anterior superior iliac spine
external iliac a
external iliac v
gluteus maximus m
internal iliac a
ventral ramus S1
internal iliac v

Section 7 from below.

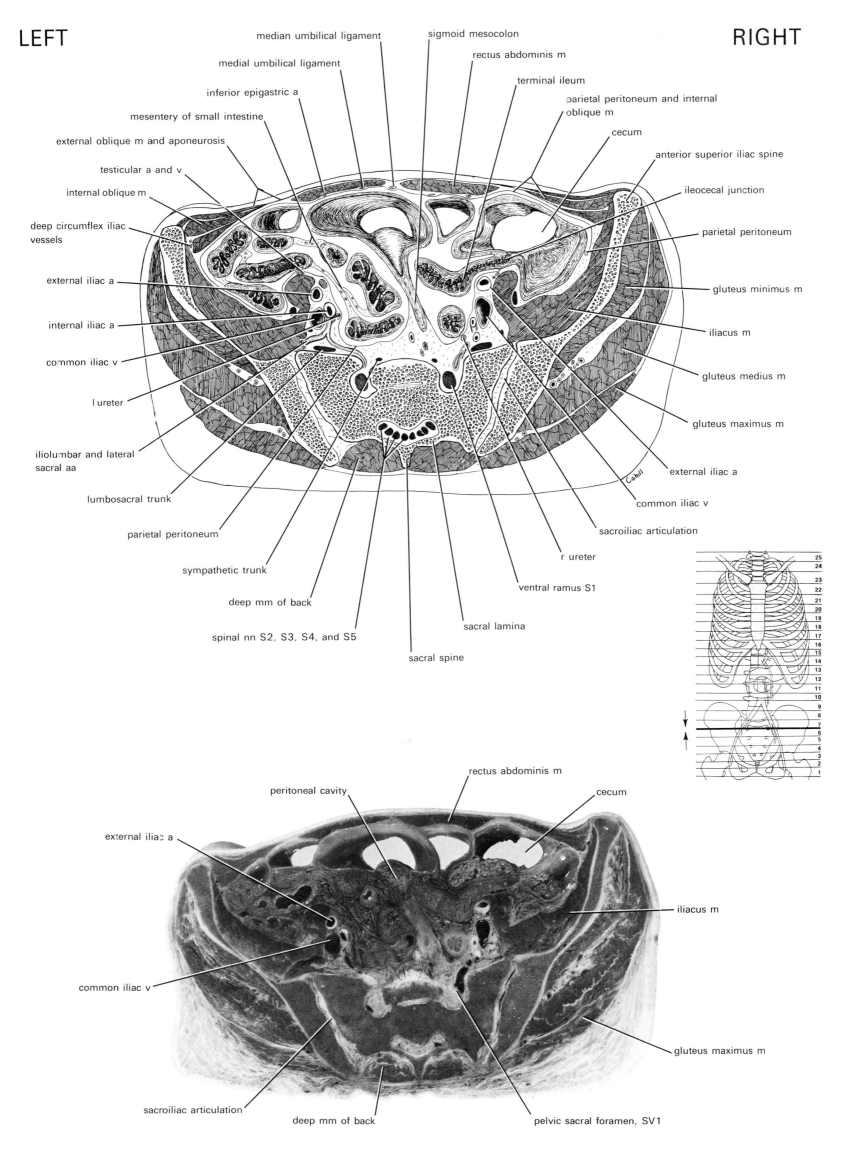

median umbilical ligament

sigmoid mesocolon

medial umbilical ligament

rectus abdominis m

inferior epigastric a

terminal ileum

mesentery of small intestine

parietal peritoneum and internal oblique m

external oblique m and aponeurosis

cecum

testicular a and v

anterior superior iliac spine

internal oblique m

ileocecal junction

deep circumflex iliac vessels

parietal peritoneum

external iliac a

gluteus minimus m

internal iliac a

iliacus m

common iliac v

gluteus medius m

l ureter

gluteus maximus m

iliolumbar and lateral sacral aa

external iliac a

lumbosacral trunk

common iliac v

parietal peritoneum

sacroiliac articulation

sympathetic trunk

r ureter

deep mm of back

ventral ramus S1

spinal nn S2, S3, S4, and S5

sacral lamina

sacral spine

Section 6 from above.

peritoneal cavity

rectus abdominis m

cecum

external iliac a

iliacus m

common iliac v

sacroiliac articulation

gluteus maximus m

deep mm of back

pelvic sacral foramen, SV1

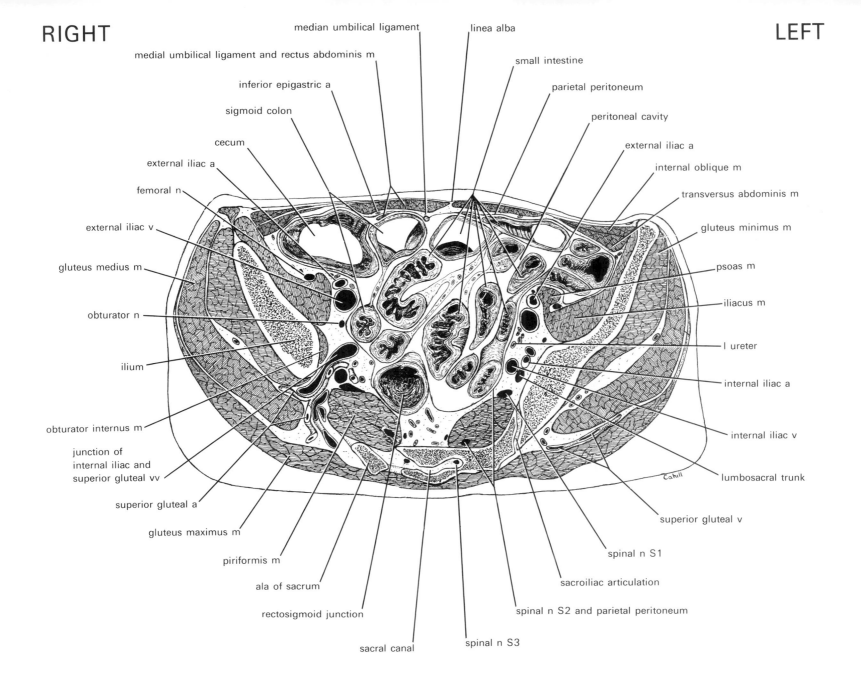

median umbilical ligament
linea alba
medial umbilical ligament and rectus abdominis m
small intestine
inferior epigastric a
parietal peritoneum
sigmoid colon
peritoneal cavity
cecum
external iliac a
external iliac a
internal oblique m
femoral n
transversus abdominis m
external iliac v
gluteus minimus m
gluteus medius m
psoas m
obturator n
iliacus m
ilium
l ureter
internal iliac a
obturator internus m
internal iliac v
junction of
internal iliac and
superior gluteal vv
lumbosacral trunk
superior gluteal a
superior gluteal v
gluteus maximus m
spinal n S1
piriformis m
sacroiliac articulation
ala of sacrum
spinal n S2 and parietal peritoneum
rectosigmoid junction
sacral canal
spinal n S3

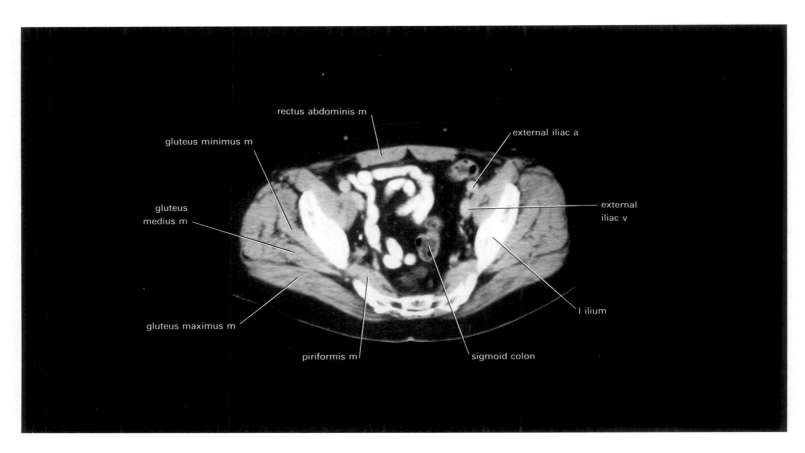

rectus abdominis m
gluteus minimus m
external iliac a
gluteus
medius m
external
iliac v
gluteus maximus m
l ilium
piriformis m
sigmoid colon

Section 6 from below.

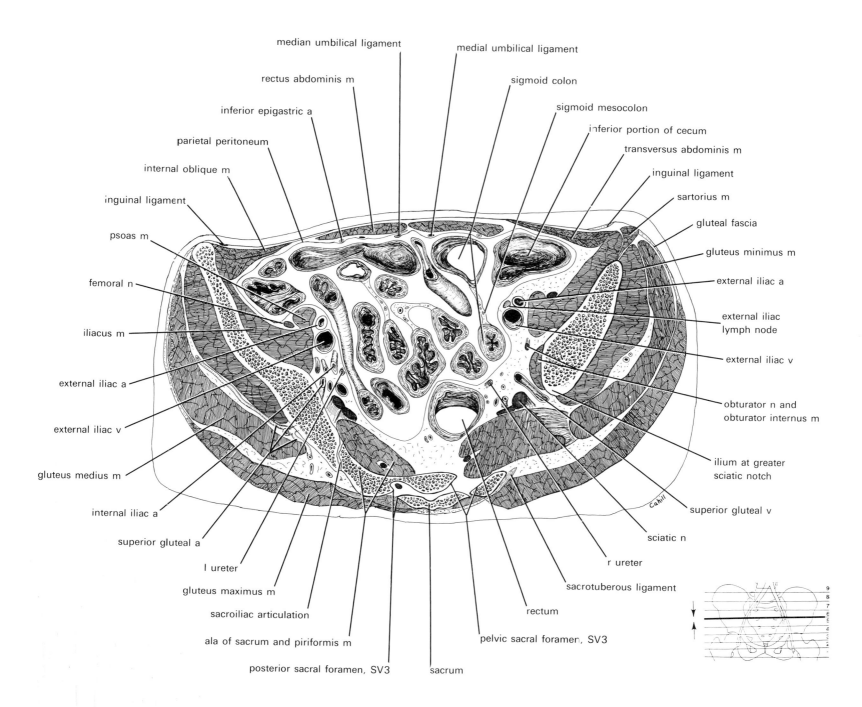

median umbilical ligament

medial umbilical ligament

rectus abdominis m

sigmoid colon

inferior epigastric a

sigmoid mesocolon

parietal peritoneum

inferior portion of cecum

internal oblique m

transversus abdominis m

inguinal ligament

inguinal ligament

sartorius m

psoas m

gluteal fascia

gluteus minimus m

femoral n

external iliac a

iliacus m

external iliac
lymph node

external iliac a

external iliac v

external iliac v

obturator n and
obturator internus m

gluteus medius m

ilium at greater
sciatic notch

internal iliac a

superior gluteal v

superior gluteal a

sciatic n

l ureter

r ureter

gluteus maximus m

sacrotuberous ligament

sacroiliac articulation

rectum

ala of sacrum and piriformis m

pelvic sacral foramen, SV3

posterior sacral foramen, SV3

sacrum

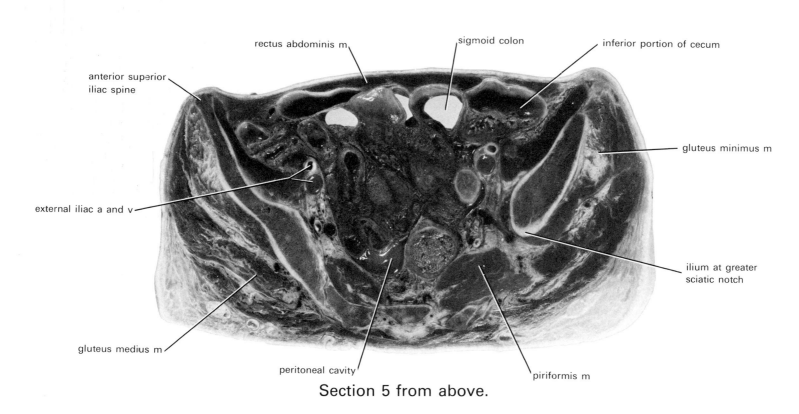

rectus abdominis m

sigmoid colon

inferior portion of cecum

anterior superior
iliac spine

gluteus minimus m

external iliac a and v

ilium at greater
sciatic notch

gluteus medius m

peritoneal cavity

piriformis m

Section 5 from above.

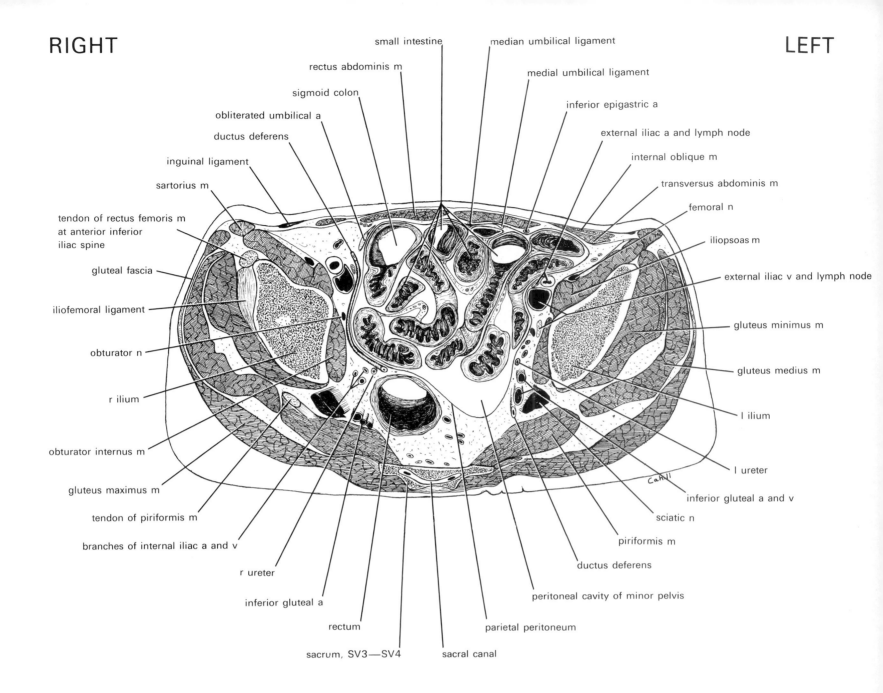

small intestine
median umbilical ligament
rectus abdominis m
medial umbilical ligament
sigmoid colon
inferior epigastric a
obliterated umbilical a
external iliac a and lymph node
ductus deferens
internal oblique m
inguinal ligament
transversus abdominis m
sartorius m
femoral n
tendon of rectus femoris m
at anterior inferior
iliac spine
iliopsoas m
gluteal fascia
external iliac v and lymph node
iliofemoral ligament
gluteus minimus m
obturator n
gluteus medius m
r ilium
l ilium
obturator internus m
l ureter
gluteus maximus m
inferior gluteal a and v
tendon of piriformis m
sciatic n
branches of internal iliac a and v
piriformis m
ductus deferens
r ureter
peritoneal cavity of minor pelvis
inferior gluteal a
parietal peritoneum
rectum
sacrum, SV3—SV4
sacral canal

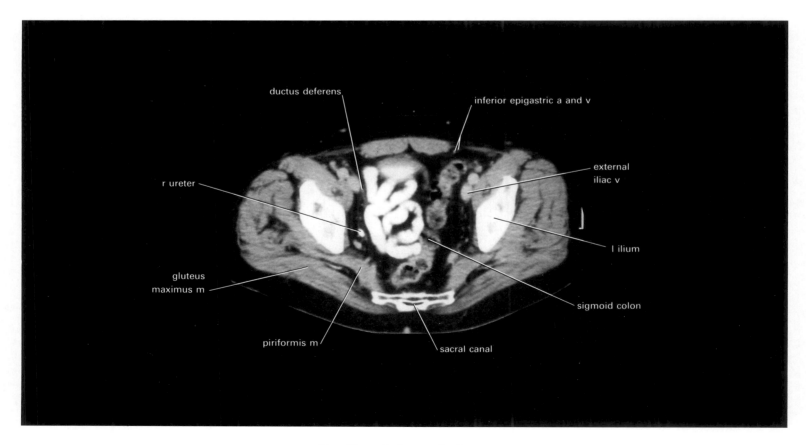

ductus deferens
inferior epigastric a and v
r ureter
external
iliac v
gluteus
maximus m
l ilium
piriformis m
sigmoid colon
sacral canal

Section 5 from below.

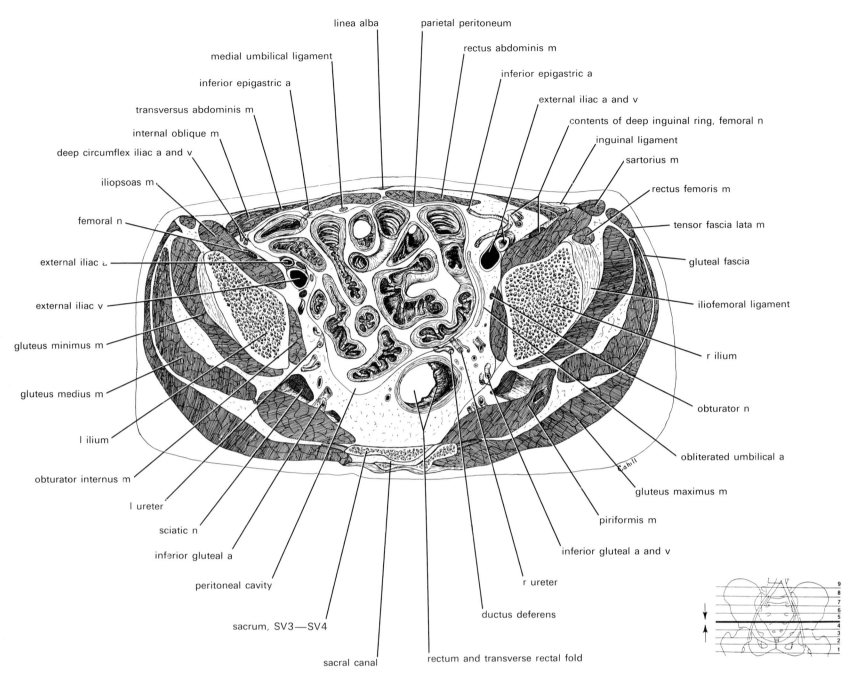

linea alba
parietal peritoneum
rectus abdominis m
medial umbilical ligament
inferior epigastric a
inferior epigastric a
transversus abdominis m
external iliac a and v
internal oblique m
contents of deep inguinal ring, femoral n
deep circumflex iliac a and v
inguinal ligament
iliopsoas m
sartorius m
rectus femoris m
femoral n
tensor fascia lata m
external iliac a
gluteal fascia
external iliac v
iliofemoral ligament
gluteus minimus m
r ilium
gluteus medius m
obturator n
l ilium
obturator internus m
obliterated umbilical a
l ureter
gluteus maximus m
sciatic n
piriformis m
inferior gluteal a
inferior gluteal a and v
peritoneal cavity
r ureter
sacrum, SV3—SV4
ductus deferens
sacral canal
rectum and transverse rectal fold

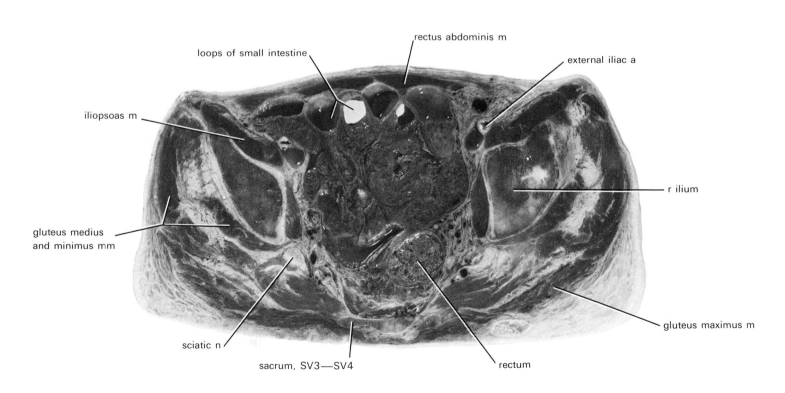

loops of small intestine
rectus abdominis m
external iliac a
iliopsoas m
r ilium
gluteus medius
and minimus mm
gluteus maximus m
sciatic n
sacrum, SV3—SV4
rectum

Section 4 from above.

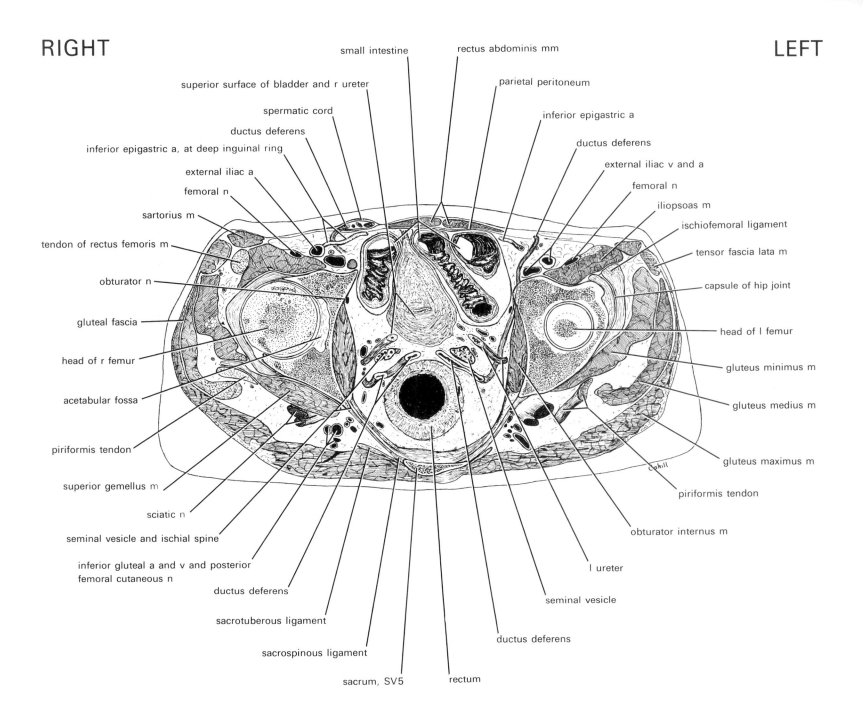

small intestine

rectus abdominis mm

superior surface of bladder and r ureter

parietal peritoneum

spermatic cord

inferior epigastric a

ductus deferens

ductus deferens

inferior epigastric a, at deep inguinal ring

external iliac v and a

external iliac a

femoral n

femoral n

iliopsoas m

sartorius m

ischiofemoral ligament

tendon of rectus femoris m

tensor fascia lata m

obturator n

capsule of hip joint

gluteal fascia

head of l femur

head of r femur

gluteus minimus m

acetabular fossa

gluteus medius m

piriformis tendon

gluteus maximus m

superior gemellus m

piriformis tendon

sciatic n

obturator internus m

seminal vesicle and ischial spine

l ureter

inferior gluteal a and v and posterior
femoral cutaneous n

seminal vesicle

ductus deferens

ductus deferens

sacrotuberous ligament

sacrospinous ligament

rectum

sacrum, SV5

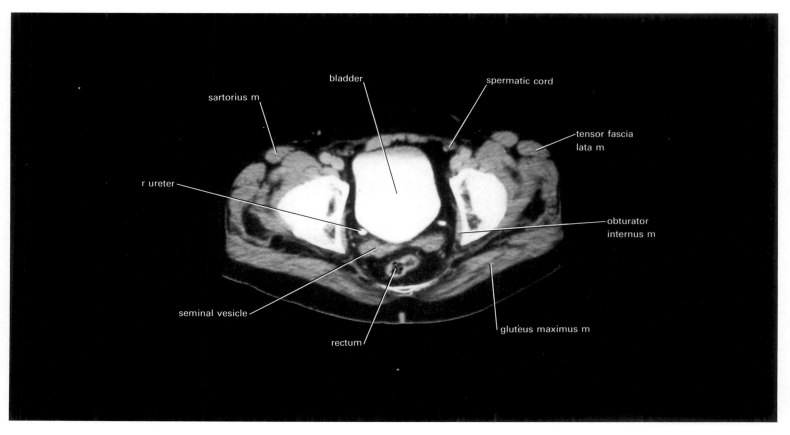

bladder

spermatic cord

sartorius m

tensor fascia
lata m

r ureter

obturator
internus m

seminal vesicle

gluteus maximus m

rectum

Section 4 from below.

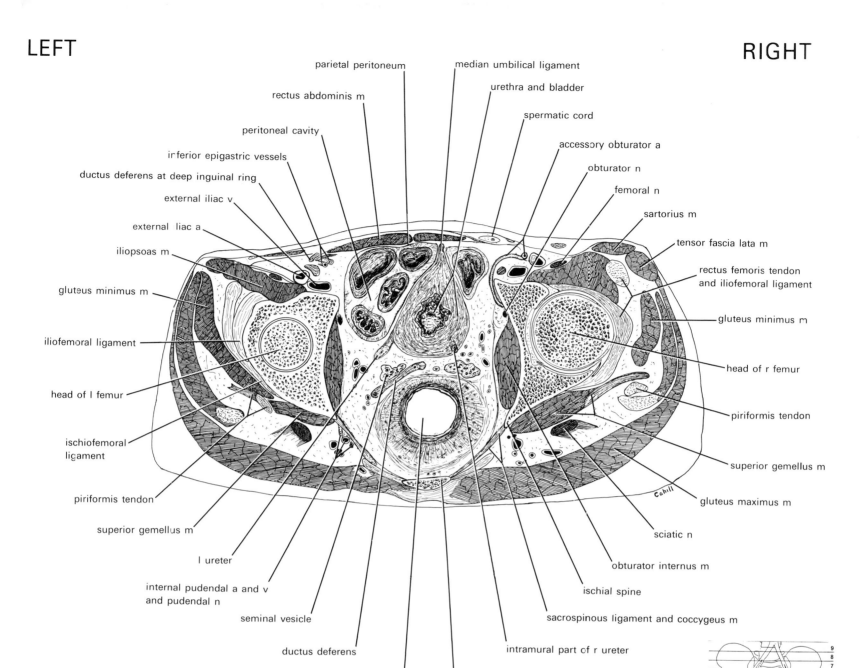

parietal peritoneum

median umbilical ligament

rectus abdominis m

urethra and bladder

spermatic cord

peritoneal cavity

accessory obturator a

inferior epigastric vessels

obturator n

ductus deferens at deep inguinal ring

femoral n

external iliac v

sartorius m

external liac a

tensor fascia lata m

iliopsoas m

rectus femoris tendon
and iliofemoral ligament

gluteus minimus m

gluteus minimus m

iliofemoral ligament

head of r femur

head of l femur

piriformis tendon

ischiofemoral
ligament

superior gemellus m

piriformis tendon

gluteus maximus m

superior gemellus m

sciatic n

l ureter

obturator internus m

internal pudendal a and v
and pudendal n

ischial spine

seminal vesicle

sacrospinous ligament and coccygeus m

ductus deferens

intramural part of r ureter

rectum

inferior aspect of sacrum

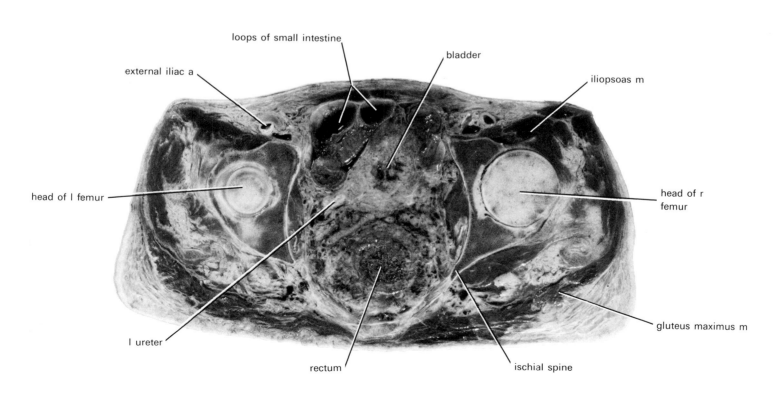

loops of small intestine

bladder

external iliac a

iliopsoas m

head of l femur

head of r
femur

gluteus maximus m

l ureter

rectum

ischial spine

Section 3 from above.

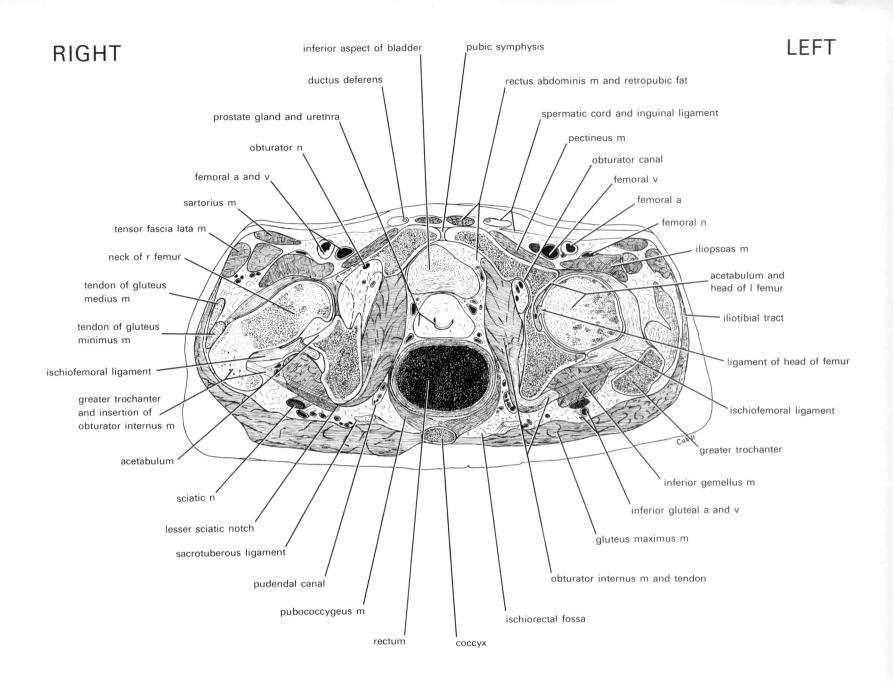

inferior aspect of bladder

pubic symphysis

ductus deferens

rectus abdominis m and retropubic fat

prostate gland and urethra

spermatic cord and inguinal ligament

obturator n

pectineus m

femoral a and v

obturator canal

sartorius m

femoral v

tensor fascia lata m

femoral a

neck of r femur

femoral n

tendon of gluteus
medius m

iliopsoas m

tendon of gluteus
minimus m

acetabulum and
head of l femur

ischiofemoral ligament

iliotibial tract

greater trochanter
and insertion of
obturator internus m

ligament of head of femur

acetabulum

ischiofemoral ligament

sciatic n

greater trochanter

lesser sciatic notch

inferior gemellus m

sacrotuberous ligament

inferior gluteal a and v

pudendal canal

gluteus maximus m

pubococcygeus m

obturator internus m and tendon

rectum

ischiorectal fossa

coccyx

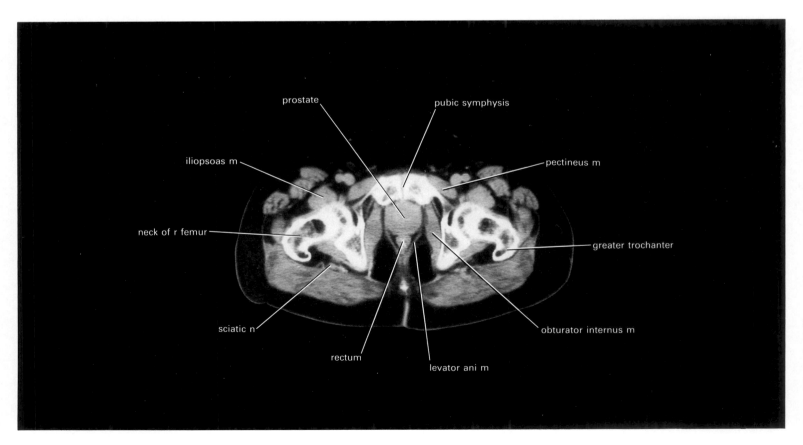

prostate

pubic symphysis

iliopsoas m

pectineus m

neck of r femur

greater trochanter

sciatic n

obturator internus m

rectum

levator ani m

Section 3 from below.

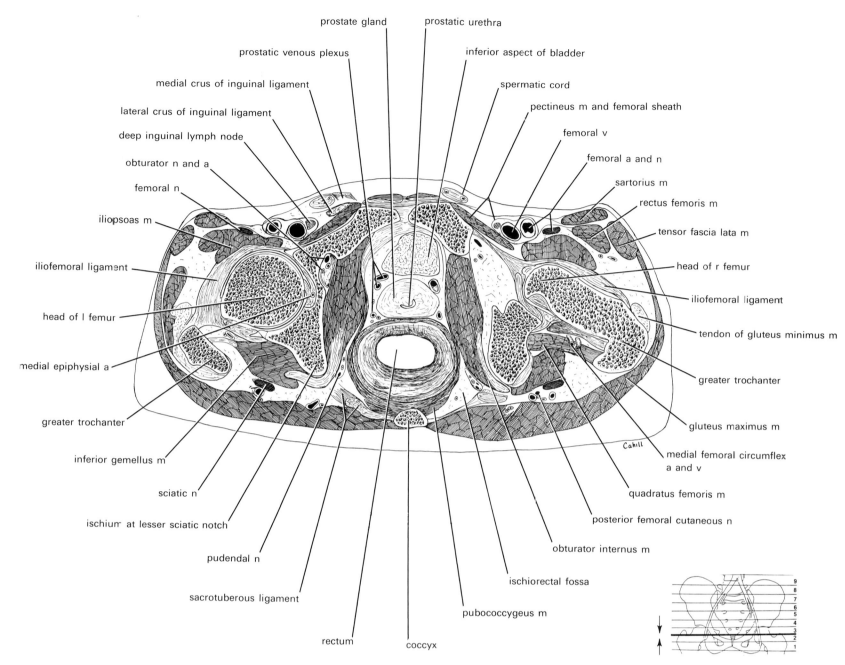

prostate gland
prostatic urethra
prostatic venous plexus
inferior aspect of bladder
medial crus of inguinal ligament
spermatic cord
lateral crus of inguinal ligament
pectineus m and femoral sheath
deep inguinal lymph node
femoral v
obturator n and a
femoral a and n
femoral n
sartorius m
iliopsoas m
rectus femoris m
tensor fascia lata m
iliofemoral ligament
head of r femur
head of l femur
iliofemoral ligament
medial epiphysial a
tendon of gluteus minimus m
greater trochanter
greater trochanter
gluteus maximus m
inferior gemellus m
medial femoral circumflex a and v
sciatic n
quadratus femoris m
ischium at lesser sciatic notch
posterior femoral cutaneous n
pudendal n
obturator internus m
sacrotuberous ligament
ischiorectal fossa
rectum
pubococcygeus m
coccyx

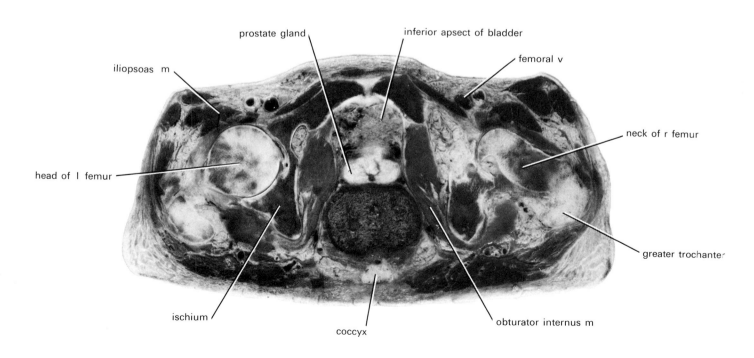

prostate gland
inferior apsect of bladder
femoral v
iliopsoas m
head of l femur
neck of r femur
ischium
greater trochanter
coccyx
obturator internus m

Section 2 from above.

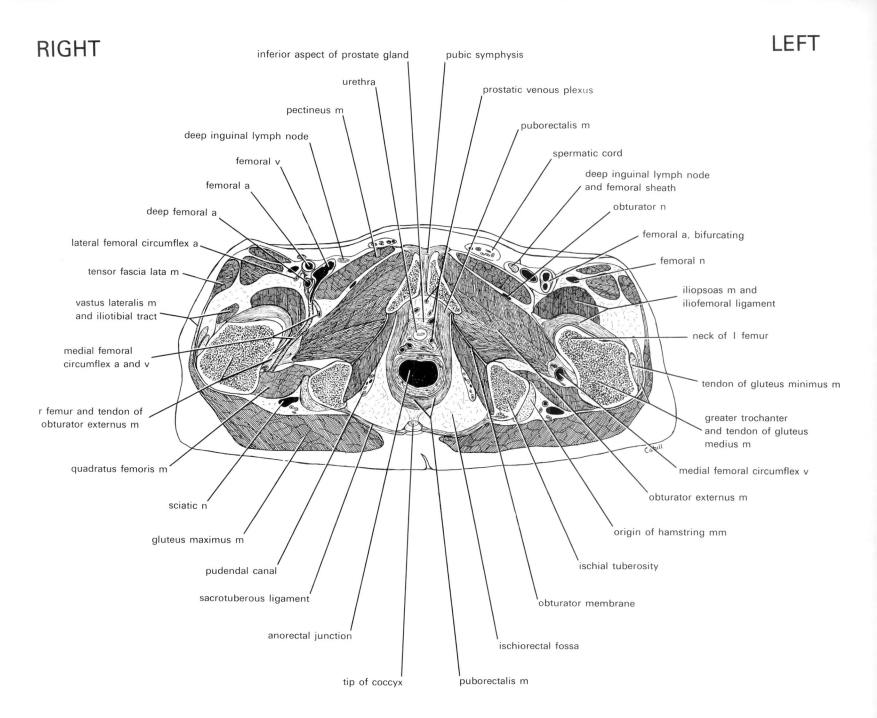

inferior aspect of prostate gland
pubic symphysis
urethra
prostatic venous plexus
pectineus m
puborectalis m
deep inguinal lymph node
spermatic cord
femoral v
deep inguinal lymph node
and femoral sheath
femoral a
obturator n
deep femoral a
femoral a, bifurcating
lateral femoral circumflex a
femoral n
tensor fascia lata m
iliopsoas m and
iliofemoral ligament
vastus lateralis m
and iliotibial tract
neck of l femur
medial femoral
circumflex a and v
tendon of gluteus minimus m
r femur and tendon of
obturator externus m
greater trochanter
and tendon of gluteus
medius m
quadratus femoris m
medial femoral circumflex v
sciatic n
obturator externus m
gluteus maximus m
origin of hamstring mm
pudendal canal
ischial tuberosity
sacrotuberous ligament
obturator membrane
anorectal junction
ischiorectal fossa
tip of coccyx
puborectalis m

Cahill

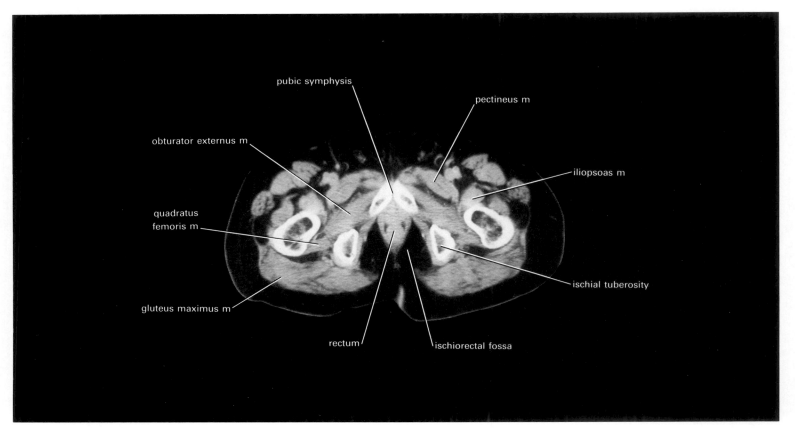

pubic symphysis
pectineus m
obturator externus m
iliopsoas m
quadratus
femoris m
ischial tuberosity
gluteus maximus m
rectum
ischiorectal fossa

Section 2 from below.

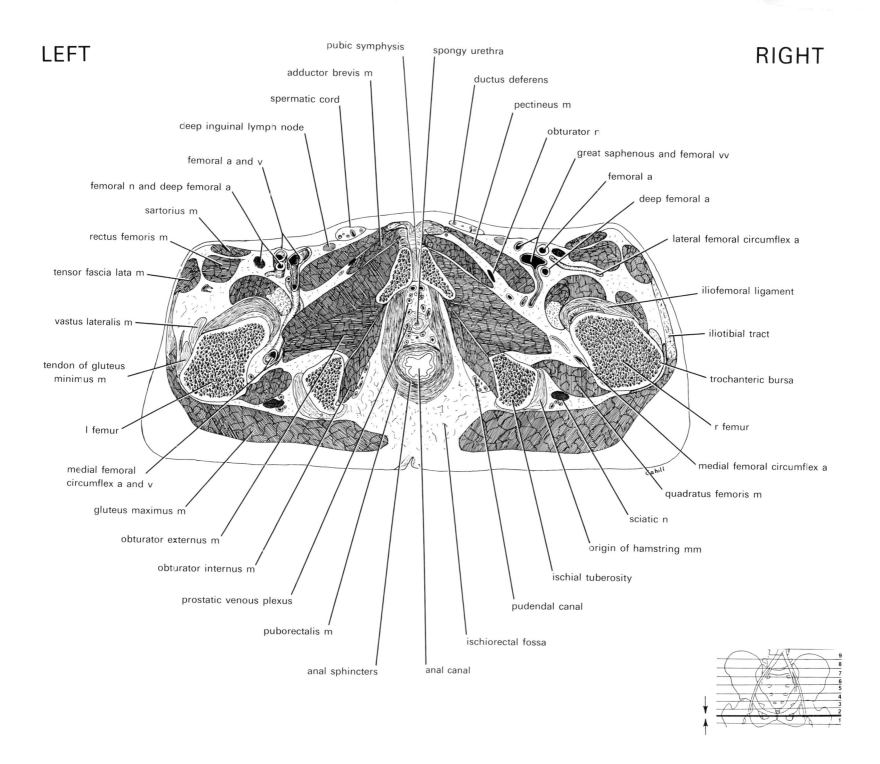

pubic symphysis

adductor brevis m

spermatic cord

deep inguinal lymph node

femoral a and v

femoral n and deep femoral a

sartorius m

rectus femoris m

tensor fascia lata m

vastus lateralis m

tendon of gluteus
minimus m

l femur

medial femoral
circumflex a and v

gluteus maximus m

obturator externus m

obturator internus m

prostatic venous plexus

puborectalis m

anal sphincters

spongy urethra

ductus deferens

pectineus m

obturator n

great saphenous and femoral vv

femoral a

deep femoral a

lateral femoral circumflex a

iliofemoral ligament

iliotibial tract

trochanteric bursa

r femur

medial femoral circumflex a

quadratus femoris m

sciatic n

origin of hamstring mm

ischial tuberosity

pudendal canal

ischiorectal fossa

anal canal

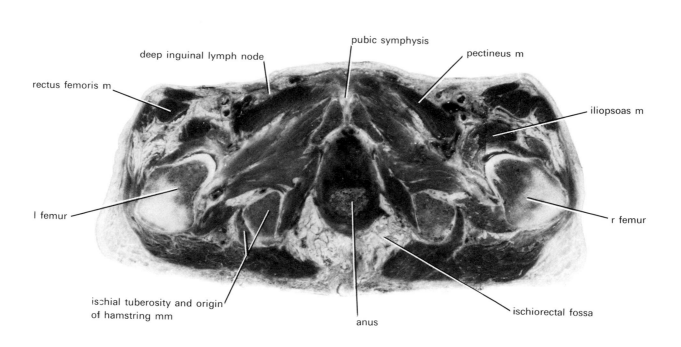

pubic symphysis

deep inguinal lymph node

pectineus m

rectus femoris m

iliopsoas m

l femur

r femur

ischial tuberosity and origin
of hamstring mm

anus

ischiorectal fossa

Section 1 from above.

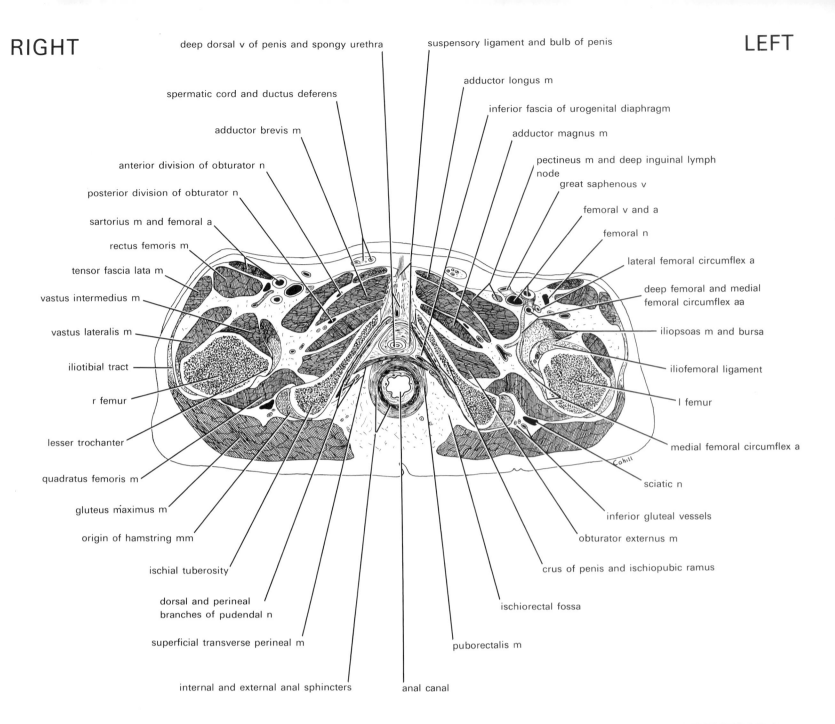

deep dorsal v of penis and spongy urethra

suspensory ligament and bulb of penis

spermatic cord and ductus deferens

adductor longus m

inferior fascia of urogenital diaphragm

adductor brevis m

adductor magnus m

anterior division of obturator n

pectineus m and deep inguinal lymph node

posterior division of obturator n

great saphenous v

sartorius m and femoral a

femoral v and a

rectus femoris m

femoral n

tensor fascia lata m

lateral femoral circumflex a

vastus intermedius m

deep femoral and medial femoral circumflex aa

vastus lateralis m

iliopsoas m and bursa

iliotibial tract

iliofemoral ligament

r femur

l femur

lesser trochanter

medial femoral circumflex a

quadratus femoris m

sciatic n

gluteus maximus m

inferior gluteal vessels

origin of hamstring mm

obturator externus m

ischial tuberosity

crus of penis and ischiopubic ramus

dorsal and perineal branches of pudendal n

ischiorectal fossa

superficial transverse perineal m

puborectalis m

internal and external anal sphincters

anal canal

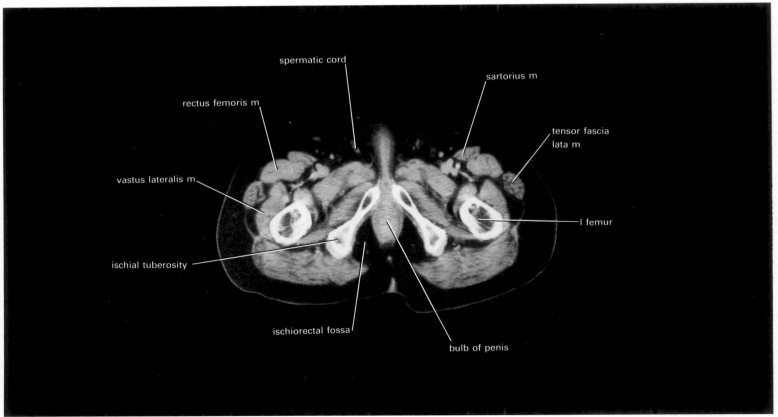

spermatic cord

sartorius m

rectus femoris m

tensor fascia lata m

vastus lateralis m

l femur

ischial tuberosity

ischiorectal fossa

bulb of penis

Section 1 from below.

The Female Pelvis

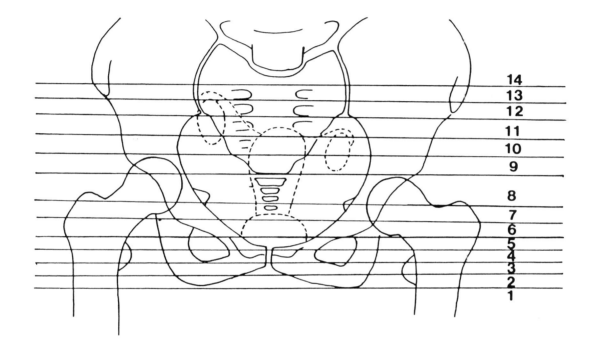

14
13
12
11
10
9
8
7
6
5
4
3
2
1

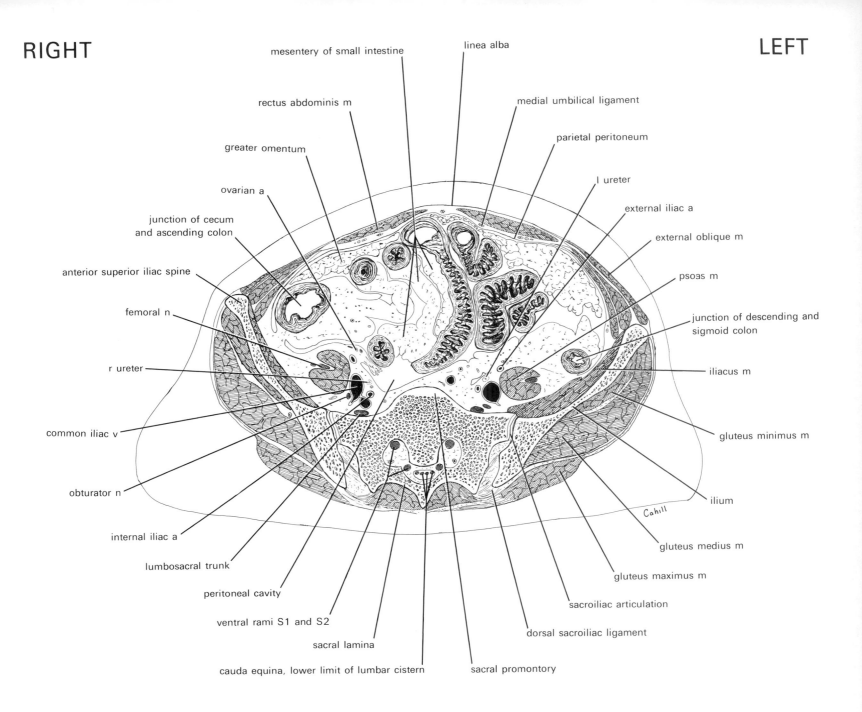

mesentery of small intestine

linea alba

rectus abdominis m

medial umbilical ligament

greater omentum

parietal peritoneum

ovarian a

l ureter

junction of cecum
and ascending colon

external iliac a

external oblique m

anterior superior iliac spine

psoas m

femoral n

junction of descending and
sigmoid colon

r ureter

iliacus m

common iliac v

gluteus minimus m

obturator n

ilium

internal iliac a

gluteus medius m

lumbosacral trunk

gluteus maximus m

peritoneal cavity

sacroiliac articulation

ventral rami S1 and S2

dorsal sacroiliac ligament

sacral lamina

cauda equina, lower limit of lumbar cistern

sacral promontory

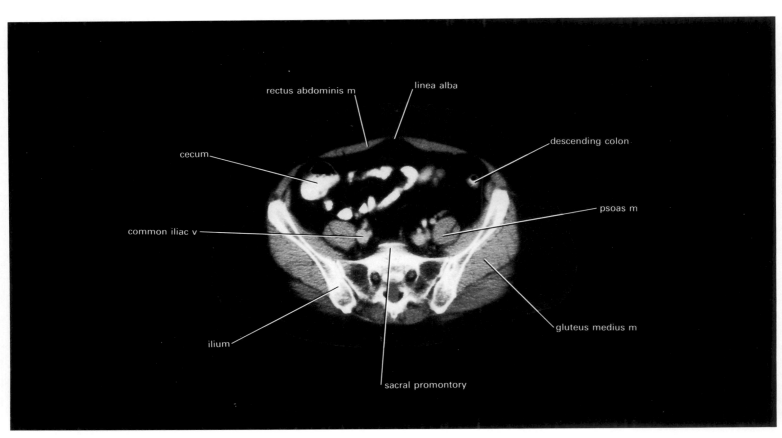

rectus abdominis m

linea alba

cecum

descending colon

psoas m

common iliac v

ilium

sacral promontory

gluteus medius m

Section 14 from below.

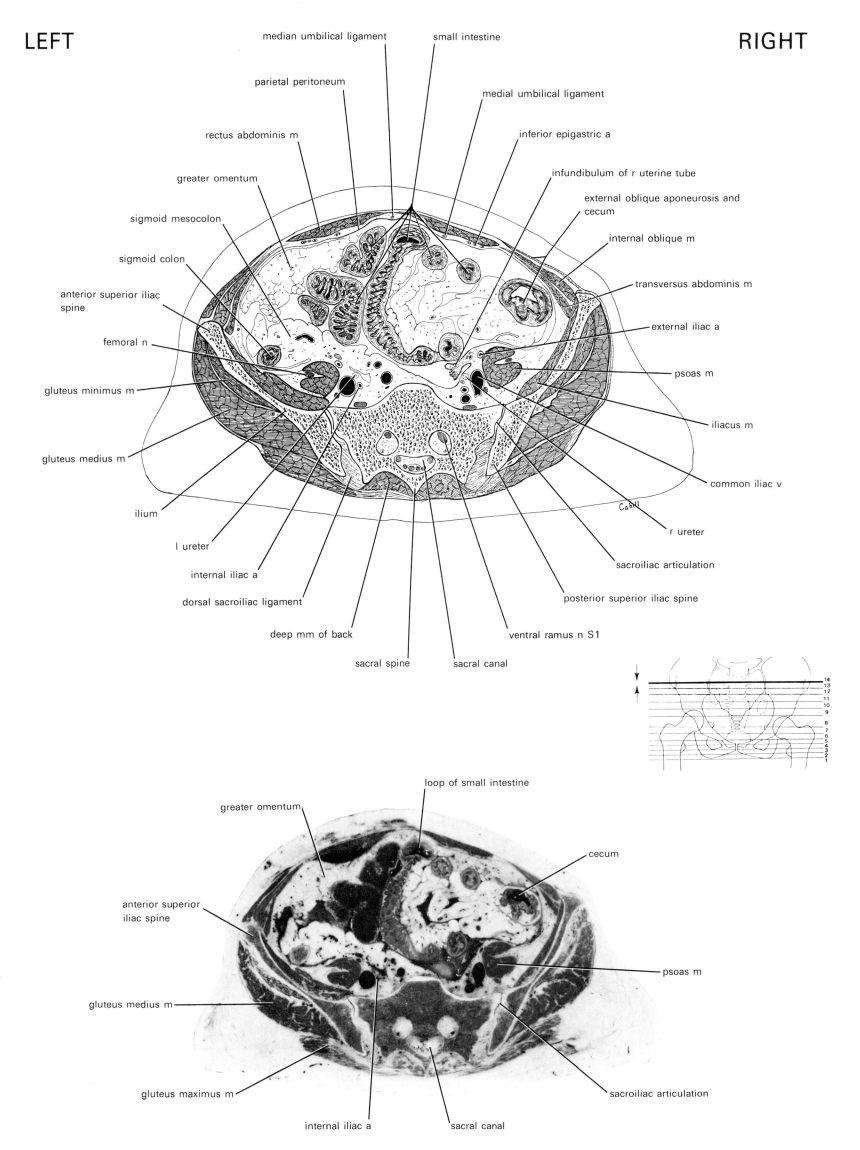

median umbilical ligament
small intestine
parietal peritoneum
medial umbilical ligament
rectus abdominis m
inferior epigastric a
greater omentum
infundibulum of r uterine tube
sigmoid mesocolon
external oblique aponeurosis and cecum
sigmoid colon
internal oblique m
anterior superior iliac spine
transversus abdominis m
femoral n
external iliac a
gluteus minimus m
psoas m
gluteus medius m
iliacus m
ilium
common iliac v
l ureter
r ureter
internal iliac a
sacroiliac articulation
dorsal sacroiliac ligament
posterior superior iliac spine
deep mm of back
ventral ramus n S1
sacral spine
sacral canal

Cahll

loop of small intestine
greater omentum
cecum
anterior superior iliac spine
psoas m
gluteus medius m
gluteus maximus m
sacroiliac articulation
internal iliac a
sacral canal

Section 13 from above.

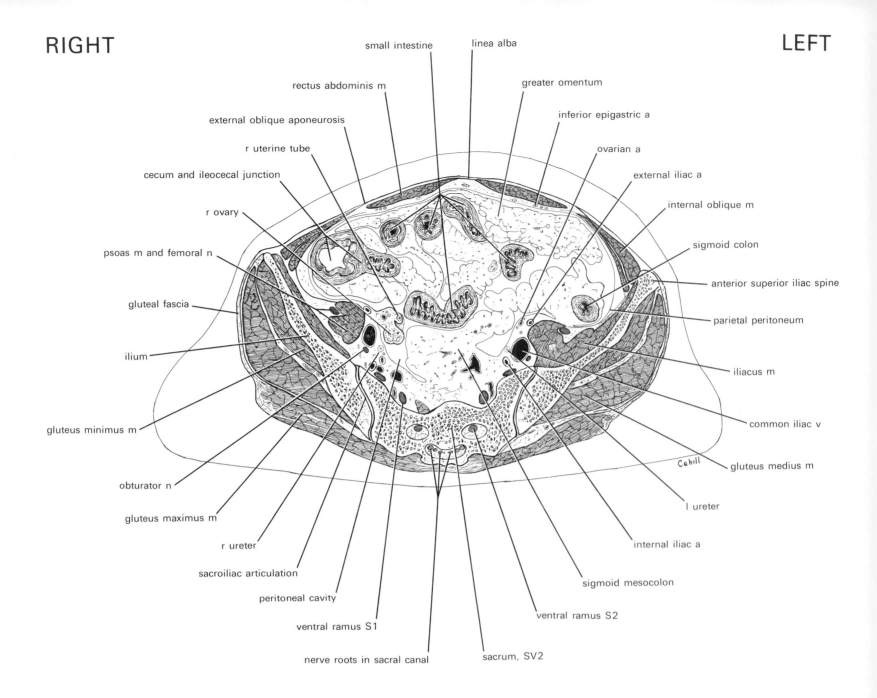

small intestine
linea alba
rectus abdominis m
greater omentum
external oblique aponeurosis
inferior epigastric a
r uterine tube
ovarian a
cecum and ileocecal junction
external iliac a
r ovary
internal oblique m
psoas m and femoral n
sigmoid colon
gluteal fascia
anterior superior iliac spine
ilium
parietal peritoneum
iliacus m
gluteus minimus m
common iliac v
obturator n
gluteus medius m
gluteus maximus m
l ureter
r ureter
internal iliac a
sacroiliac articulation
sigmoid mesocolon
peritoneal cavity
ventral ramus S2
ventral ramus S1
nerve roots in sacral canal
sacrum, SV2

Cahill

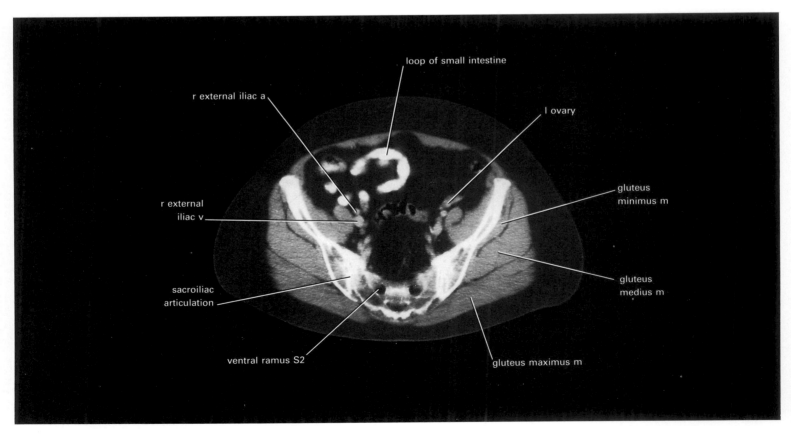

loop of small intestine
r external iliac a
l ovary
r external
iliac v
gluteus
minimus m
sacroiliac
articulation
gluteus
medius m
ventral ramus S2
gluteus maximus m

Section 13 from below.

LEFT   RIGHT

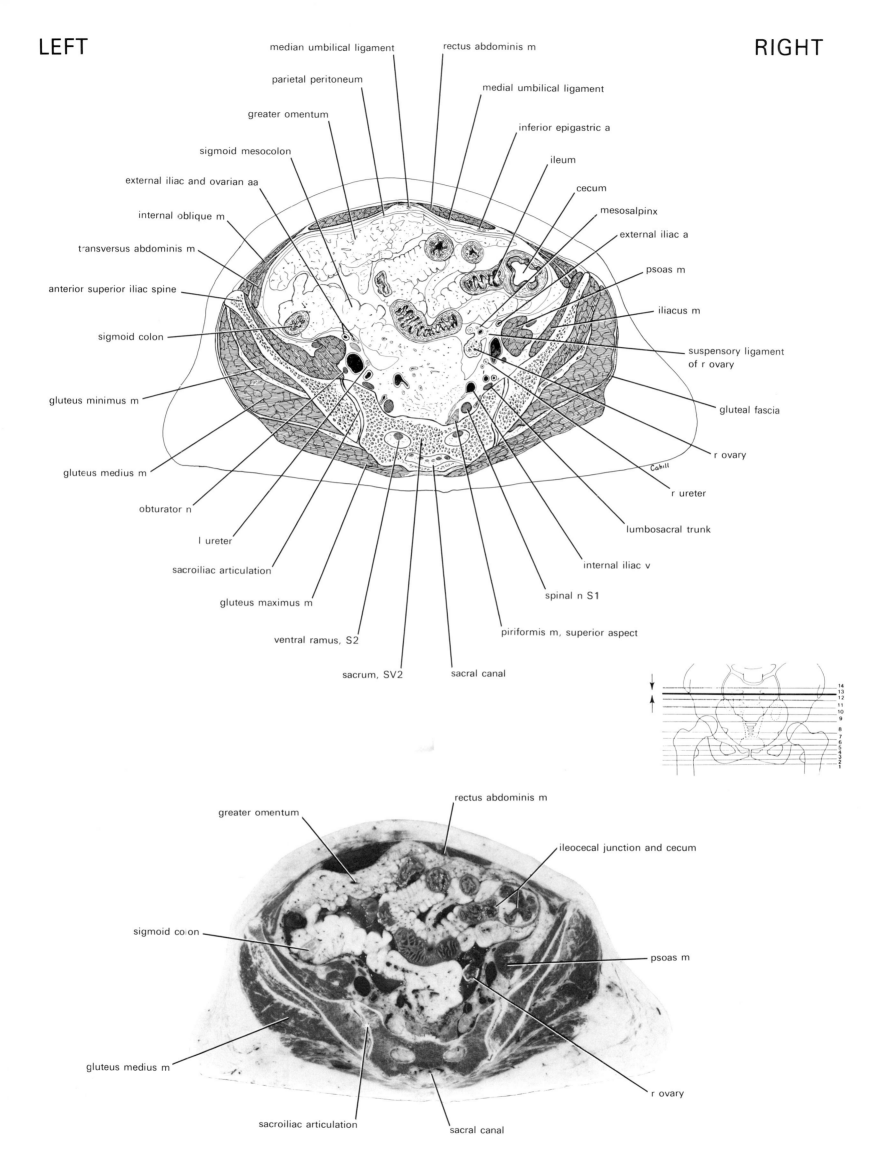

median umbilical ligament
parietal peritoneum
greater omentum
sigmoid mesocolon
external iliac and ovarian aa
internal oblique m
transversus abdominis m
anterior superior iliac spine
sigmoid colon
gluteus minimus m
gluteus medius m
obturator n
l ureter
sacroiliac articulation
gluteus maximus m
ventral ramus, S2
sacrum, SV2

rectus abdominis m
medial umbilical ligament
inferior epigastric a
ileum
cecum
mesosalpinx
external iliac a
psoas m
iliacus m
suspensory ligament of r ovary
gluteal fascia
r ovary
r ureter
lumbosacral trunk
internal iliac v
spinal n S1
piriformis m, superior aspect
sacral canal

Cahill

greater omentum
sigmoid colon
gluteus medius m
sacroiliac articulation

rectus abdominis m
ileocecal junction and cecum
psoas m
r ovary
sacral canal

Section 12 from above.

ATLAS OF HUMAN CROSS-SECTIONAL ANATOMY   71

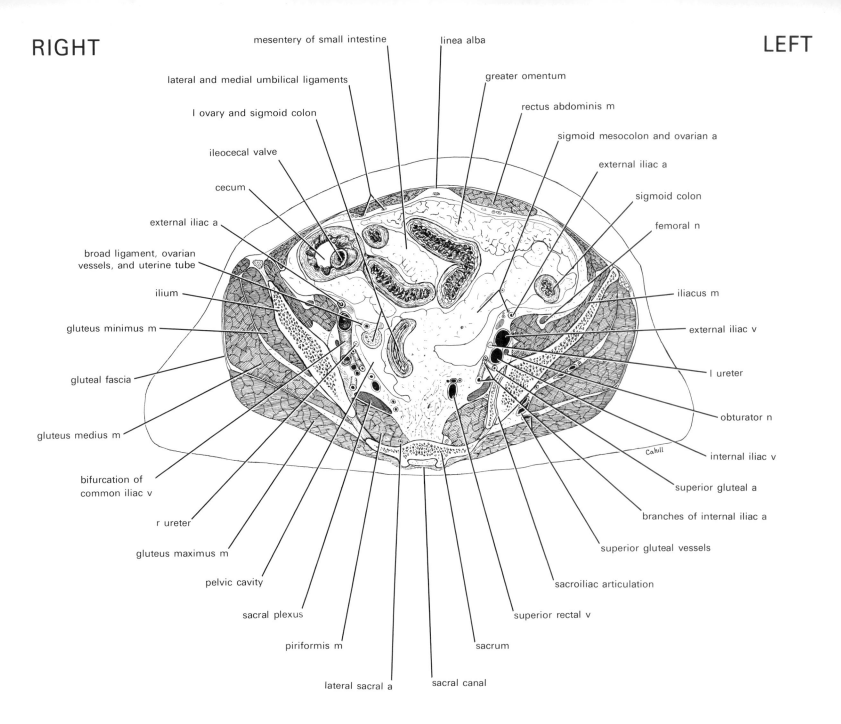

mesentery of small intestine
linea alba
lateral and medial umbilical ligaments
greater omentum
l ovary and sigmoid colon
rectus abdominis m
ileocecal valve
sigmoid mesocolon and ovarian a
cecum
external iliac a
external iliac a
sigmoid colon
broad ligament, ovarian vessels, and uterine tube
femoral n
ilium
iliacus m
gluteus minimus m
external iliac v
gluteal fascia
l ureter
gluteus medius m
obturator n
internal iliac v
bifurcation of common iliac v
superior gluteal a
r ureter
branches of internal iliac a
gluteus maximus m
superior gluteal vessels
pelvic cavity
sacroiliac articulation
sacral plexus
superior rectal v
piriformis m
sacrum
lateral sacral a
sacral canal

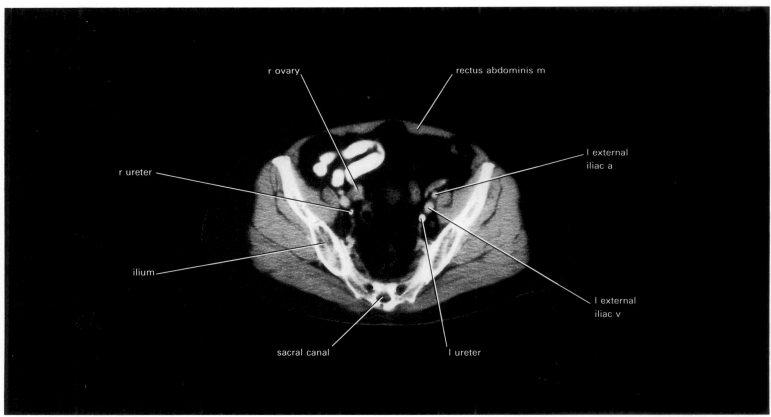

r ovary
rectus abdominis m
l external iliac a
r ureter
ilium
l external iliac v
sacral canal
l ureter

Section 12 from below.

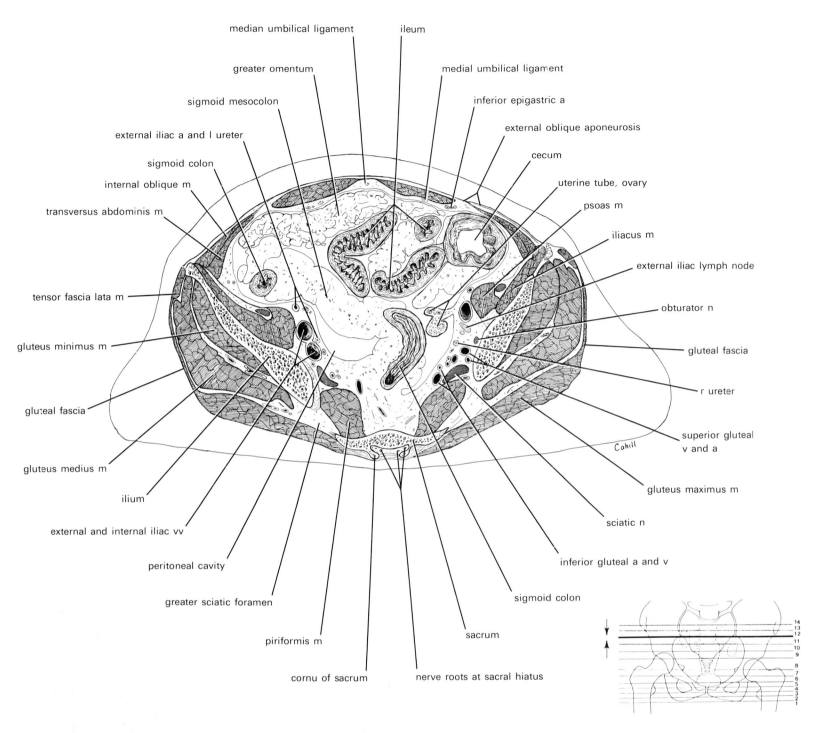

median umbilical ligament

ileum

greater omentum

medial umbilical ligament

sigmoid mesocolon

inferior epigastric a

external iliac a and l ureter

external oblique aponeurosis

sigmoid colon

cecum

internal oblique m

uterine tube, ovary

transversus abdominis m

psoas m

iliacus m

external iliac lymph node

tensor fascia lata m

obturator n

gluteus minimus m

gluteal fascia

gluteal fascia

r ureter

gluteus medius m

superior gluteal
v and a

ilium

gluteus maximus m

external and internal iliac vv

sciatic n

peritoneal cavity

inferior gluteal a and v

greater sciatic foramen

sigmoid colon

piriformis m

sacrum

cornu of sacrum

nerve roots at sacral hiatus

Cahill

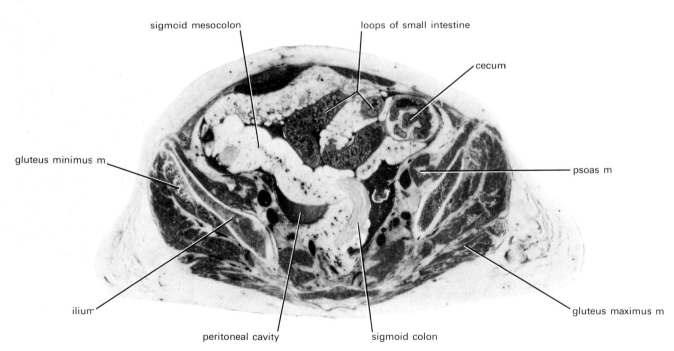

sigmoid mesocolon

loops of small intestine

cecum

gluteus minimus m

psoas m

ilium

gluteus maximus m

peritoneal cavity

sigmoid colon

Section 11 from above.

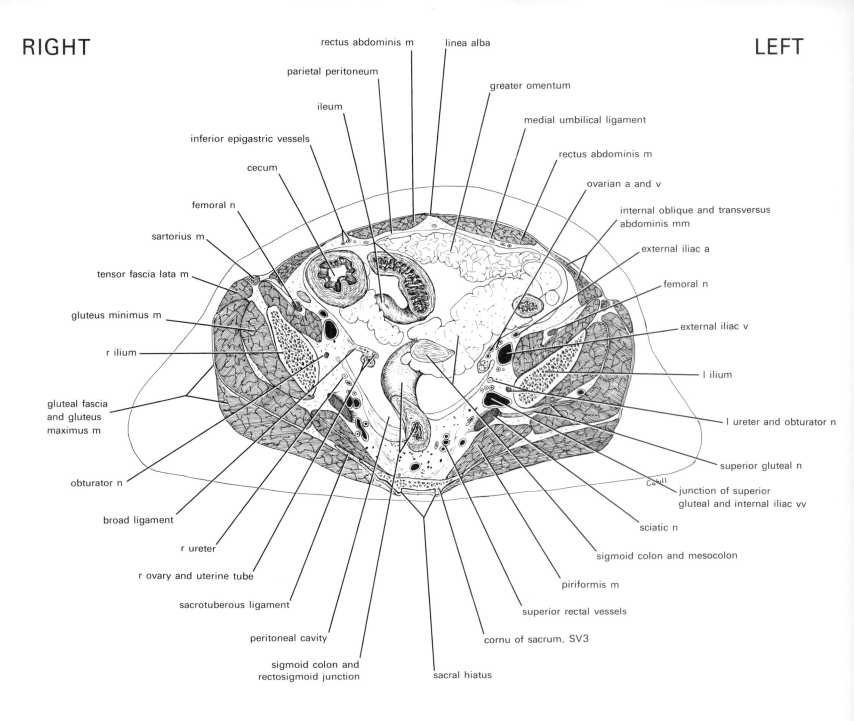

rectus abdominis m — linea alba

parietal peritoneum

greater omentum

ileum

medial umbilical ligament

inferior epigastric vessels

rectus abdominis m

cecum

ovarian a and v

femoral n

internal oblique and transversus abdominis mm

sartorius m

external iliac a

tensor fascia lata m

femoral n

gluteus minimus m

external iliac v

r ilium

l ilium

gluteal fascia and gluteus maximus m

l ureter and obturator n

obturator n

superior gluteal n

broad ligament

junction of superior gluteal and internal iliac vv

r ureter

sciatic n

r ovary and uterine tube

sigmoid colon and mesocolon

sacrotuberous ligament

piriformis m

peritoneal cavity

superior rectal vessels

sigmoid colon and rectosigmoid junction

cornu of sacrum, SV3

sacral hiatus

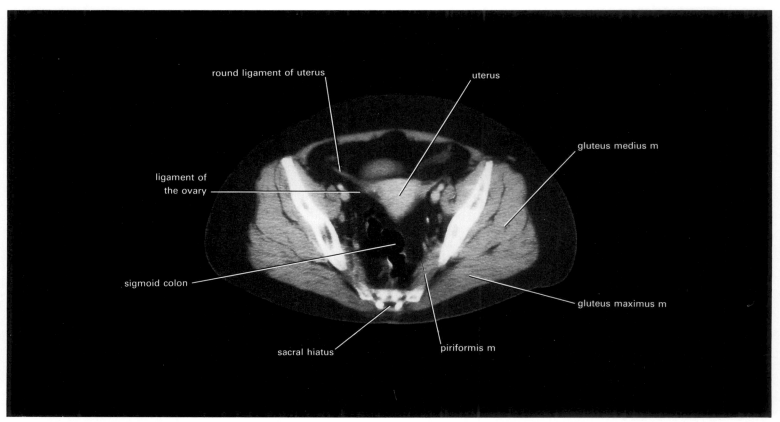

round ligament of uterus

uterus

gluteus medius m

ligament of the ovary

sigmoid colon

gluteus maximus m

sacral hiatus

piriformis m

Section 11 from below.

LEFT   RIGHT

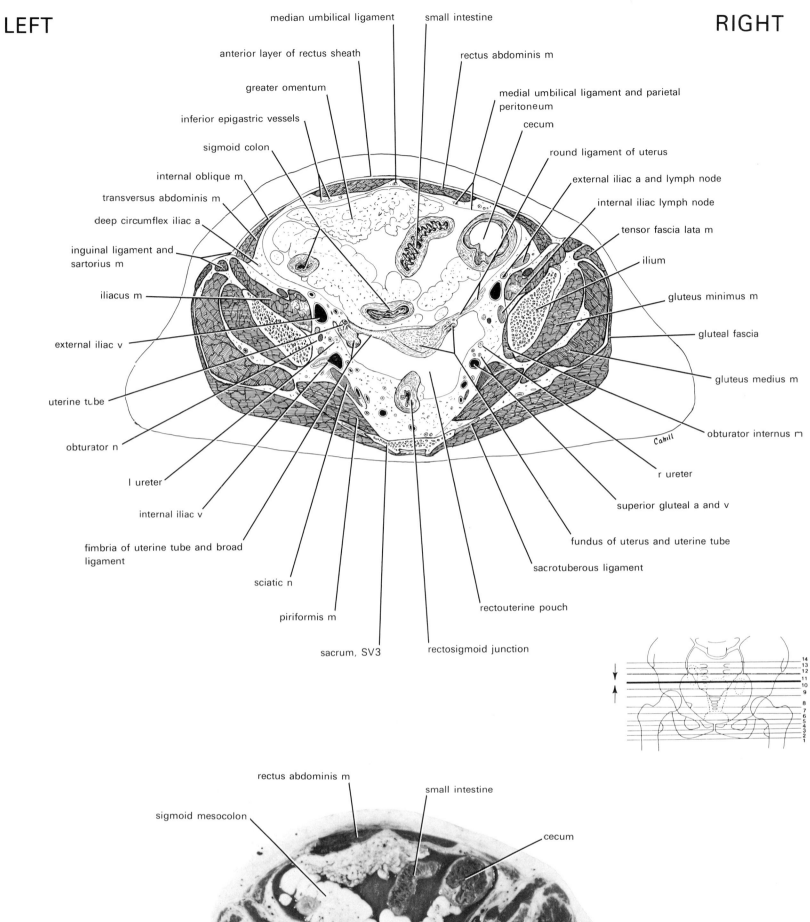

median umbilical ligament
anterior layer of rectus sheath
greater omentum
inferior epigastric vessels
sigmoid colon
internal oblique m
transversus abdominis m
deep circumflex iliac a
inguinal ligament and sartorius m
iliacus m
external iliac v
uterine tube
obturator n
l ureter
internal iliac v
fimbria of uterine tube and broad ligament
sciatic n
piriformis m
sacrum, SV3
rectosigmoid junction
rectouterine pouch
sacrotuberous ligament
fundus of uterus and uterine tube
superior gluteal a and v
r ureter

small intestine
rectus abdominis m
medial umbilical ligament and parietal peritoneum
cecum
round ligament of uterus
external iliac a and lymph node
internal iliac lymph node
tensor fascia lata m
ilium
gluteus minimus m
gluteal fascia
gluteus medius m
obturator internus m

Cahill

rectus abdominis m
sigmoid mesocolon
small intestine
cecum
external iliac v
gluteus minimus m
superior gluteal v
rectouterine pouch
fundus of uterus
gluteus maximus m

Section 10 from above.

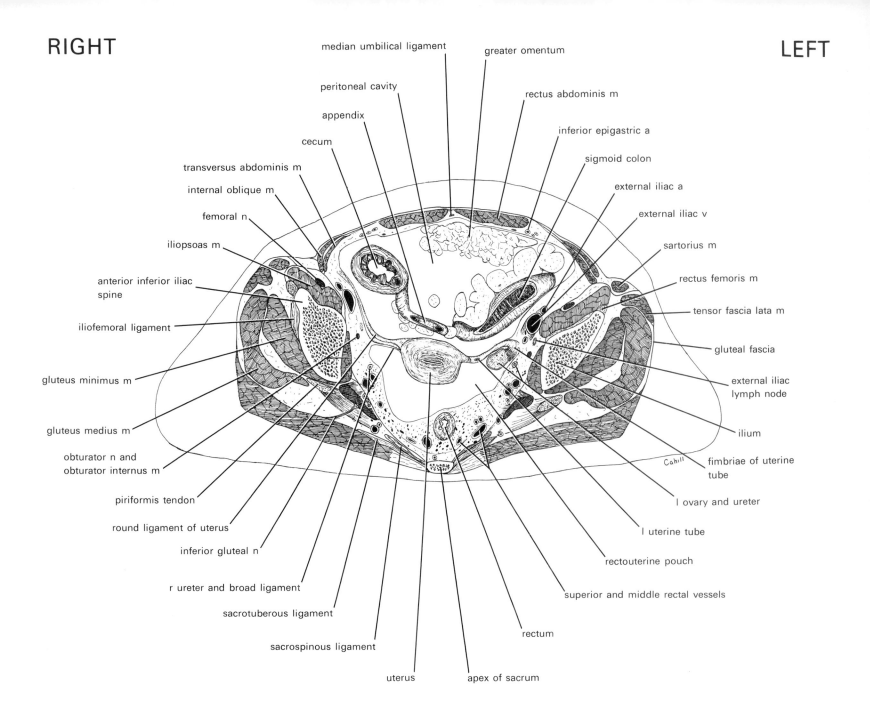

median umbilical ligament
greater omentum
peritoneal cavity
rectus abdominis m
appendix
inferior epigastric a
cecum
sigmoid colon
transversus abdominis m
external iliac a
internal oblique m
external iliac v
femoral n
sartorius m
iliopsoas m
rectus femoris m
anterior inferior iliac spine
tensor fascia lata m
iliofemoral ligament
gluteal fascia
gluteus minimus m
external iliac lymph node
gluteus medius m
ilium
obturator n and obturator internus m
fimbriae of uterine tube
piriformis tendon
l ovary and ureter
round ligament of uterus
l uterine tube
inferior gluteal n
rectouterine pouch
r ureter and broad ligament
superior and middle rectal vessels
sacrotuberous ligament
rectum
sacrospinous ligament
uterus
apex of sacrum

Cahill

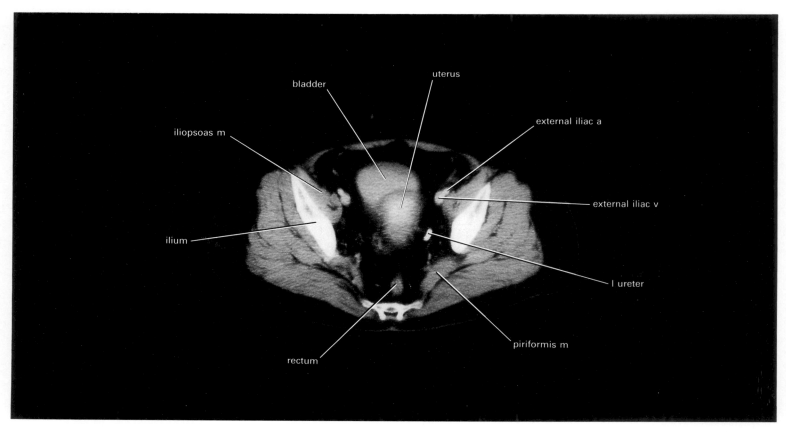

bladder
uterus
iliopsoas m
external iliac a
ilium
external iliac v
l ureter
piriformis m
rectum

Section 10 from below.

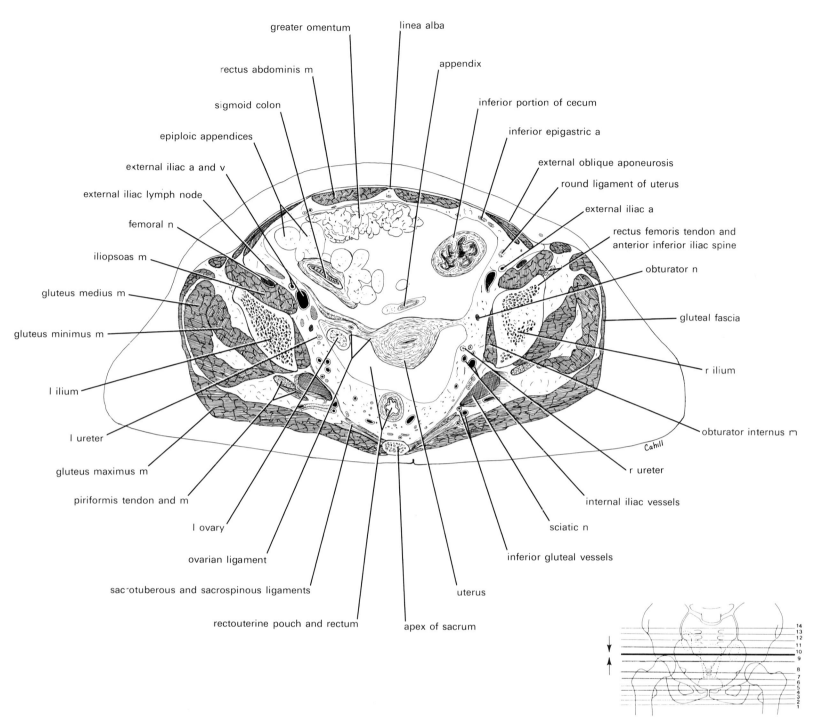

greater omentum
linea alba
rectus abdominis m
appendix
sigmoid colon
inferior portion of cecum
epiploic appendices
inferior epigastric a
external iliac a and v
external oblique aponeurosis
external iliac lymph node
round ligament of uterus
femoral n
external iliac a
iliopsoas m
rectus femoris tendon and
anterior inferior iliac spine
gluteus medius m
obturator n
gluteus minimus m
gluteal fascia
l ilium
r ilium
l ureter
obturator internus m
gluteus maximus m
r ureter
piriformis tendon and m
internal iliac vessels
l ovary
sciatic n
ovarian ligament
inferior gluteal vessels
sacrotuberous and sacrospinous ligaments
uterus
rectouterine pouch and rectum
apex of sacrum

Cahill

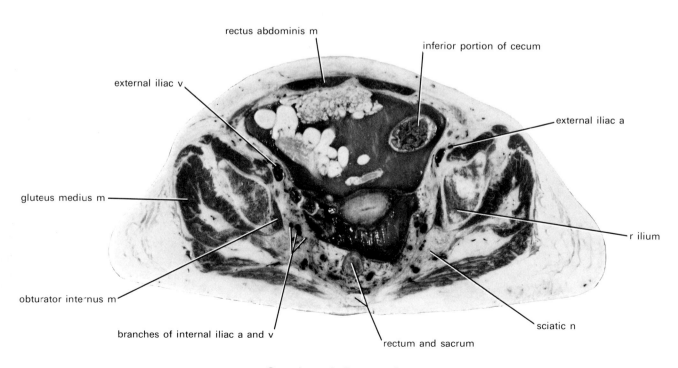

rectus abdominis m
inferior portion of cecum
external iliac v
external iliac a
gluteus medius m
r ilium
obturator internus m
sciatic n
branches of internal iliac a and v
rectum and sacrum

Section 9 from above.

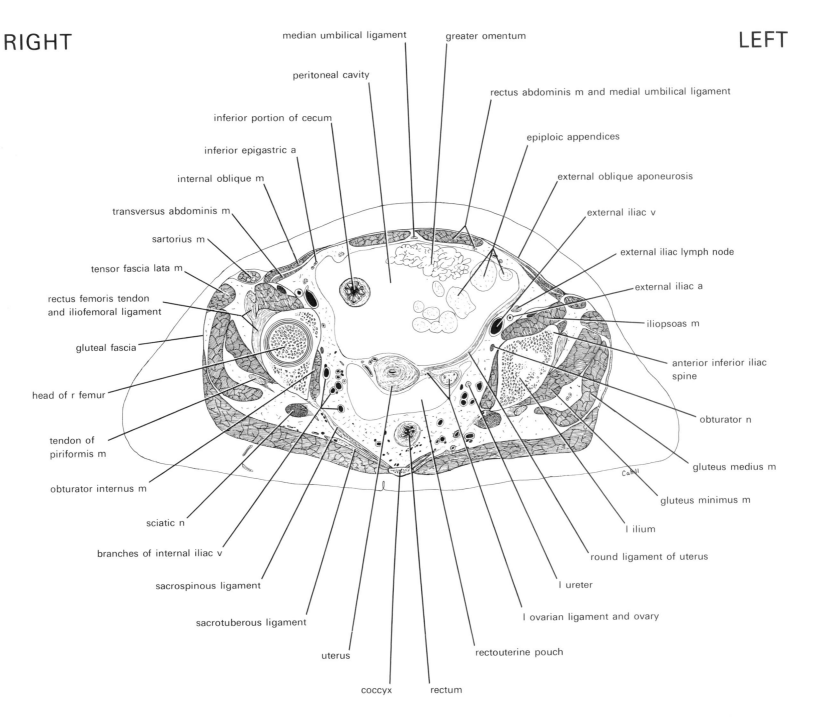

median umbilical ligament
greater omentum
peritoneal cavity
rectus abdominis m and medial umbilical ligament
inferior portion of cecum
epiploic appendices
inferior epigastric a
external oblique aponeurosis
internal oblique m
external iliac v
transversus abdominis m
external iliac lymph node
sartorius m
external iliac a
tensor fascia lata m
iliopsoas m
rectus femoris tendon and iliofemoral ligament
anterior inferior iliac spine
gluteal fascia
head of r femur
obturator n
tendon of piriformis m
gluteus medius m
obturator internus m
gluteus minimus m
sciatic n
l ilium
branches of internal iliac v
round ligament of uterus
sacrospinous ligament
l ureter
sacrotuberous ligament
l ovarian ligament and ovary
uterus
rectouterine pouch
coccyx   rectum

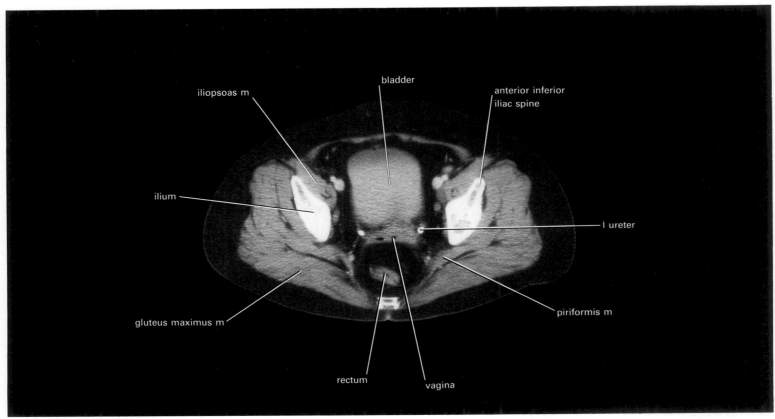

iliopsoas m
bladder
anterior inferior iliac spine
ilium
l ureter
piriformis m
gluteus maximus m
rectum   vagina

Section 9 from below.

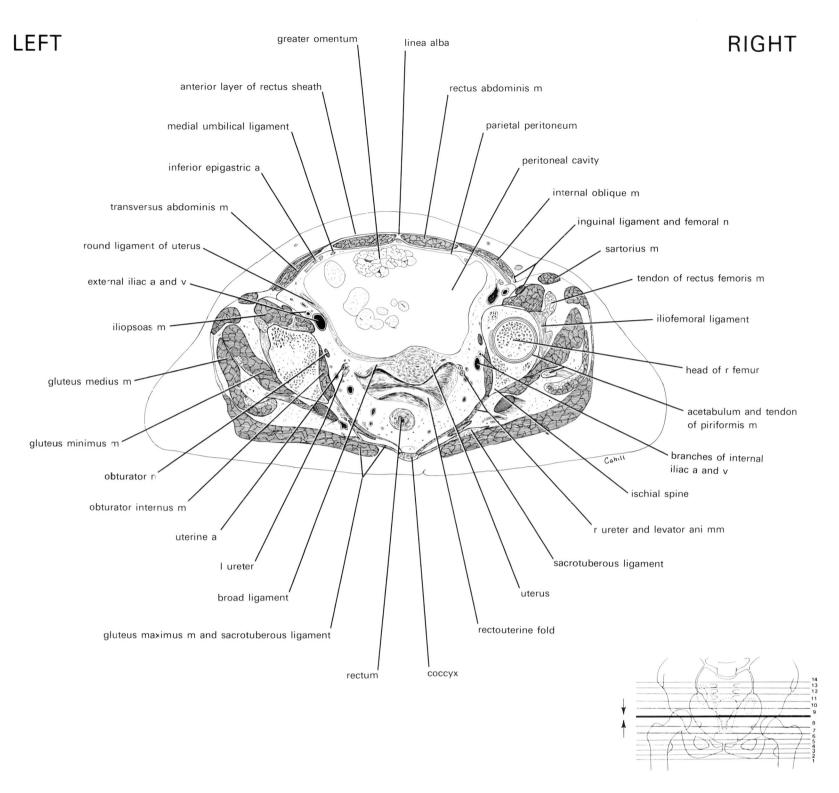

greater omentum
linea alba
anterior layer of rectus sheath
rectus abdominis m
medial umbilical ligament
parietal peritoneum
inferior epigastric a
peritoneal cavity
transversus abdominis m
internal oblique m
round ligament of uterus
inguinal ligament and femoral n
external iliac a and v
sartorius m
iliopsoas m
tendon of rectus femoris m
iliofemoral ligament
gluteus medius m
head of r femur
gluteus minimus m
acetabulum and tendon
of piriformis m
obturator n
branches of internal
iliac a and v
obturator internus m
ischial spine
uterine a
r ureter and levator ani mm
l ureter
sacrotuberous ligament
broad ligament
uterus
gluteus maximus m and sacrotuberous ligament
rectouterine fold
rectum   coccyx

Cahill

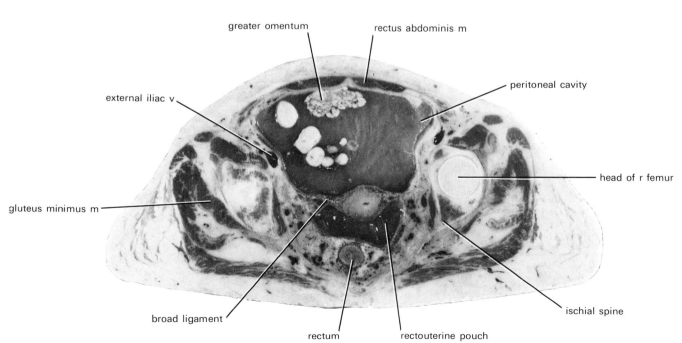

greater omentum   rectus abdominis m
external iliac v
peritoneal cavity
gluteus minimus m
head of r femur
broad ligament
ischial spine
rectum   rectouterine pouch

Section 8 from above.

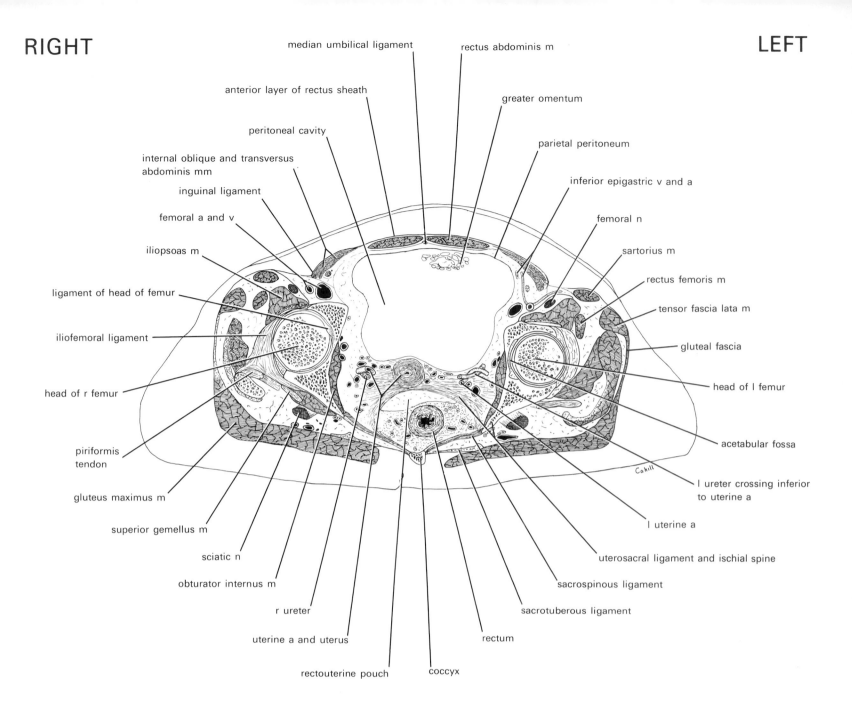

median umbilical ligament
rectus abdominis m
anterior layer of rectus sheath
greater omentum
peritoneal cavity
parietal peritoneum
internal oblique and transversus abdominis mm
inferior epigastric v and a
inguinal ligament
femoral n
femoral a and v
sartorius m
iliopsoas m
rectus femoris m
ligament of head of femur
tensor fascia lata m
iliofemoral ligament
gluteal fascia
head of r femur
head of l femur
piriformis tendon
acetabular fossa
gluteus maximus m
l ureter crossing inferior to uterine a
superior gemellus m
l uterine a
sciatic n
uterosacral ligament and ischial spine
obturator internus m
sacrospinous ligament
r ureter
sacrotuberous ligament
uterine a and uterus
rectum
rectouterine pouch
coccyx

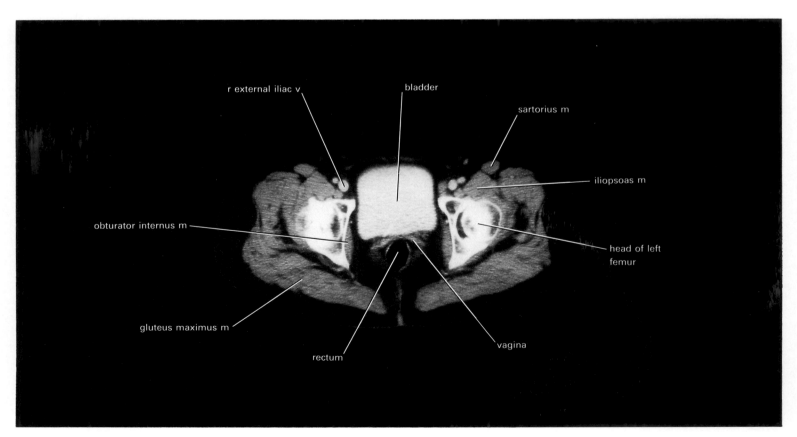

r external iliac v
bladder
sartorius m
iliopsoas m
obturator internus m
head of left femur
gluteus maximus m
vagina
rectum

Section 8 from below.

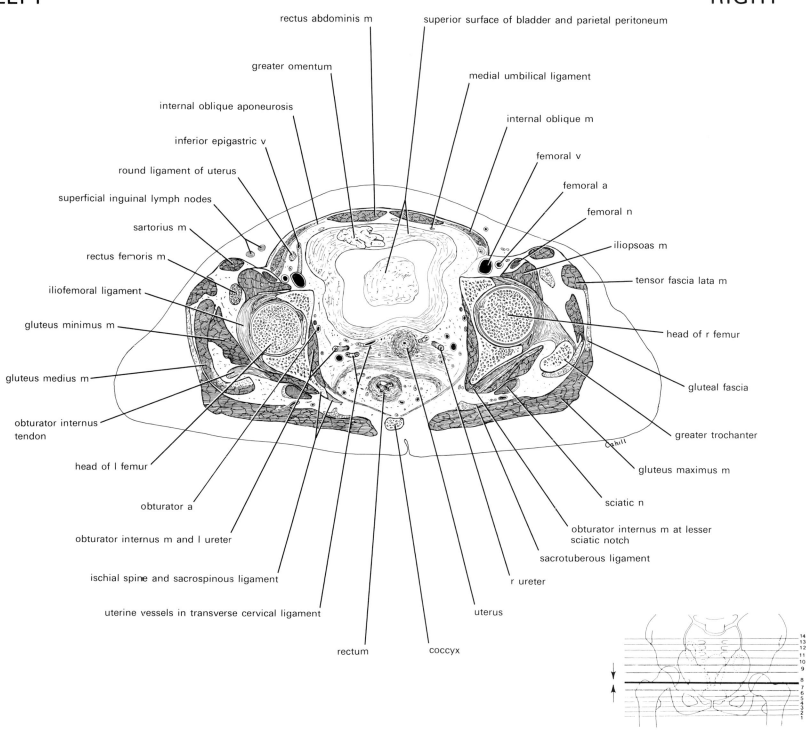

rectus abdominis m

superior surface of bladder and parietal peritoneum

greater omentum

medial umbilical ligament

internal oblique aponeurosis

internal oblique m

inferior epigastric v

femoral v

round ligament of uterus

femoral a

superficial inguinal lymph nodes

femoral n

sartorius m

iliopsoas m

rectus femoris m

tensor fascia lata m

iliofemoral ligament

gluteus minimus m

head of r femur

gluteus medius m

obturator internus
tendon

gluteal fascia

head of l femur

greater trochanter

gluteus maximus m

obturator a

sciatic n

obturator internus m and l ureter

obturator internus m at lesser
sciatic notch

ischial spine and sacrospinous ligament

sacrotuberous ligament

uterine vessels in transverse cervical ligament

r ureter

uterus

rectum

coccyx

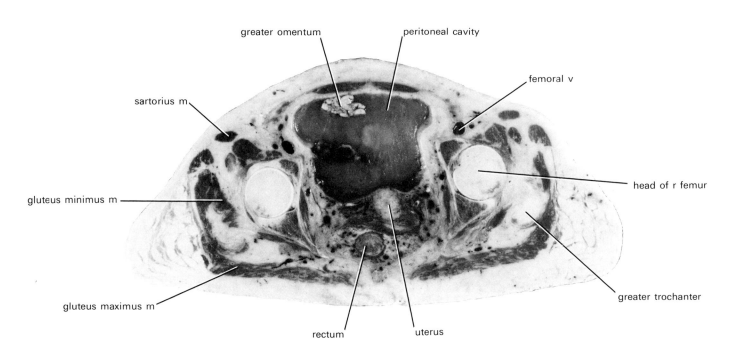

greater omentum

peritoneal cavity

femoral v

sartorius m

gluteus minimus m

head of r femur

greater trochanter

gluteus maximus m

rectum

uterus

Section 7 from above.

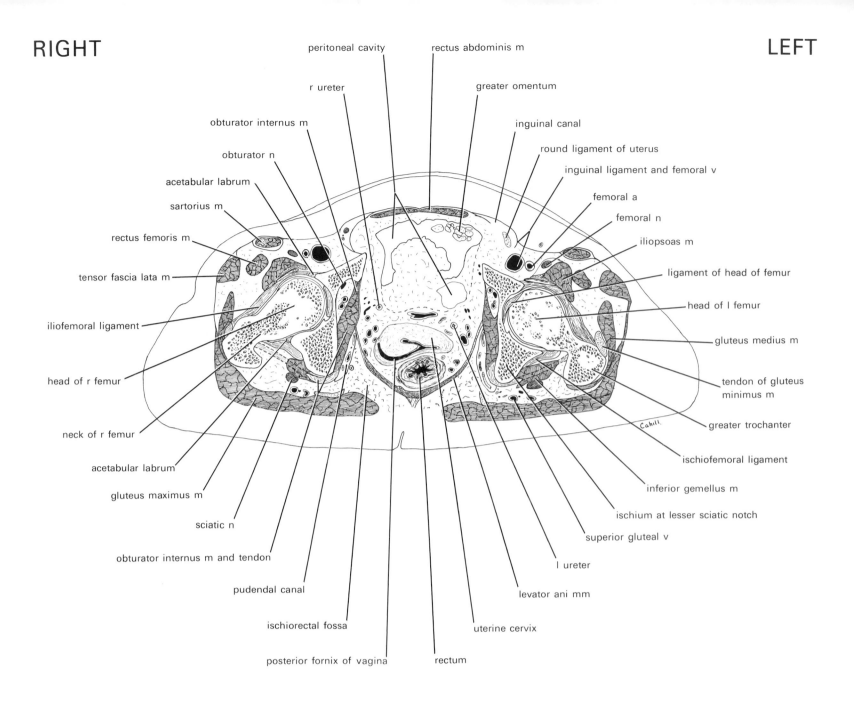

peritoneal cavity

rectus abdominis m

r ureter

greater omentum

obturator internus m

inguinal canal

obturator n

round ligament of uterus

acetabular labrum

inguinal ligament and femoral v

sartorius m

femoral a

rectus femoris m

femoral n

tensor fascia lata m

iliopsoas m

ligament of head of femur

iliofemoral ligament

head of l femur

gluteus medius m

head of r femur

tendon of gluteus minimus m

neck of r femur

greater trochanter

acetabular labrum

ischiofemoral ligament

gluteus maximus m

inferior gemellus m

sciatic n

ischium at lesser sciatic notch

obturator internus m and tendon

superior gluteal v

pudendal canal

l ureter

levator ani mm

ischiorectal fossa

uterine cervix

posterior fornix of vagina

rectum

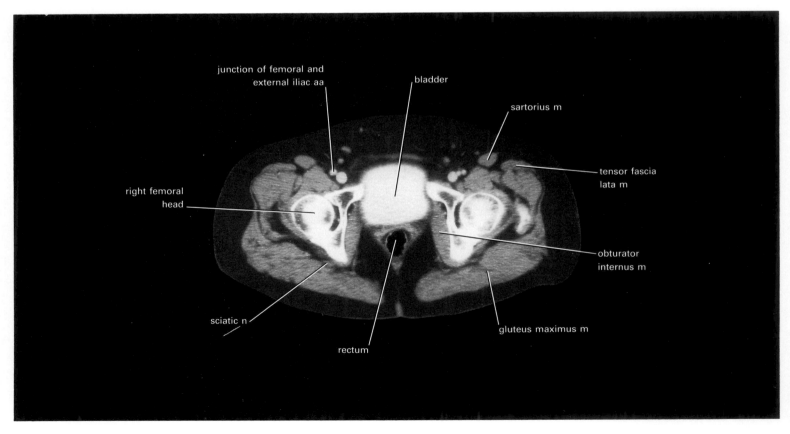

junction of femoral and external iliac aa

bladder

sartorius m

right femoral head

tensor fascia lata m

obturator internus m

sciatic n

gluteus maximus m

rectum

Section 7 from below.

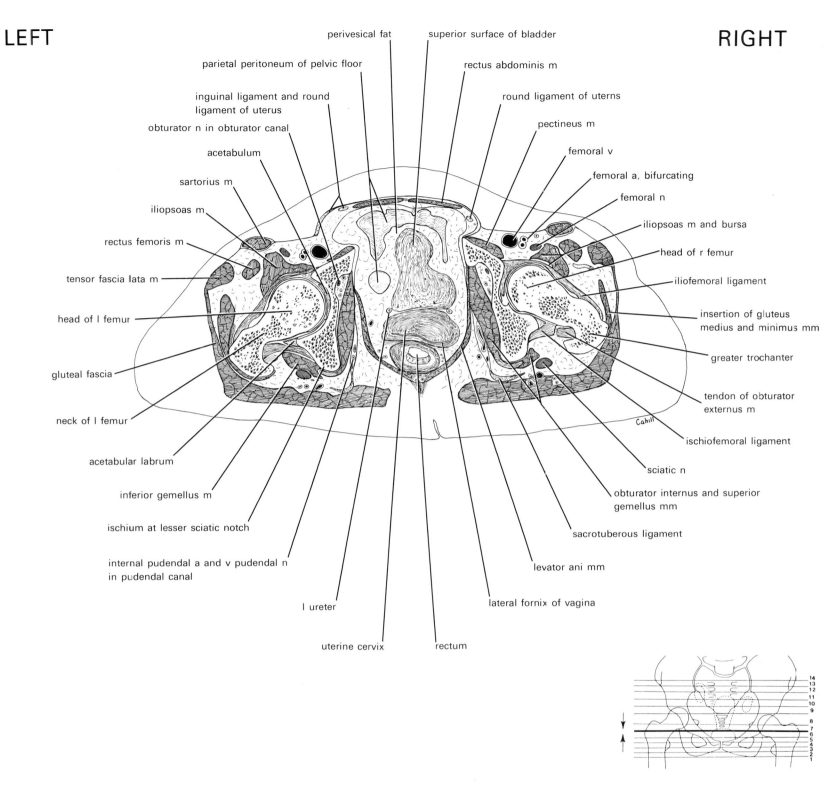

perivesical fat

superior surface of bladder

parietal peritoneum of pelvic floor

rectus abdominis m

inguinal ligament and round
ligament of uterus

round ligament of uterns

obturator n in obturator canal

pectineus m

acetabulum

femoral v

sartorius m

femoral a, bifurcating

iliopsoas m

femoral n

rectus femoris m

iliopsoas m and bursa

tensor fascia lata m

head of r femur

head of l femur

iliofemoral ligament

insertion of gluteus
medius and minimus mm

gluteal fascia

greater trochanter

neck of l femur

tendon of obturator
externus m

acetabular labrum

ischiofemoral ligament

inferior gemellus m

sciatic n

ischium at lesser sciatic notch

obturator internus and superior
gemellus mm

internal pudendal a and v pudendal n
in pudendal canal

sacrotuberous ligament

levator ani mm

l ureter

lateral fornix of vagina

uterine cervix

rectum

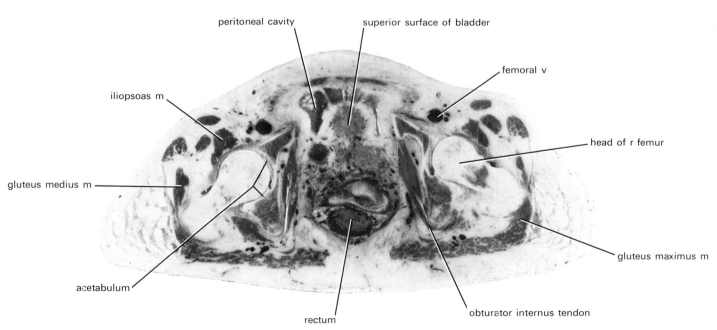

peritoneal cavity

superior surface of bladder

femoral v

iliopsoas m

head of r femur

gluteus medius m

gluteus maximus m

acetabulum

obturator internus tendon

rectum

Section 6 from above.

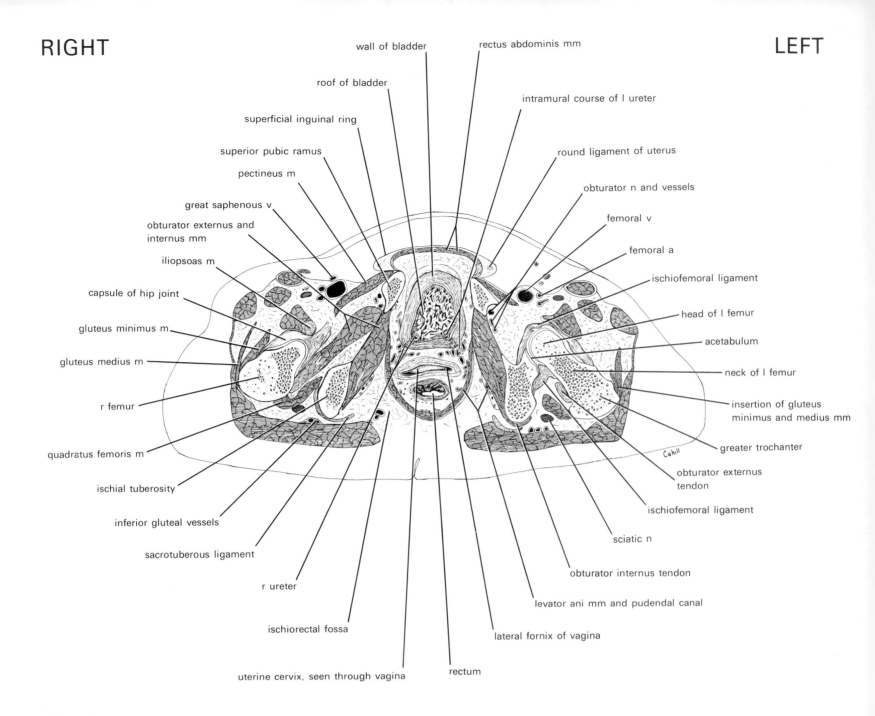

wall of bladder

rectus abdominis mm

roof of bladder

intramural course of l ureter

superficial inguinal ring

round ligament of uterus

superior pubic ramus

obturator n and vessels

pectineus m

femoral v

great saphenous v

femoral a

obturator externus and
internus mm

ischiofemoral ligament

iliopsoas m

head of l femur

capsule of hip joint

acetabulum

gluteus minimus m

neck of l femur

gluteus medius m

insertion of gluteus
minimus and medius mm

r femur

greater trochanter

quadratus femoris m

obturator externus
tendon

ischial tuberosity

ischiofemoral ligament

inferior gluteal vessels

sciatic n

sacrotuberous ligament

obturator internus tendon

r ureter

levator ani mm and pudendal canal

ischiorectal fossa

lateral fornix of vagina

uterine cervix, seen through vagina

rectum

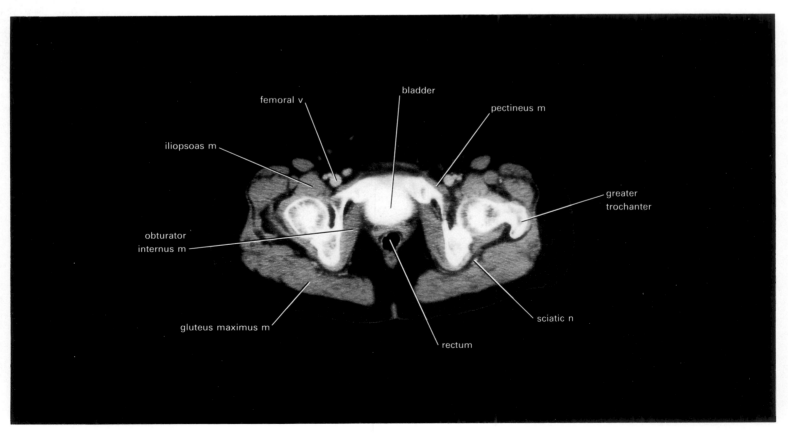

femoral v

bladder

pectineus m

iliopsoas m

greater
trochanter

obturator
internus m

gluteus maximus m

sciatic n

rectum

Section 6 from below.

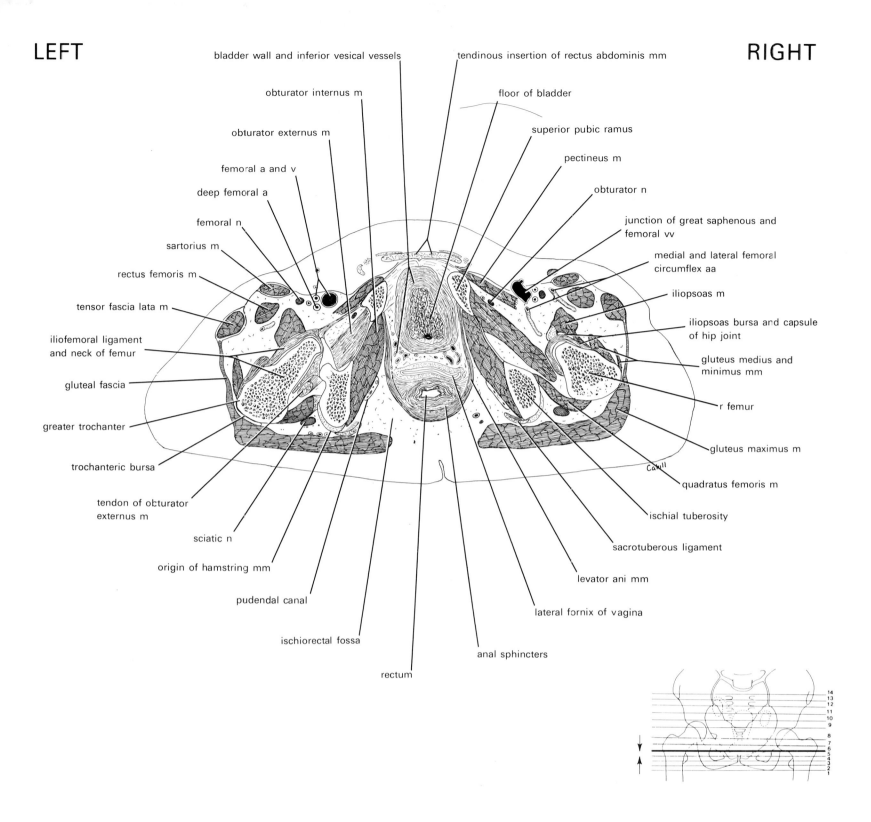

bladder wall and inferior vesical vessels

obturator internus m

obturator externus m

femoral a and v

deep femoral a

femoral n

sartorius m

rectus femoris m

tensor fascia lata m

iliofemoral ligament and neck of femur

gluteal fascia

greater trochanter

trochanteric bursa

tendon of obturator externus m

sciatic n

origin of hamstring mm

pudendal canal

ischiorectal fossa

rectum

tendinous insertion of rectus abdominis mm

floor of bladder

superior pubic ramus

pectineus m

obturator n

junction of great saphenous and femoral vv

medial and lateral femoral circumflex aa

iliopsoas m

iliopsoas bursa and capsule of hip joint

gluteus medius and minimus mm

r femur

gluteus maximus m

quadratus femoris m

ischial tuberosity

sacrotuberous ligament

levator ani mm

lateral fornix of vagina

anal sphincters

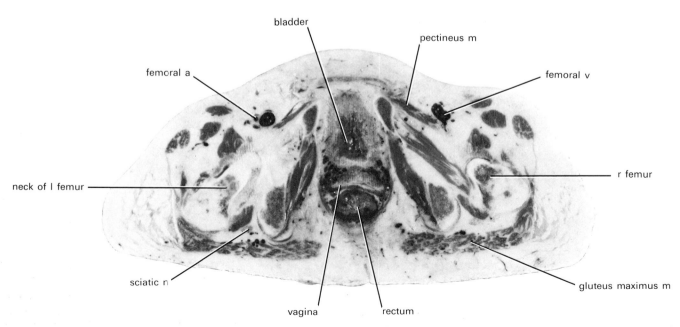

bladder

pectineus m

femoral a

femoral v

neck of l femur

r femur

sciatic n

gluteus maximus m

vagina

rectum

Section 5 from above.

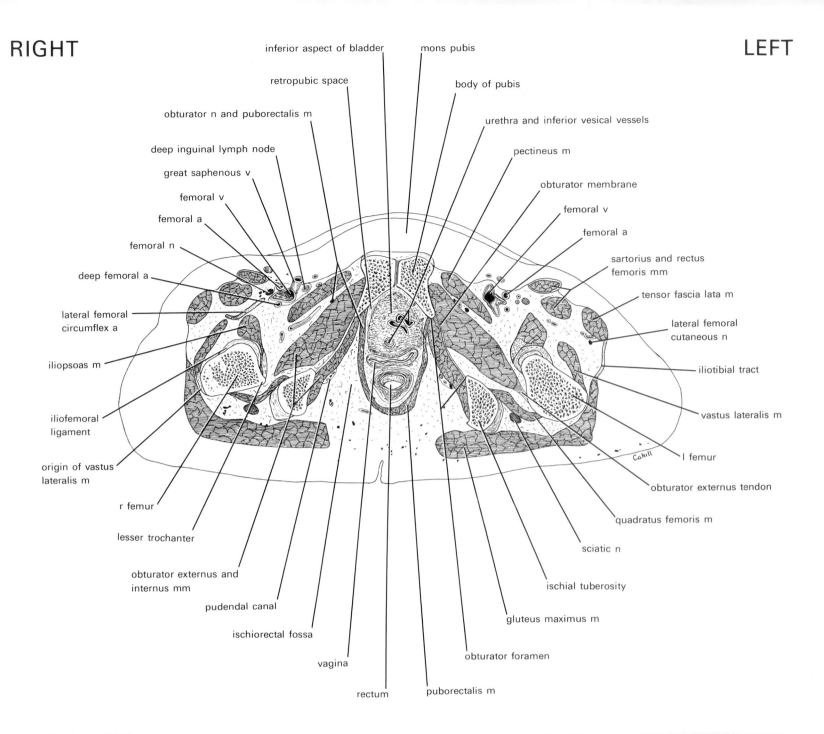

inferior aspect of bladder

mons pubis

retropubic space

body of pubis

obturator n and puborectalis m

urethra and inferior vesical vessels

deep inguinal lymph node

pectineus m

great saphenous v

obturator membrane

femoral v

femoral v

femoral a

femoral a

femoral n

sartorius and rectus femoris mm

deep femoral a

tensor fascia lata m

lateral femoral circumflex a

lateral femoral cutaneous n

iliopsoas m

iliotibial tract

iliofemoral ligament

vastus lateralis m

origin of vastus lateralis m

l femur

r femur

obturator externus tendon

lesser trochanter

quadratus femoris m

sciatic n

obturator externus and internus mm

ischial tuberosity

pudendal canal

gluteus maximus m

ischiorectal fossa

obturator foramen

vagina

puborectalis m

rectum

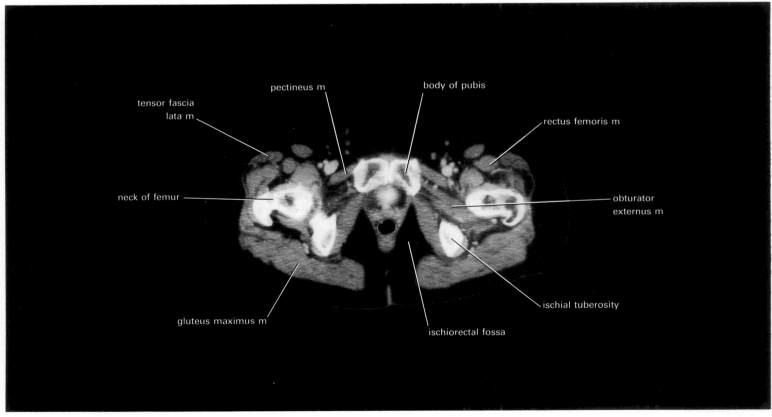

tensor fascia lata m

pectineus m

body of pubis

rectus femoris m

neck of femur

obturator externus m

gluteus maximus m

ischiorectal fossa

ischial tuberosity

Section 5 from below.

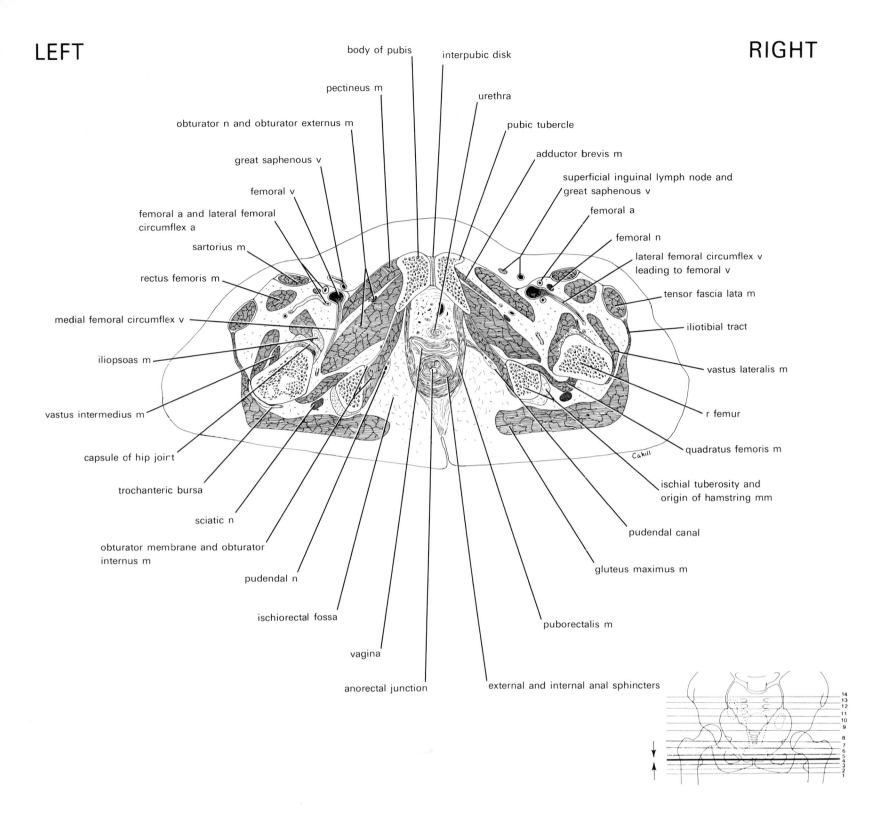

body of pubis
interpubic disk
pectineus m
urethra
obturator n and obturator externus m
pubic tubercle
great saphenous v
adductor brevis m
femoral v
superficial inguinal lymph node and
great saphenous v
femoral a and lateral femoral
circumflex a
femoral a
sartorius m
femoral n
rectus femoris m
lateral femoral circumflex v
leading to femoral v
medial femoral circumflex v
tensor fascia lata m
iliotibial tract
iliopsoas m
vastus lateralis m
vastus intermedius m
r femur
capsule of hip joint
quadratus femoris m
trochanteric bursa
ischial tuberosity and
origin of hamstring mm
sciatic n
pudendal canal
obturator membrane and obturator
internus m
gluteus maximus m
pudendal n
ischiorectal fossa
puborectalis m
vagina
external and internal anal sphincters
anorectal junction

Cahill

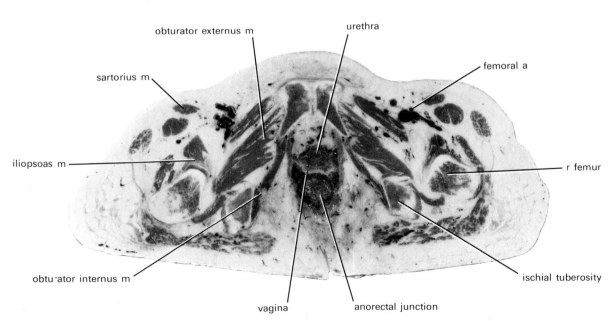

obturator externus m
urethra
sartorius m
femoral a
iliopsoas m
r femur
obturator internus m
ischial tuberosity
vagina
anorectal junction

Section 4 from above.

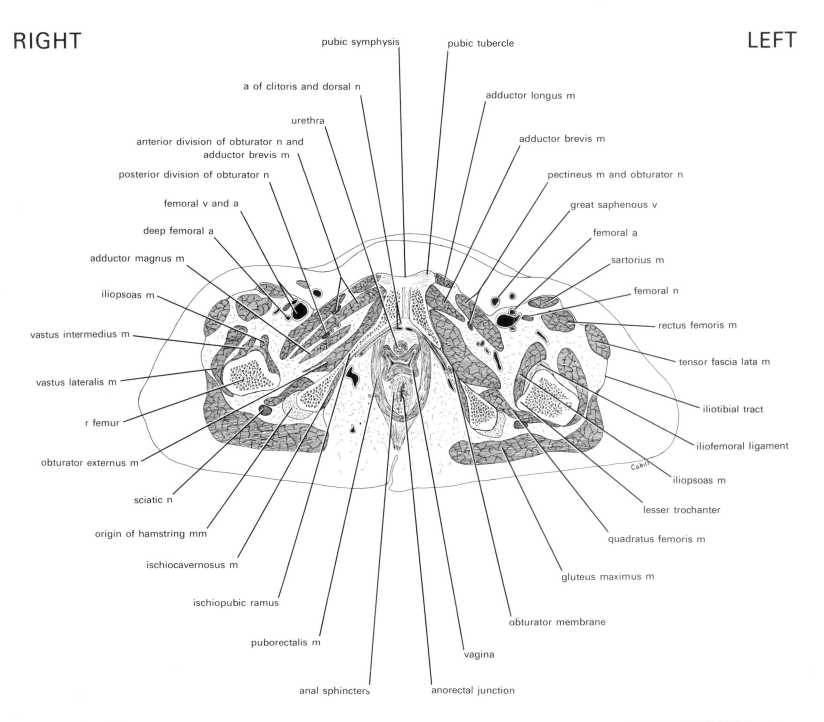

pubic symphysis

pubic tubercle

a of clitoris and dorsal n

adductor longus m

urethra

adductor brevis m

anterior division of obturator n and
adductor brevis m

pectineus m and obturator n

posterior division of obturator n

great saphenous v

femoral v and a

femoral a

deep femoral a

sartorius m

adductor magnus m

femoral n

iliopsoas m

rectus femoris m

vastus intermedius m

tensor fascia lata m

vastus lateralis m

iliotibial tract

r femur

iliofemoral ligament

obturator externus m

iliopsoas m

sciatic n

lesser trochanter

origin of hamstring mm

quadratus femoris m

ischiocavernosus m

gluteus maximus m

ischiopubic ramus

obturator membrane

puborectalis m

vagina

anal sphincters

anorectal junction

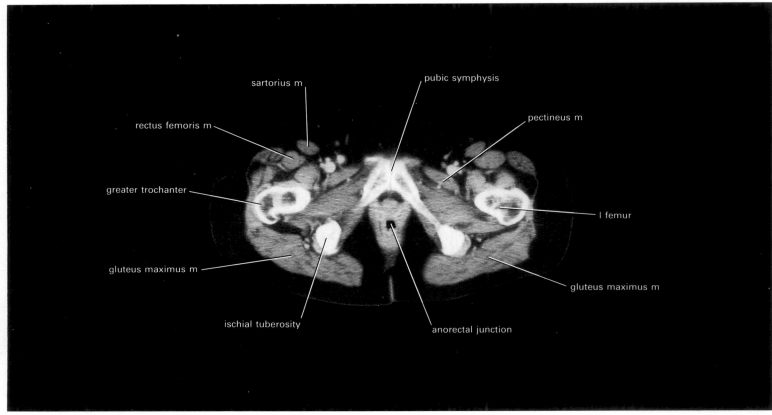

sartorius m

pubic symphysis

rectus femoris m

pectineus m

greater trochanter

l femur

gluteus maximus m

gluteus maximus m

ischial tuberosity

anorectal junction

Section 4 from below.

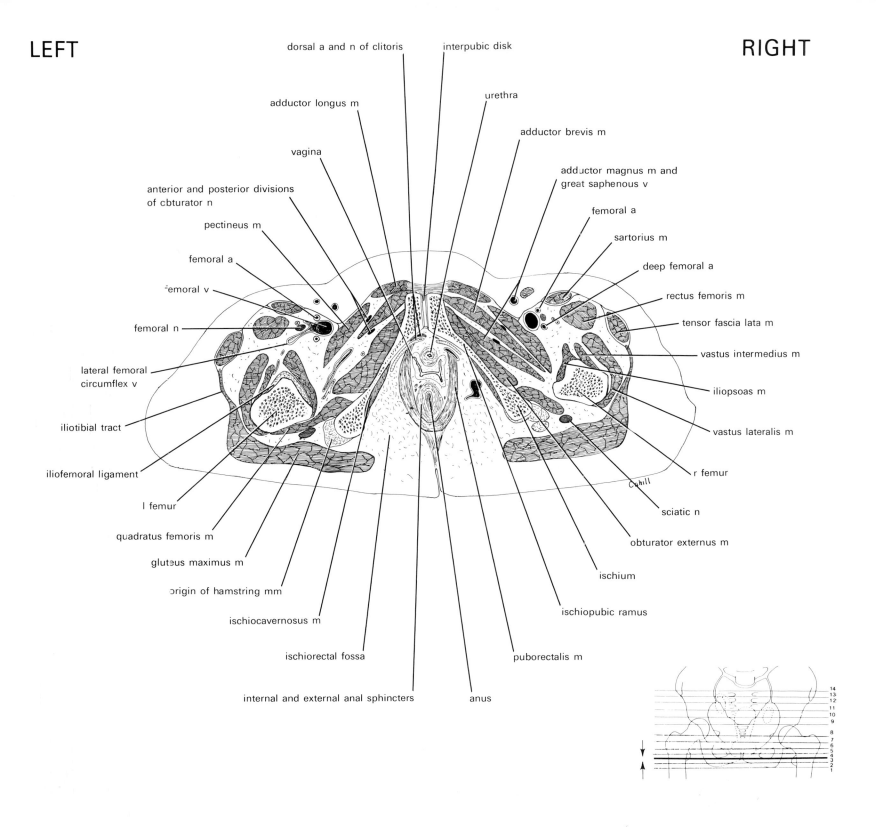

dorsal a and n of clitoris

interpubic disk

urethra

adductor longus m

adductor brevis m

vagina

adductor magnus m and
great saphenous v

anterior and posterior divisions
of obturator n

femoral a

pectineus m

sartorius m

femoral a

deep femoral a

femoral v

rectus femoris m

femoral n

tensor fascia lata m

vastus intermedius m

lateral femoral
circumflex v

iliopsoas m

iliotibial tract

vastus lateralis m

iliofemoral ligament

r femur

l femur

sciatic n

quadratus femoris m

obturator externus m

gluteus maximus m

ischium

origin of hamstring mm

ischiopubic ramus

ischiocavernosus m

puborectalis m

ischiorectal fossa

internal and external anal sphincters

anus

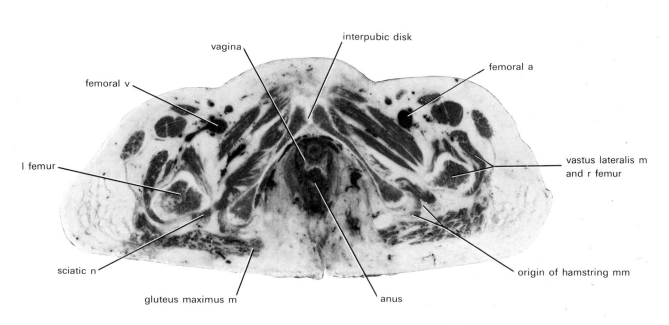

vagina

interpubic disk

femoral v

femoral a

l femur

vastus lateralis m
and r femur

sciatic n

origin of hamstring mm

gluteus maximus m

anus

Section 3 from above.

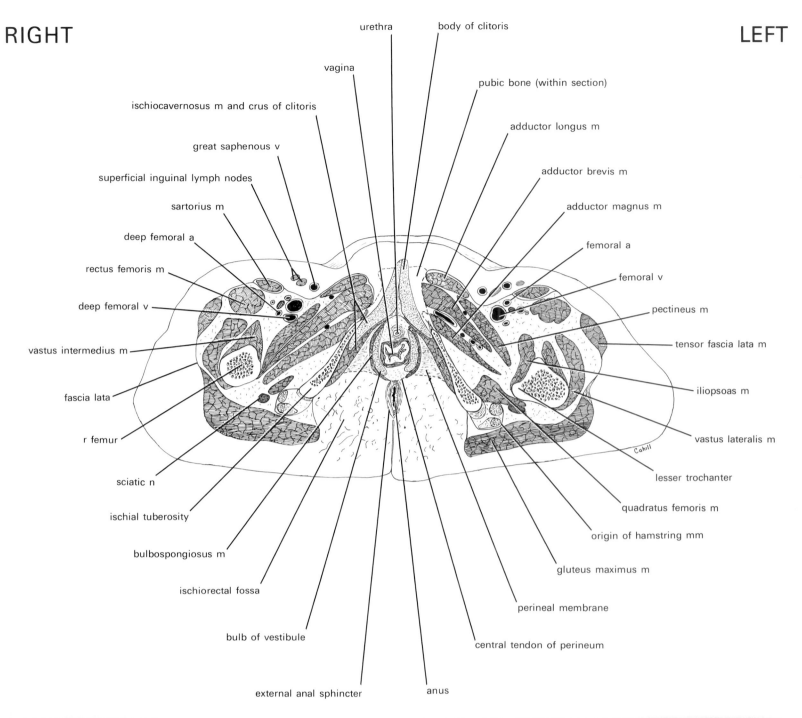

urethra
body of clitoris

vagina

pubic bone (within section)

ischiocavernosus m and crus of clitoris

adductor longus m

great saphenous v

adductor brevis m

superficial inguinal lymph nodes

adductor magnus m

sartorius m

femoral a

deep femoral a

femoral v

rectus femoris m

pectineus m

deep femoral v

tensor fascia lata m

vastus intermedius m

iliopsoas m

fascia lata

vastus lateralis m

r femur

lesser trochanter

sciatic n

quadratus femoris m

ischial tuberosity

origin of hamstring mm

bulbospongiosus m

gluteus maximus m

ischiorectal fossa

perineal membrane

bulb of vestibule

central tendon of perineum

external anal sphincter
anus

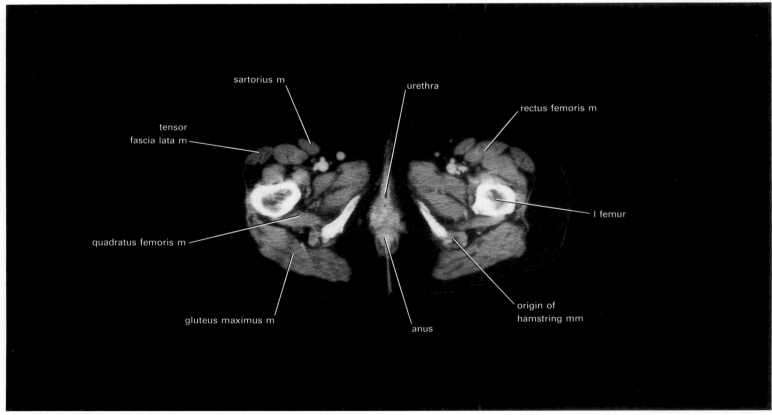

sartorius m
urethra

rectus femoris m

tensor
fascia lata m

l femur

quadratus femoris m

origin of
hamstring mm

gluteus maximus m
anus

Section 3 from below.

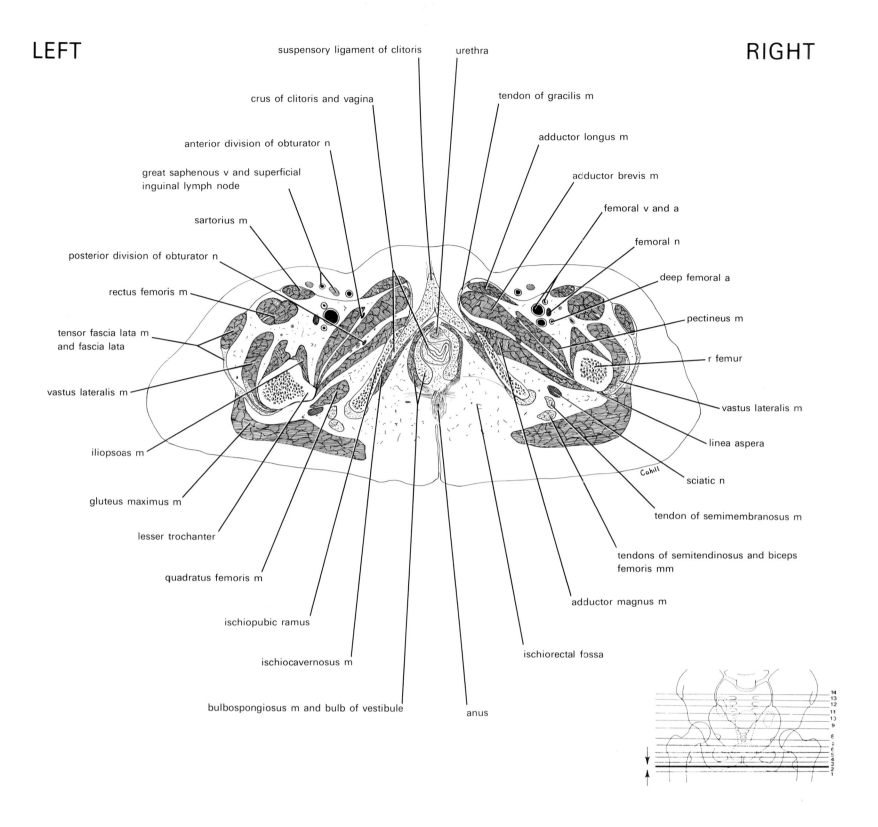

suspensory ligament of clitoris
urethra
crus of clitoris and vagina
tendon of gracilis m
anterior division of obturator n
adductor longus m
great saphenous v and superficial
inguinal lymph node
adductor brevis m
sartorius m
femoral v and a
posterior division of obturator n
femoral n
rectus femoris m
deep femoral a
pectineus m
tensor fascia lata m
and fascia lata
r femur
vastus lateralis m
vastus lateralis m
linea aspera
iliopsoas m
sciatic n
gluteus maximus m
tendon of semimembranosus m
lesser trochanter
tendons of semitendinosus and biceps
femoris mm
quadratus femoris m
adductor magnus m
ischiopubic ramus
ischiocavernosus m
ischiorectal fossa
bulbospongiosus m and bulb of vestibule
anus

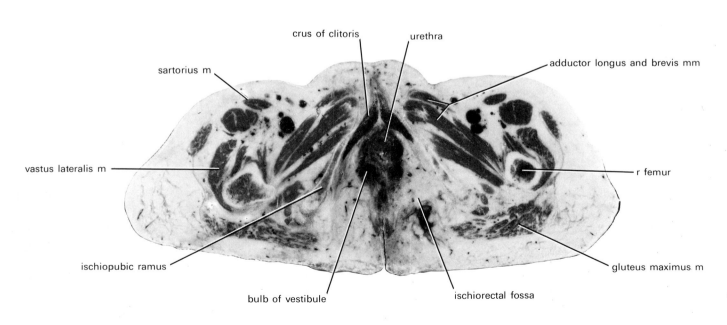

crus of clitoris
urethra
sartorius m
adductor longus and brevis mm
vastus lateralis m
r femur
ischiopubic ramus
gluteus maximus m
bulb of vestibule
ischiorectal fossa

Section 2 from above.

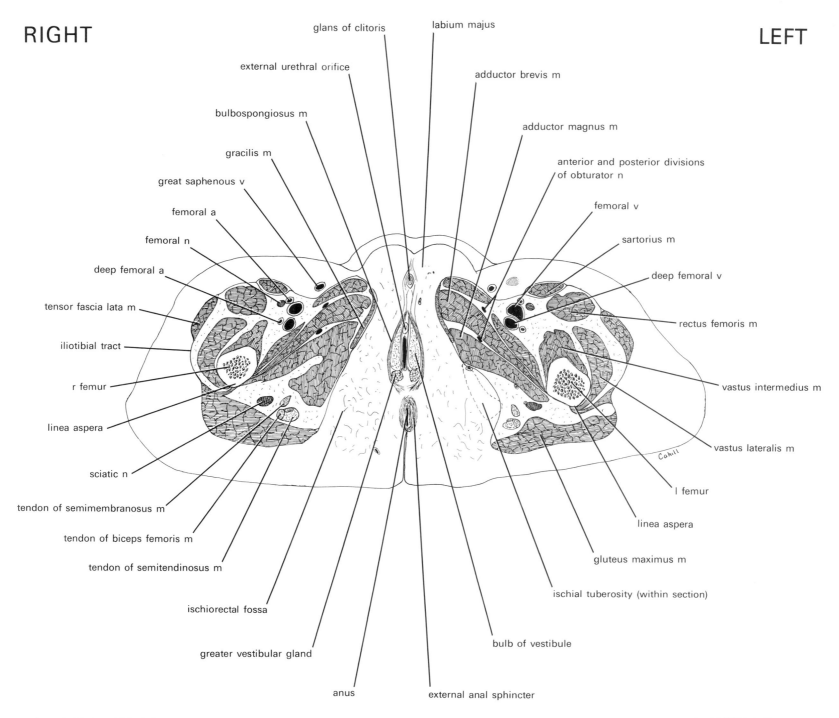

glans of clitoris

labium majus

external urethral orifice

adductor brevis m

bulbospongiosus m

adductor magnus m

gracilis m

anterior and posterior divisions of obturator n

great saphenous v

femoral v

femoral a

sartorius m

femoral n

deep femoral v

deep femoral a

rectus femoris m

tensor fascia lata m

iliotibial tract

r femur

vastus intermedius m

linea aspera

sciatic n

vastus lateralis m

tendon of semimembranosus m

l femur

tendon of biceps femoris m

linea aspera

tendon of semitendinosus m

gluteus maximus m

ischiorectal fossa

ischial tuberosity (within section)

greater vestibular gland

bulb of vestibule

anus

external anal sphincter

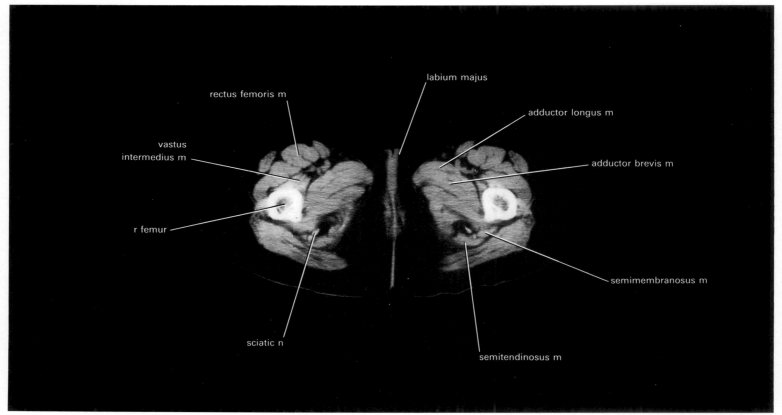

labium majus

rectus femoris m

adductor longus m

vastus intermedius m

adductor brevis m

r femur

semimembranosus m

sciatic n

semitendinosus m

Section 2 from below.

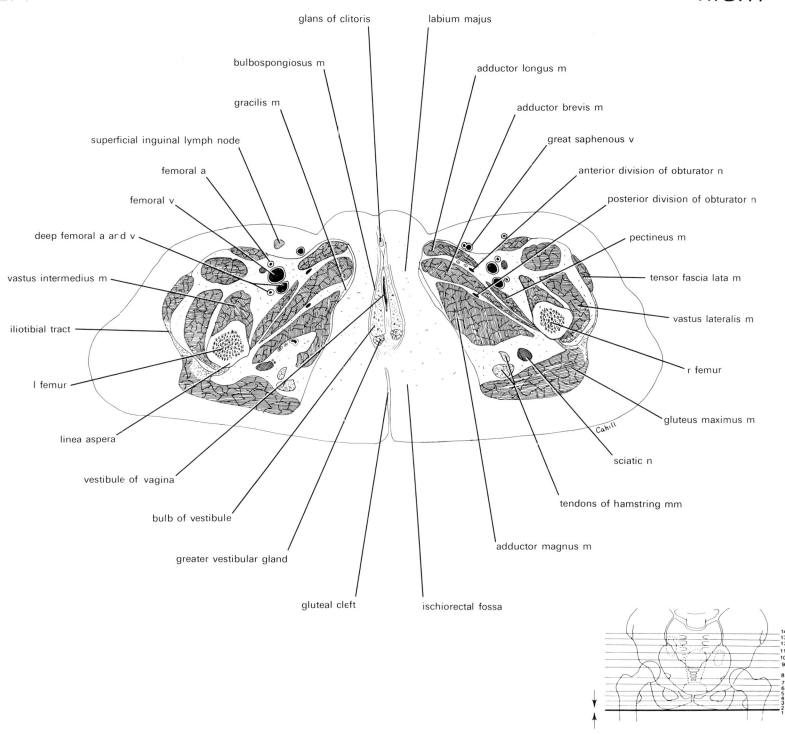

glans of clitoris

labium majus

bulbospongiosus m

adductor longus m

gracilis m

adductor brevis m

superficial inguinal lymph node

great saphenous v

femoral a

anterior division of obturator n

femoral v

posterior division of obturator n

deep femoral a and v

pectineus m

vastus intermedius m

tensor fascia lata m

iliotibial tract

vastus lateralis m

l femur

r femur

linea aspera

gluteus maximus m

vestibule of vagina

sciatic n

bulb of vestibule

tendons of hamstring mm

greater vestibular gland

adductor magnus m

gluteal cleft

ischiorectal fossa

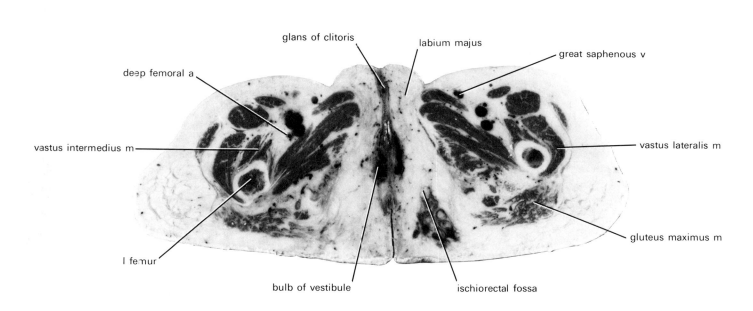

glans of clitoris

labium majus

great saphenous v

deep femoral a

vastus intermedius m

vastus lateralis m

l femur

gluteus maximus m

bulb of vestibule

ischiorectal fossa

Section 1 from above.

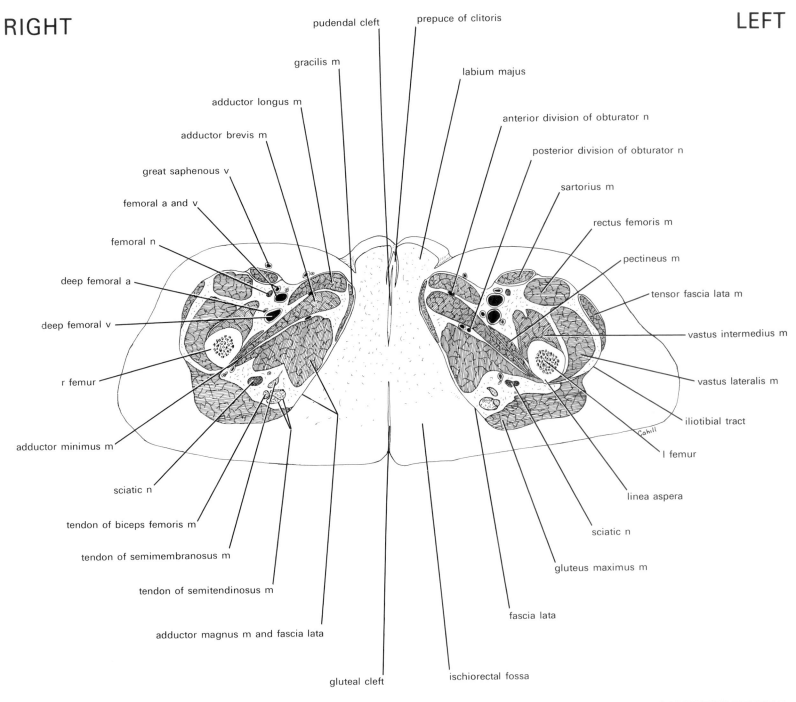

pudendal cleft

prepuce of clitoris

gracilis m

labium majus

adductor longus m

anterior division of obturator n

adductor brevis m

posterior division of obturator n

great saphenous v

sartorius m

femoral a and v

rectus femoris m

femoral n

pectineus m

deep femoral a

tensor fascia lata m

deep femoral v

vastus intermedius m

r femur

vastus lateralis m

iliotibial tract

adductor minimus m

l femur

linea aspera

sciatic n

sciatic n

tendon of biceps femoris m

gluteus maximus m

tendon of semimembranosus m

fascia lata

tendon of semitendinosus m

adductor magnus m and fascia lata

gluteal cleft

ischiorectal fossa

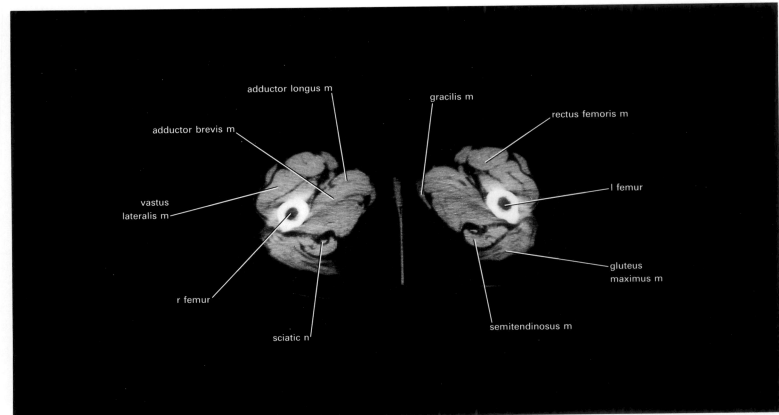

adductor longus m

gracilis m

rectus femoris m

adductor brevis m

vastus
lateralis m

l femur

r femur

gluteus
maximus m

sciatic n

semitendinosus m

Section 1 from below.

The Right Thigh, Knee, and Leg

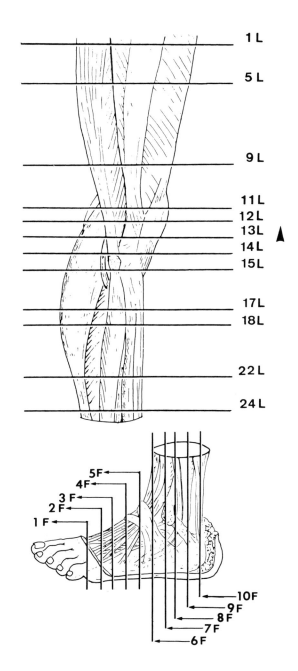

1 L
5 L
9 L
11 L
12 L
13 L
14 L
15 L
17 L
18 L
22 L
24 L

5 F
4 F
3 F
2 F
1 F
10 F
9 F
8 F
7 F
6 F

The Left Ankle and Foot

1 L
5 L
9 L
11 L
12 L
13 L
14 L
15 L
17 L
18 L
22 L
24 L

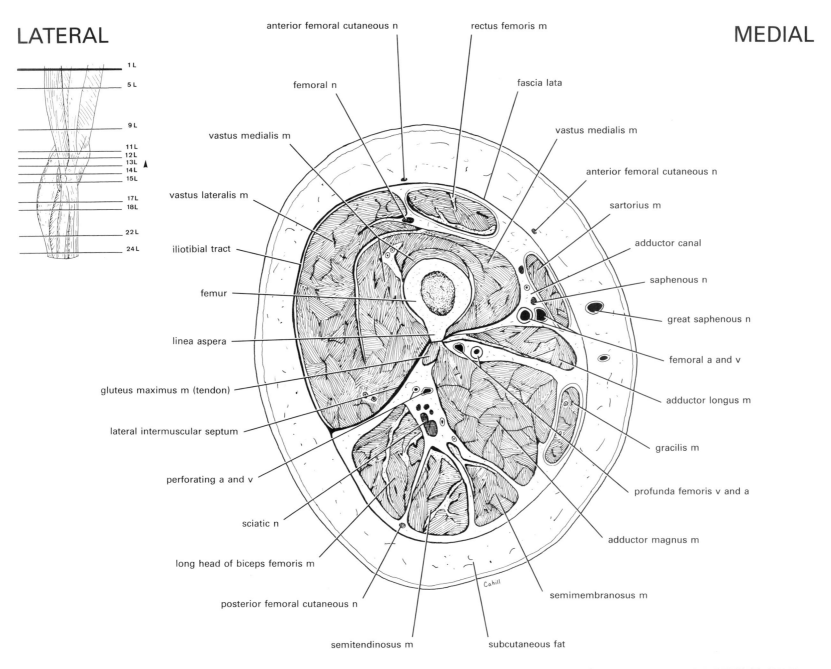

anterior femoral cutaneous n

rectus femoris m

femoral n

fascia lata

vastus medialis m

vastus medialis m

anterior femoral cutaneous n

vastus lateralis m

sartorius m

iliotibial tract

adductor canal

saphenous n

femur

great saphenous n

linea aspera

femoral a and v

gluteus maximus m (tendon)

adductor longus m

lateral intermuscular septum

gracilis m

perforating a and v

profunda femoris v and a

sciatic n

adductor magnus m

long head of biceps femoris m

semimembranosus m

posterior femoral cutaneous n

semitendinosus m

subcutaneous fat

Cahill

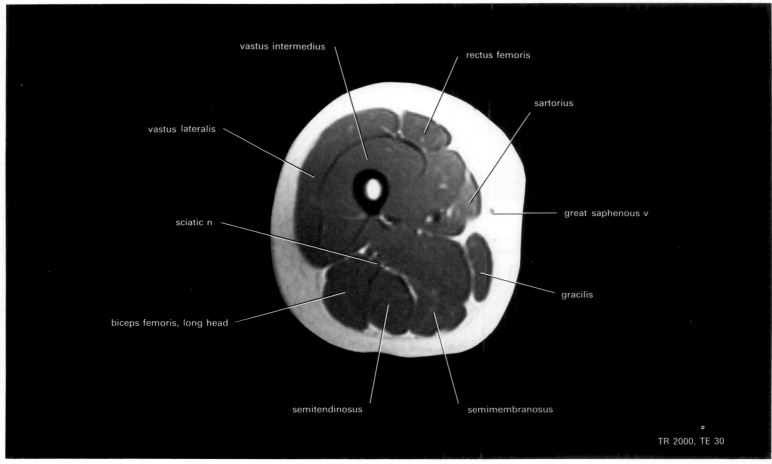

vastus intermedius

rectus femoris

vastus lateralis

sartorius

great saphenous v

sciatic n

gracilis

biceps femoris, long head

semitendinosus

semimembranosus

TR 2000, TE 30

Section 1L from below.

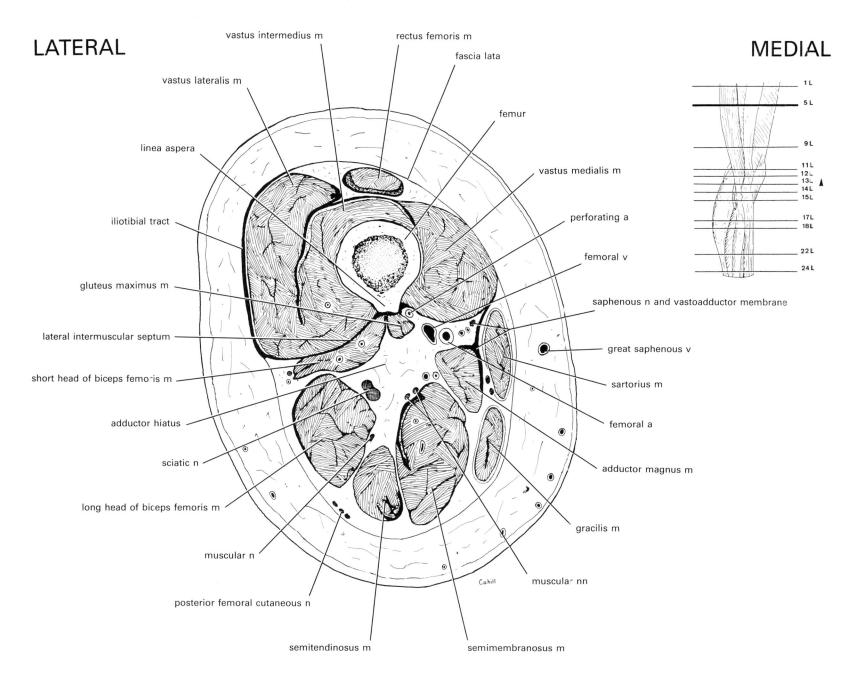

vastus intermedius m

rectus femoris m

fascia lata

femur

vastus lateralis m

vastus medialis m

linea aspera

perforating a

iliotibial tract

femoral v

saphenous n and vastoadductor membrane

gluteus maximus m

great saphenous v

lateral intermuscular septum

sartorius m

short head of biceps femoris m

femoral a

adductor hiatus

adductor magnus m

sciatic n

long head of biceps femoris m

gracilis m

muscular n

muscular nn

posterior femoral cutaneous n

semitendinosus m

semimembranosus m

1 L
5 L
9 L
11 L
12 L
13 L
14 L
15 L
17 L
18 L
22 L
24 L

Cahill

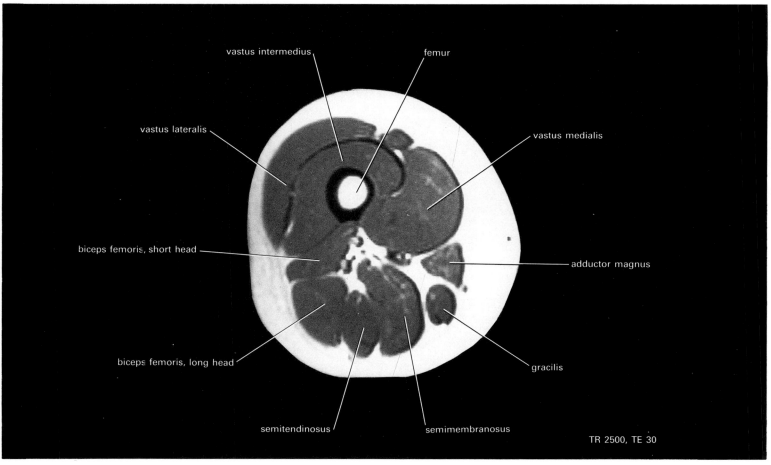

vastus intermedius

femur

vastus lateralis

vastus medialis

biceps femoris, short head

adductor magnus

biceps femoris, long head

gracilis

semitendinosus

semimembranosus

TR 2500, TE 30

Section 5L from below.

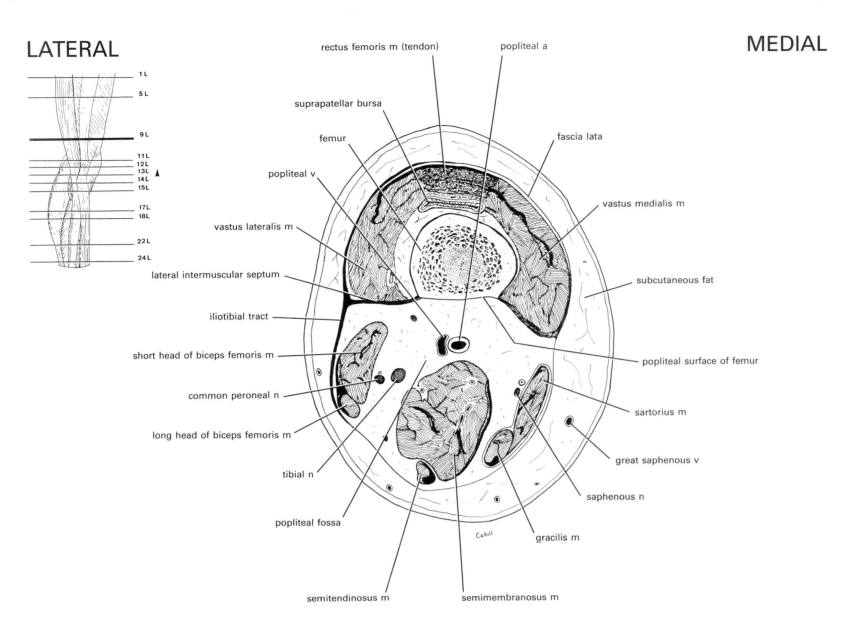

rectus femoris m (tendon)

popliteal a

suprapatellar bursa

fascia lata

femur

popliteal v

vastus medialis m

vastus lateralis m

lateral intermuscular septum

subcutaneous fat

iliotibial tract

popliteal surface of femur

short head of biceps femoris m

common peroneal n

sartorius m

long head of biceps femoris m

great saphenous v

tibial n

saphenous n

popliteal fossa

gracilis m

semitendinosus m

semimembranosus m

1 L
5 L
9 L
11 L
12 L
13 L
14 L
15 L
17 L
18 L
22 L
24 L

Cahill

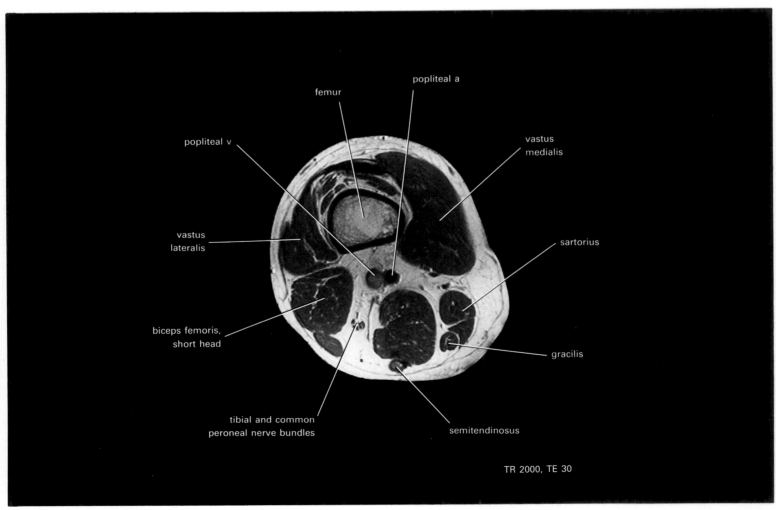

popliteal a

femur

popliteal v

vastus
medialis

vastus
lateralis

sartorius

biceps femoris,
short head

gracilis

tibial and common
peroneal nerve bundles

semitendinosus

TR 2000, TE 30

Section 9L from below.

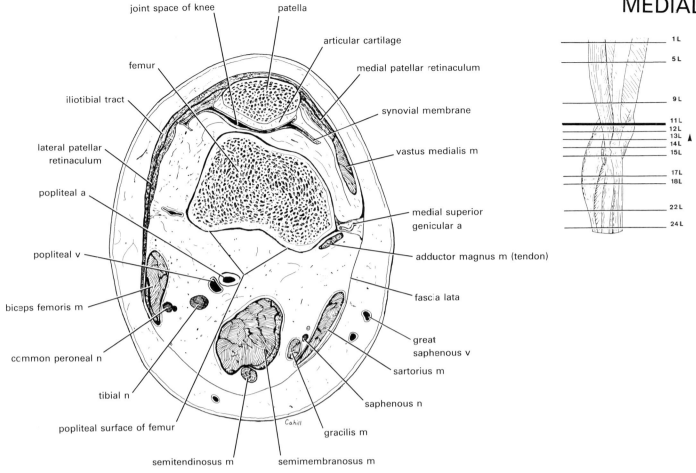

joint space of knee

patella

articular cartilage

femur

medial patellar retinaculum

iliotibial tract

synovial membrane

lateral patellar
retinaculum

vastus medialis m

popliteal a

medial superior
genicular a

popliteal v

adductor magnus m (tendon)

biceps femoris m

fascia lata

common peroneal n

great
saphenous v

tibial n

sartorius m

popliteal surface of femur

saphenous n

semitendinosus m

gracilis m

semimembranosus m

1 L
5 L
9 L
11 L
12 L
13 L
14 L
15 L
17 L
18 L
22 L
24 L

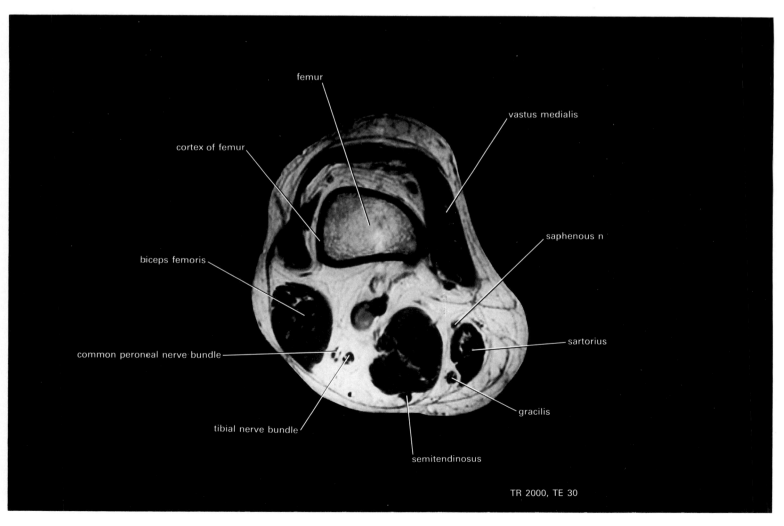

femur

vastus medialis

cortex of femur

biceps femoris

saphenous n

common peroneal nerve bundle

sartorius

tibial nerve bundle

gracilis

semitendinosus

TR 2000, TE 30

Section 11L from below.

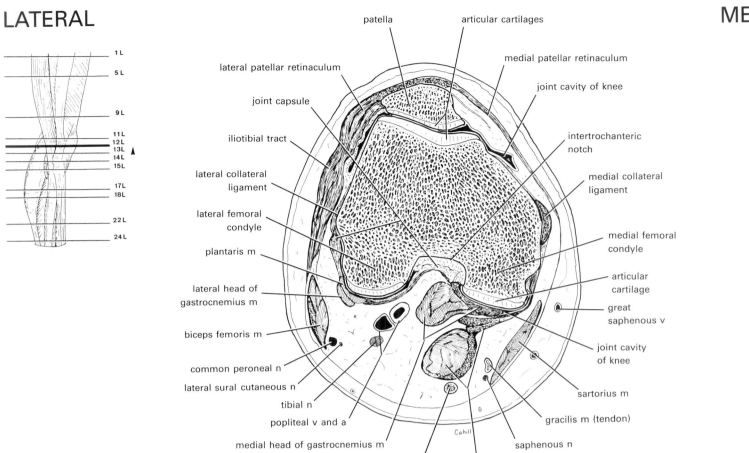

patella

articular cartilages

lateral patellar retinaculum

medial patellar retinaculum

joint capsule

joint cavity of knee

iliotibial tract

intertrochanteric notch

lateral collateral ligament

medial collateral ligament

lateral femoral condyle

medial femoral condyle

plantaris m

articular cartilage

lateral head of gastrocnemius m

great saphenous v

biceps femoris m

joint cavity of knee

common peroneal n

lateral sural cutaneous n

sartorius m

tibial n

gracilis m (tendon)

popliteal v and a

medial head of gastrocnemius m

saphenous n

semitendinosus m (tendon)

semimembranosus m

1 L
5 L
9 L
11 L
12 L
13 L
14 L
15 L
17 L
18 L
22 L
24 L

Cahill

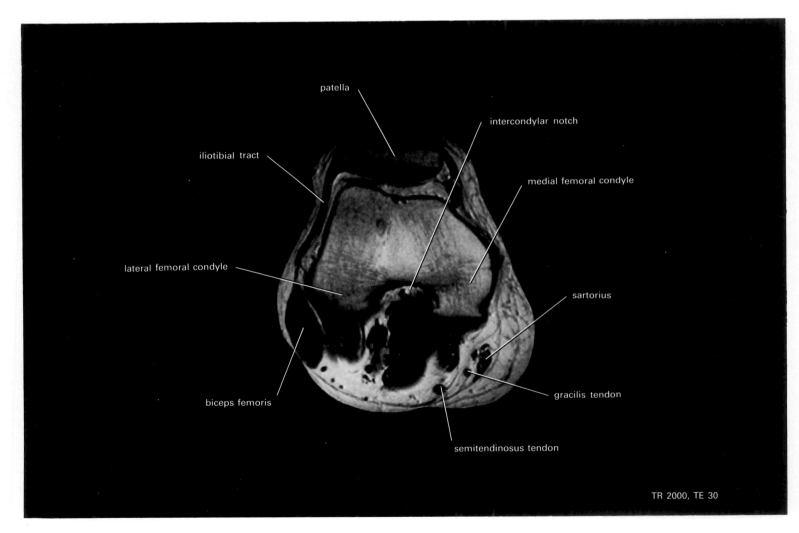

patella

intercondylar notch

iliotibial tract

medial femoral condyle

lateral femoral condyle

sartorius

gracilis tendon

biceps femoris

semitendinosus tendon

TR 2000, TE 30

Section 12L from below.

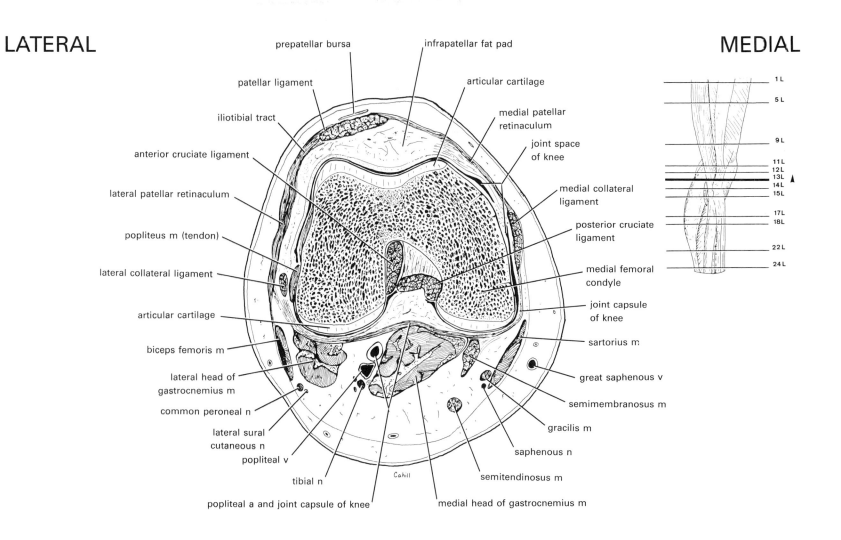

prepatellar bursa

infrapatellar fat pad

patellar ligament

articular cartilage

iliotibial tract

medial patellar retinaculum

anterior cruciate ligament

joint space of knee

lateral patellar retinaculum

medial collateral ligament

popliteus m (tendon)

posterior cruciate ligament

lateral collateral ligament

medial femoral condyle

articular cartilage

joint capsule of knee

biceps femoris m

sartorius m

lateral head of gastrocnemius m

great saphenous v

common peroneal n

semimembranosus m

lateral sural cutaneous n

gracilis m

popliteal v

saphenous n

tibial n

semitendinosus m

popliteal a and joint capsule of knee

medial head of gastrocnemius m

Cahill

1 L
5 L
9 L
11 L
12 L
13 L
14 L
15 L
17 L
18 L
22 L
24 L

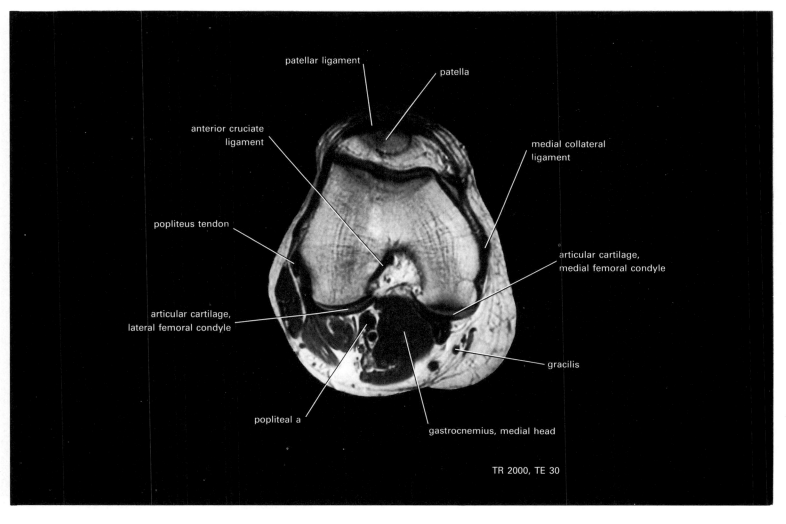

patellar ligament

patella

anterior cruciate ligament

medial collateral ligament

popliteus tendon

articular cartilage, medial femoral condyle

articular cartilage, lateral femoral condyle

gracilis

popliteal a

gastrocnemius, medial head

TR 2000, TE 30

Section 13L from below.

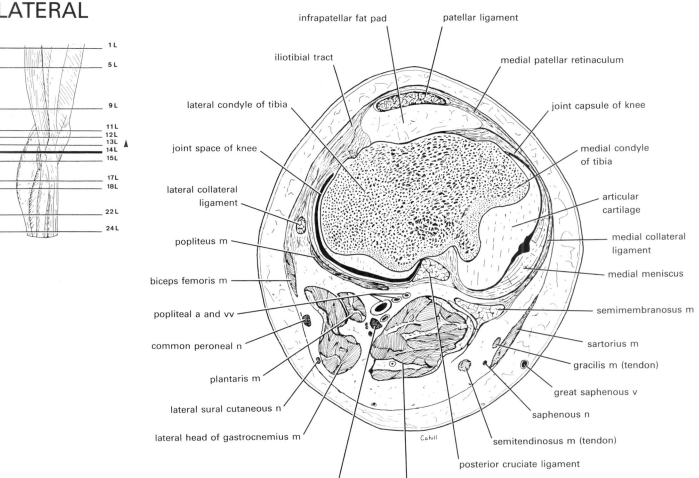

infrapatellar fat pad

patellar ligament

iliotibial tract

medial patellar retinaculum

lateral condyle of tibia

joint capsule of knee

medial condyle of tibia

joint space of knee

articular cartilage

lateral collateral ligament

medial collateral ligament

popliteus m

medial meniscus

biceps femoris m

semimembranosus m

popliteal a and vv

common peroneal n

sartorius m

gracilis m (tendon)

plantaris m

great saphenous v

lateral sural cutaneous n

saphenous n

lateral head of gastrocnemius m

semitendinosus m (tendon)

posterior cruciate ligament

tibial n

medial head of gastrocnemius m

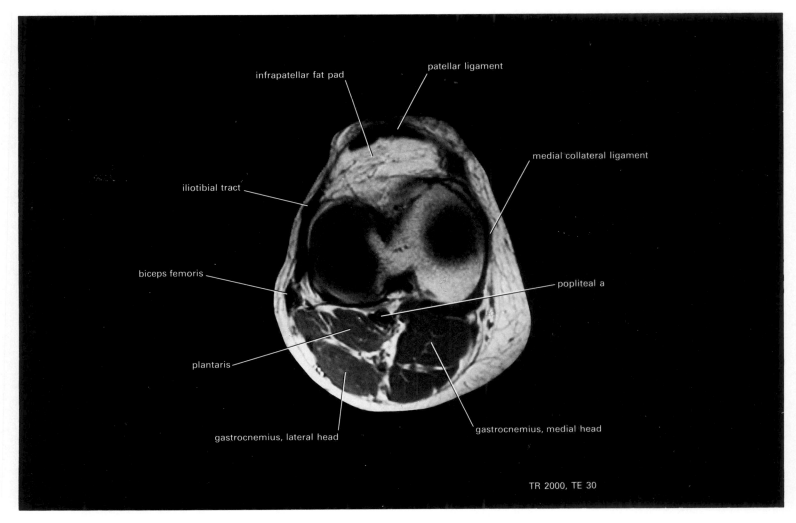

infrapatellar fat pad

patellar ligament

iliotibial tract

medial collateral ligament

biceps femoris

popliteal a

plantaris

gastrocnemius, lateral head

gastrocnemius, medial head

TR 2000, TE 30

Section 14L from below.

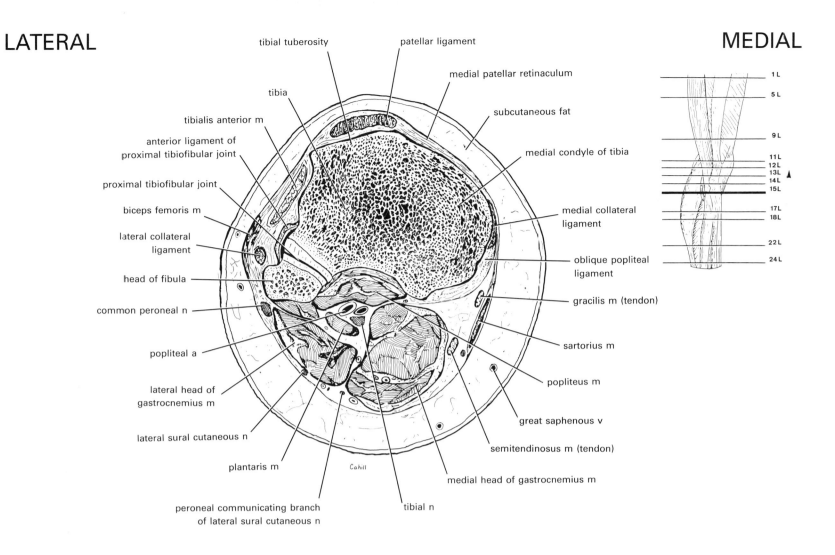

tibial tuberosity

patellar ligament

medial patellar retinaculum

tibia

subcutaneous fat

tibialis anterior m

anterior ligament of
proximal tibiofibular joint

medial condyle of tibia

proximal tibiofibular joint

medial collateral
ligament

biceps femoris m

lateral collateral
ligament

oblique popliteal
ligament

head of fibula

gracilis m (tendon)

common peroneal n

sartorius m

popliteal a

popliteus m

lateral head of
gastrocnemius m

great saphenous v

lateral sural cutaneous n

semitendinosus m (tendon)

plantaris m

medial head of gastrocnemius m

peroneal communicating branch
of lateral sural cutaneous n

tibial n

Cahill

1 L
5 L
9 L
11 L
12 L
13 L
14 L
15 L
17 L
18 L
22 L
24 L

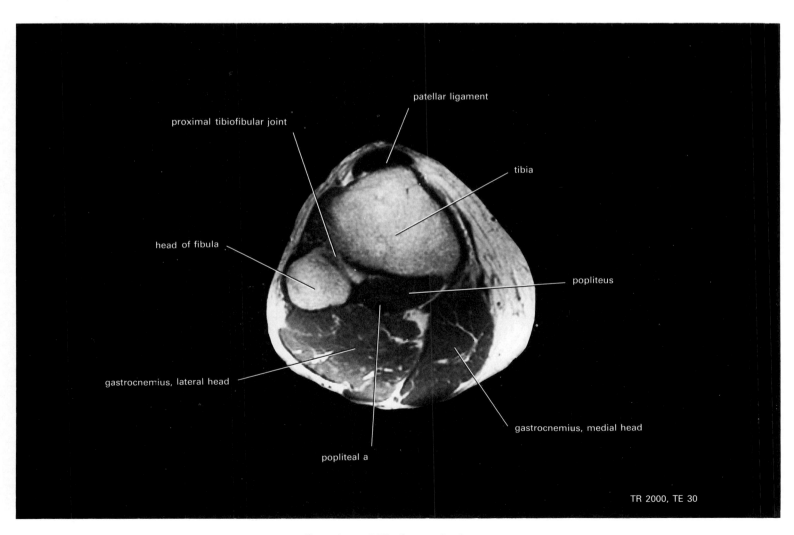

patellar ligament

proximal tibiofibular joint

tibia

head of fibula

popliteus

gastrocnemius, lateral head

gastrocnemius, medial head

popliteal a

TR 2000, TE 30

Section 15L from below.

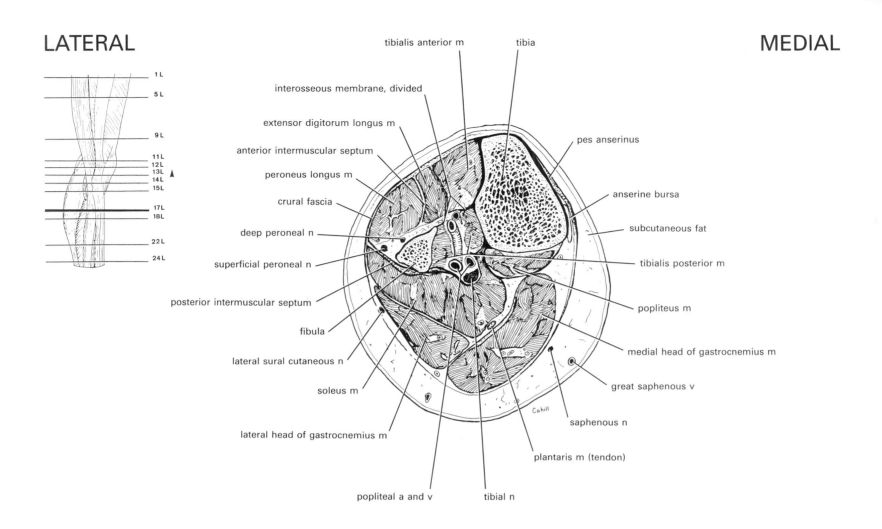

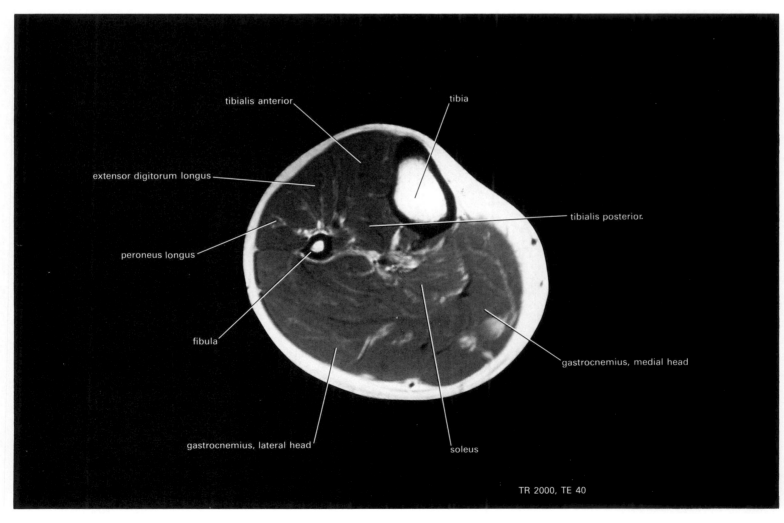

Section 17L from below.

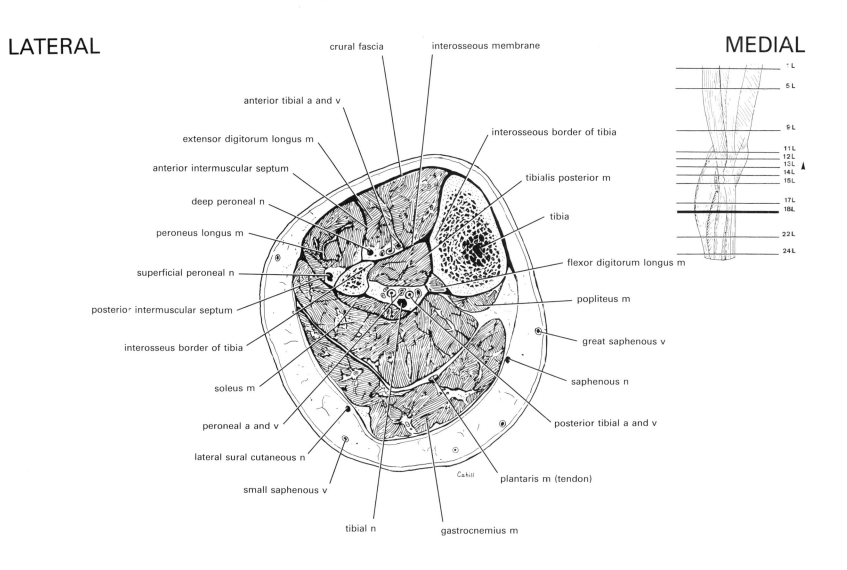

crural fascia

interosseous membrane

anterior tibial a and v

interosseous border of tibia

extensor digitorum longus m

anterior intermuscular septum

tibialis posterior m

deep peroneal n

tibia

peroneus longus m

flexor digitorum longus m

superficial peroneal n

popliteus m

posterior intermuscular septum

great saphenous v

interosseus border of tibia

saphenous n

soleus m

posterior tibial a and v

peroneal a and v

lateral sural cutaneous n

plantaris m (tendon)

small saphenous v

Cahill

tibial n

gastrocnemius m

1 L
5 L
9 L
11 L
12 L
13 L
14 L
15 L
17 L
18 L
22 L
24 L

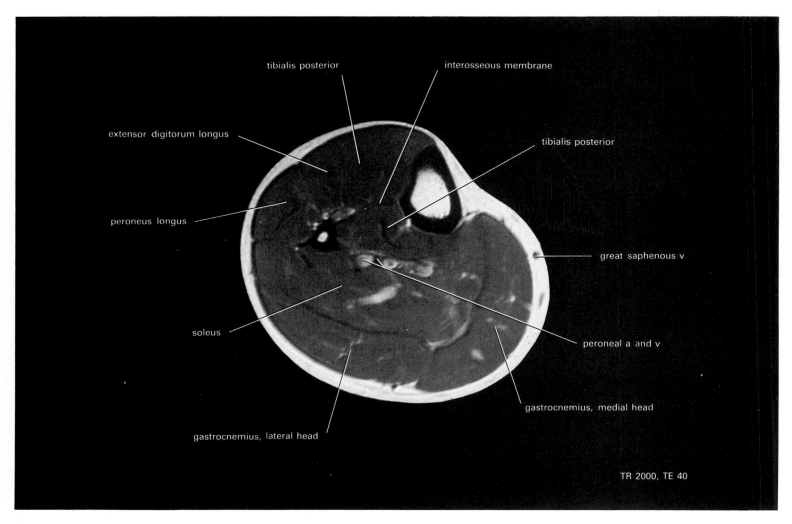

tibialis posterior

interosseous membrane

extensor digitorum longus

tibialis posterior

peroneus longus

great saphenous v

soleus

peroneal a and v

gastrocnemius, medial head

gastrocnemius, lateral head

TR 2000, TE 40

Section 18L from below.

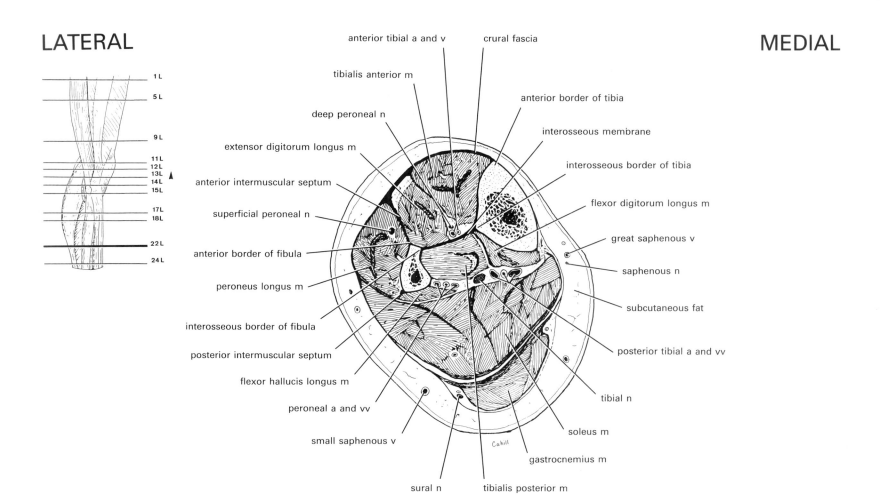

anterior tibial a and v
crural fascia
tibialis anterior m
anterior border of tibia
deep peroneal n
interosseous membrane
extensor digitorum longus m
interosseous border of tibia
anterior intermuscular septum
flexor digitorum longus m
superficial peroneal n
great saphenous v
anterior border of fibula
saphenous n
peroneus longus m
subcutaneous fat
interosseous border of fibula
posterior tibial a and vv
posterior intermuscular septum
flexor hallucis longus m
tibial n
peroneal a and vv
soleus m
small saphenous v
gastrocnemius m
sural n
tibialis posterior m

1 L
5 L
9 L
11 L
12 L
13 L
14 L
15 L
17 L
18 L
22 L
24 L

Cahill

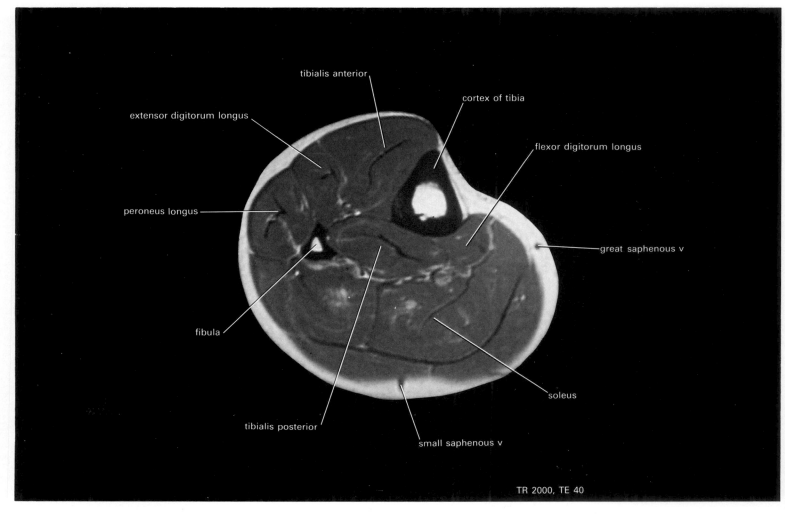

tibialis anterior
cortex of tibia
extensor digitorum longus
flexor digitorum longus
peroneus longus
great saphenous v
fibula
soleus
tibialis posterior
small saphenous v

TR 2000, TE 40

Section 22L from below.

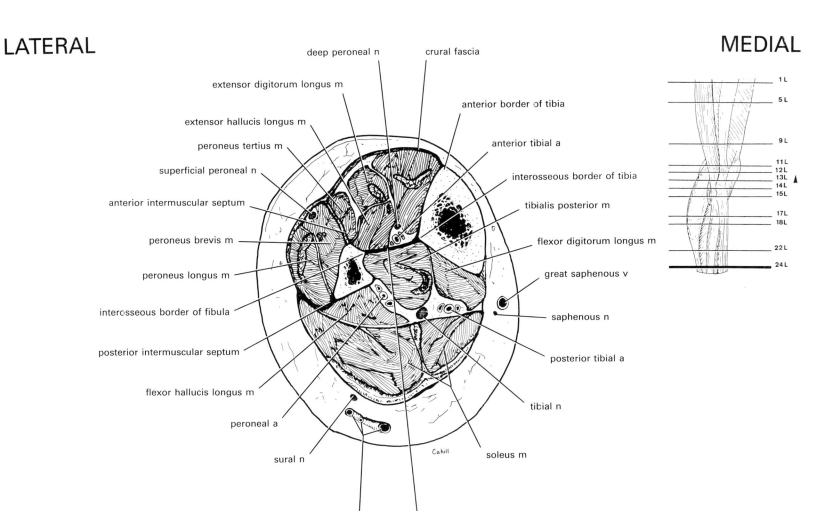

deep peroneal n

crural fascia

extensor digitorum longus m

anterior border of tibia

extensor hallucis longus m

anterior tibial a

peroneus tertius m

interosseous border of tibia

superficial peroneal n

tibialis posterior m

anterior intermuscular septum

flexor digitorum longus m

peroneus brevis m

great saphenous v

peroneus longus m

saphenous n

interosseous border of fibula

posterior tibial a

posterior intermuscular septum

tibial n

flexor hallucis longus m

peroneal a

soleus m

sural n

small saphenous v

interosseous membrane

1 L
5 L
9 L
11 L
12 L
13 L
14 L
15 L
17 L
18 L
22 L
24 L

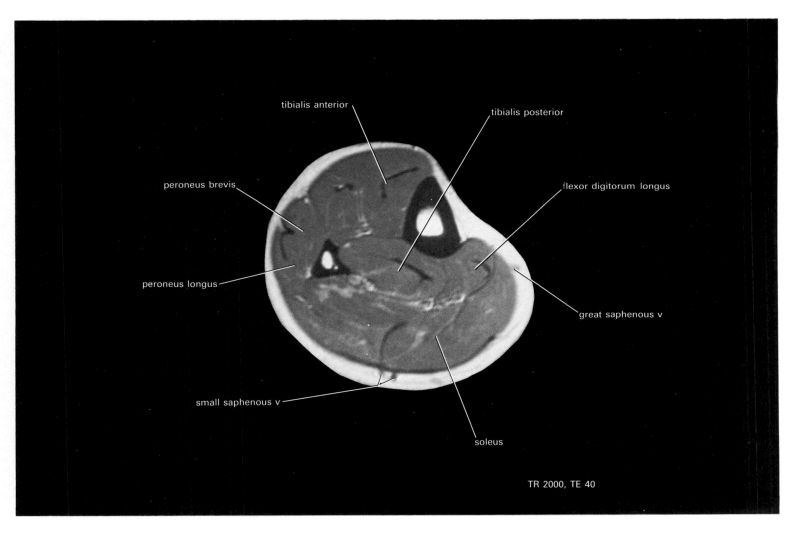

tibialis anterior

tibialis posterior

peroneus brevis

flexor digitorum longus

peroneus longus

great saphenous v

small saphenous v

soleus

TR 2000, TE 40

Section 24L from below.

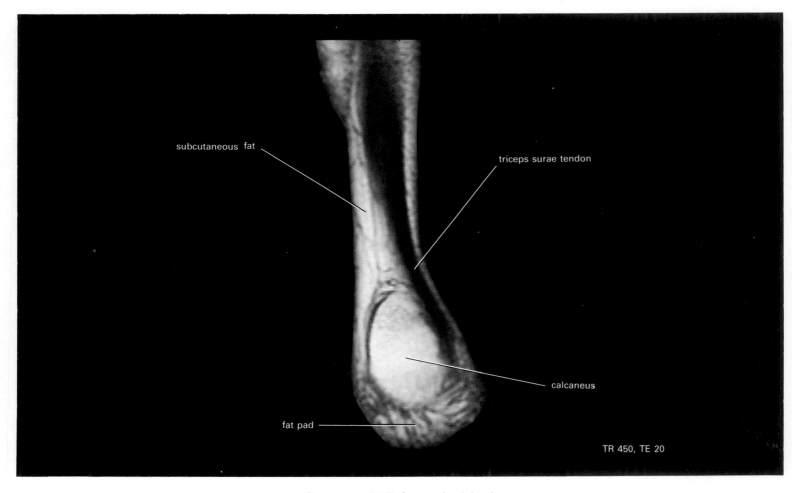

peroneus longus m

flexor hallucis longus m

peroneus brevis m

soleus m

posterior intermuscular septum

deep transverse fascia

small saphenous v

triceps surae m (tendon)

bursa tendinis calcanei

calcaneus

fat pad of heel

Cahill

subcutaneous fat

triceps surae tendon

calcaneus

fat pad

TR 450, TE 20

Section 10F from behind.

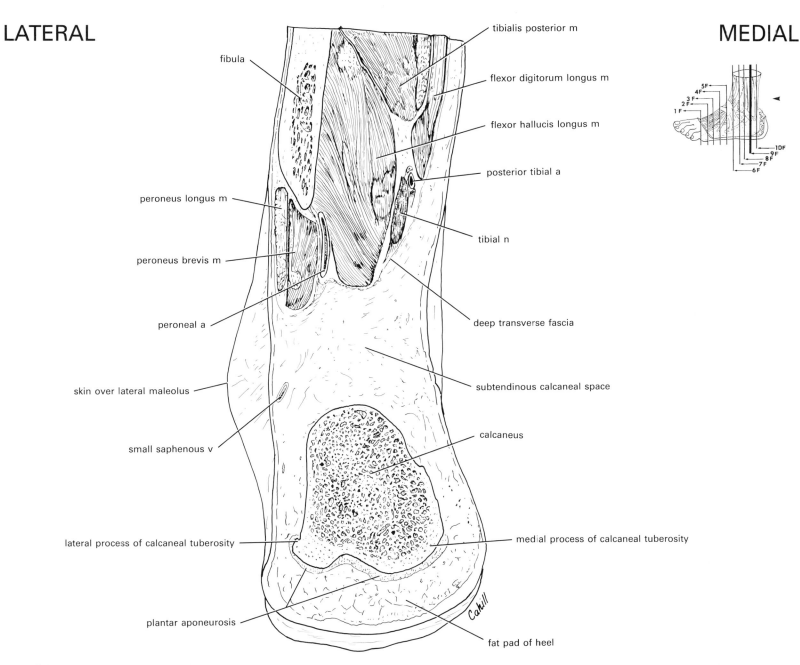

fibula

tibialis posterior m

flexor digitorum longus m

flexor hallucis longus m

posterior tibial a

peroneus longus m

peroneus brevis m

tibial n

peroneal a

deep transverse fascia

skin over lateral maleolus

subtendinous calcaneal space

calcaneus

small saphenous v

lateral process of calcaneal tuberosity

medial process of calcaneal tuberosity

plantar aponeurosis

fat pad of heel

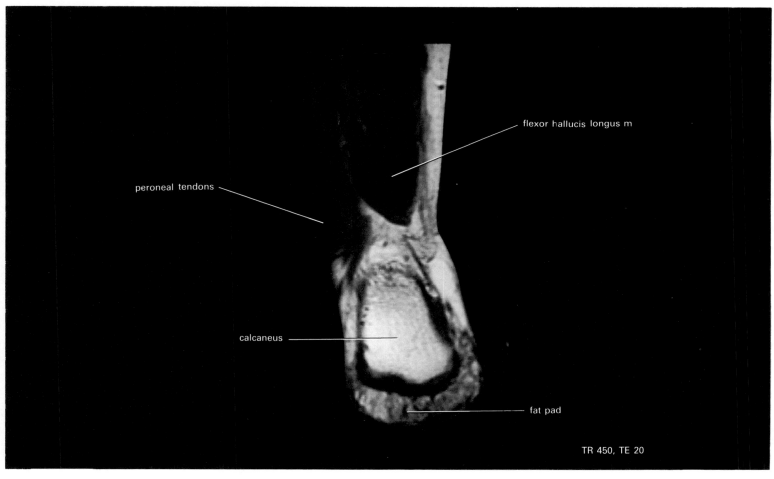

flexor hallucis longus m

peroneal tendons

calcaneus

fat pad

TR 450, TE 20

Section 9F from behind.

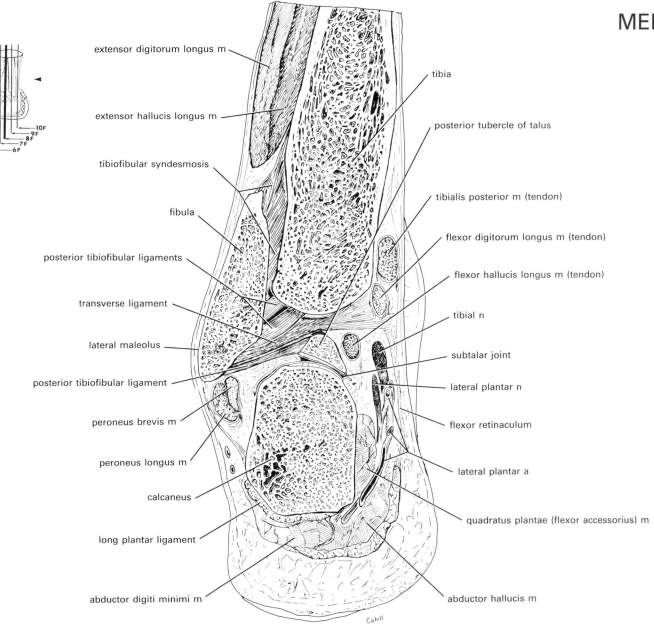

extensor digitorum longus m

tibia

extensor hallucis longus m

posterior tubercle of talus

tibiofibular syndesmosis

tibialis posterior m (tendon)

fibula

flexor digitorum longus m (tendon)

posterior tibiofibular ligaments

flexor hallucis longus m (tendon)

transverse ligament

tibial n

lateral maleolus

subtalar joint

posterior tibiofibular ligament

lateral plantar n

peroneus brevis m

flexor retinaculum

peroneus longus m

lateral plantar a

calcaneus

quadratus plantae (flexor accessorius) m

long plantar ligament

abductor digiti minimi m

abductor hallucis m

Cahill

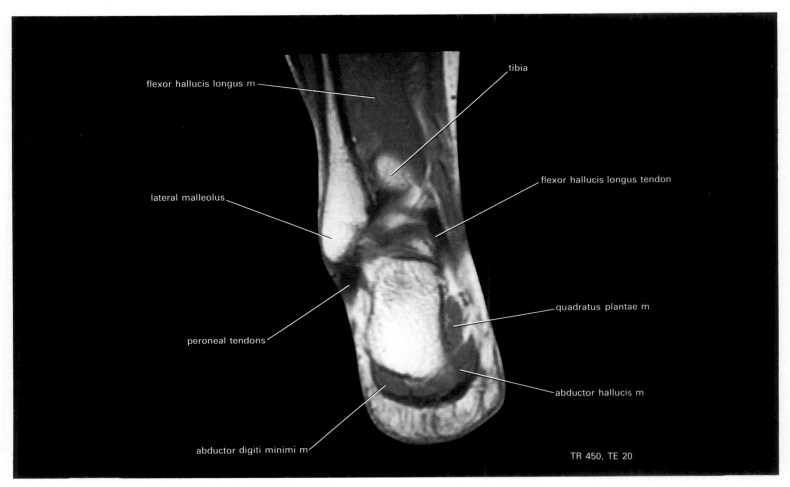

flexor hallucis longus m

tibia

flexor hallucis longus tendon

lateral malleolus

peroneal tendons

quadratus plantae m

abductor hallucis m

abductor digiti minimi m

TR 450, TE 20

Section 8F from behind.

LATERAL

MEDIAL

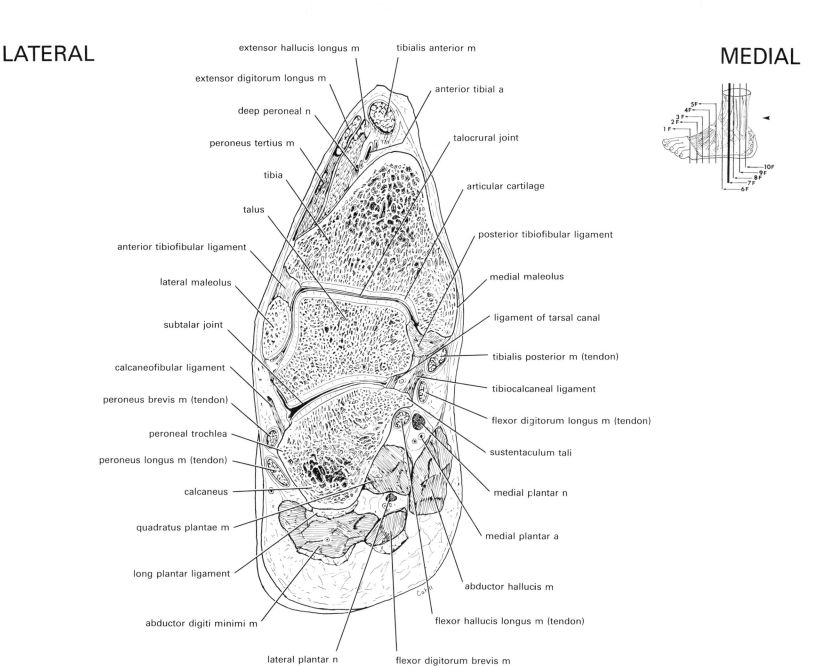

extensor hallucis longus m
extensor digitorum longus m
deep peroneal n
peroneus tertius m
tibia
talus
anterior tibiofibular ligament
lateral maleolus
subtalar joint
calcaneofibular ligament
peroneus brevis m (tendon)
peroneal trochlea
peroneus longus m (tendon)
calcaneus
quadratus plantae m
long plantar ligament
abductor digiti minimi m

tibialis anterior m
anterior tibial a
talocrural joint
articular cartilage
posterior tibiofibular ligament
medial maleolus
ligament of tarsal canal
tibialis posterior m (tendon)
tibiocalcaneal ligament
flexor digitorum longus m (tendon)
sustentaculum tali
medial plantar n
medial plantar a
abductor hallucis m
flexor hallucis longus m (tendon)

lateral plantar n
flexor digitorum brevis m

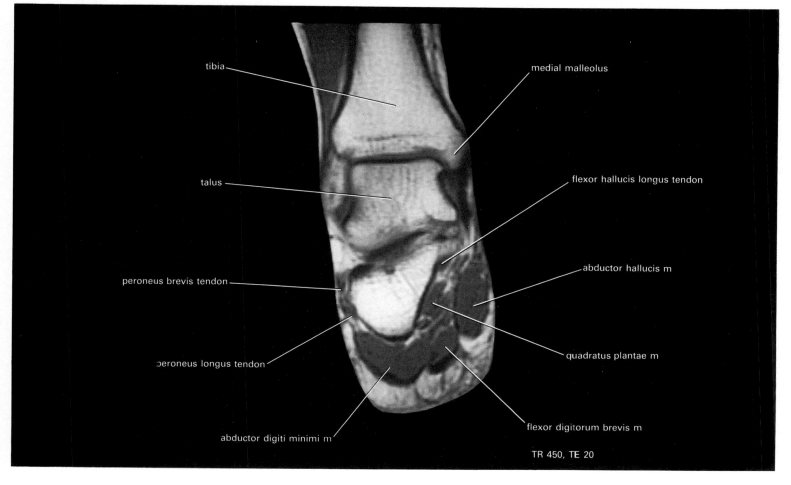

tibia
talus
peroneus brevis tendon
peroneus longus tendon
abductor digiti minimi m

medial malleolus
flexor hallucis longus tendon
abductor hallucis m
quadratus plantae m
flexor digitorum brevis m

TR 450, TE 20

Section 7F from behind.

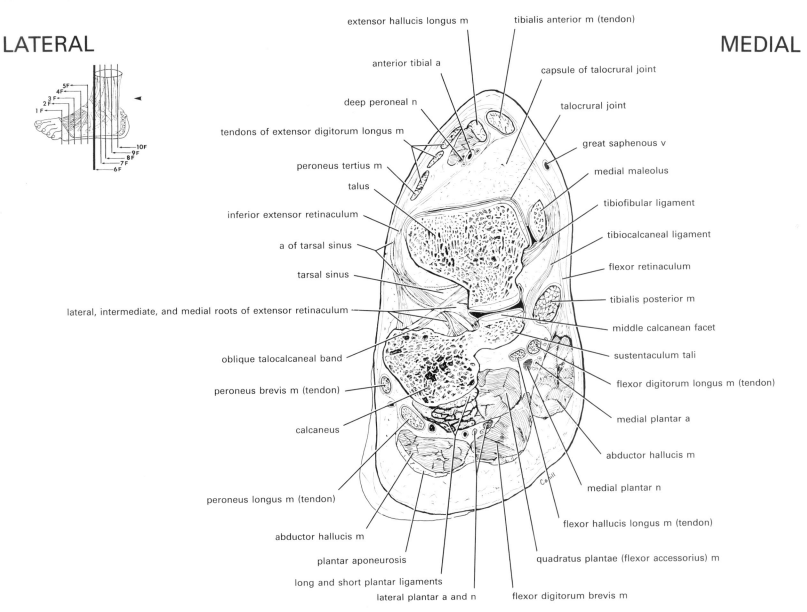

extensor hallucis longus m

tibialis anterior m (tendon)

anterior tibial a

capsule of talocrural joint

deep peroneal n

talocrural joint

tendons of extensor digitorum longus m

great saphenous v

peroneus tertius m

medial maleolus

talus

tibiofibular ligament

inferior extensor retinaculum

tibiocalcaneal ligament

a of tarsal sinus

flexor retinaculum

tarsal sinus

tibialis posterior m

lateral, intermediate, and medial roots of extensor retinaculum

middle calcanean facet

oblique talocalcaneal band

sustentaculum tali

peroneus brevis m (tendon)

flexor digitorum longus m (tendon)

calcaneus

medial plantar a

abductor hallucis m

peroneus longus m (tendon)

medial plantar n

abductor hallucis m

flexor hallucis longus m (tendon)

plantar aponeurosis

quadratus plantae (flexor accessorius) m

long and short plantar ligaments

lateral plantar a and n

flexor digitorum brevis m

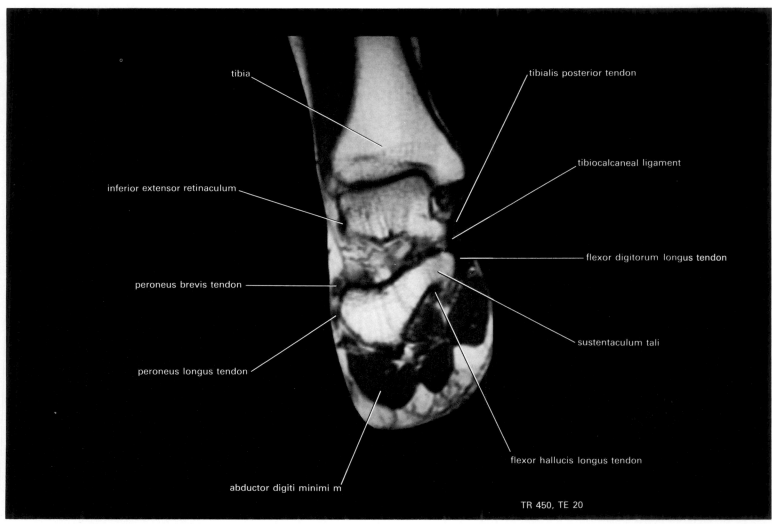

tibia

tibialis posterior tendon

inferior extensor retinaculum

tibiocalcaneal ligament

flexor digitorum longus tendon

peroneus brevis tendon

peroneus longus tendon

sustentaculum tali

flexor hallucis longus tendon

abductor digiti minimi m

TR 450, TE 20

Section 6F from behind.

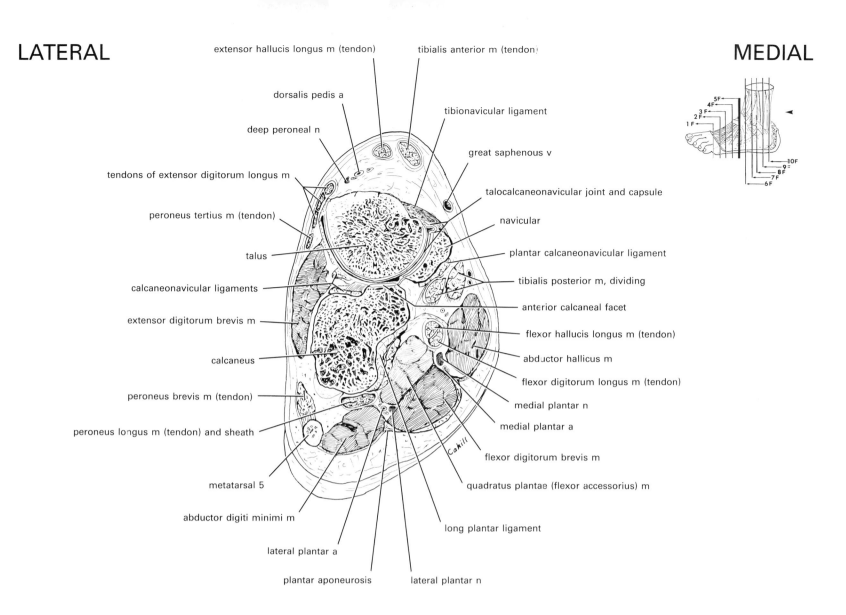

extensor hallucis longus m (tendon)

tibialis anterior m (tendon)

dorsalis pedis a

tibionavicular ligament

deep peroneal n

great saphenous v

tendons of extensor digitorum longus m

talocalcaneonavicular joint and capsule

peroneus tertius m (tendon)

navicular

talus

plantar calcaneonavicular ligament

calcaneonavicular ligaments

tibialis posterior m, dividing

extensor digitorum brevis m

anterior calcaneal facet

flexor hallucis longus m (tendon)

calcaneus

abductor hallicus m

peroneus brevis m (tendon)

flexor digitorum longus m (tendon)

peroneus longus m (tendon) and sheath

medial plantar n

medial plantar a

flexor digitorum brevis m

metatarsal 5

quadratus plantae (flexor accessorius) m

abductor digiti minimi m

long plantar ligament

lateral plantar a

plantar aponeurosis

lateral plantar n

Cahill

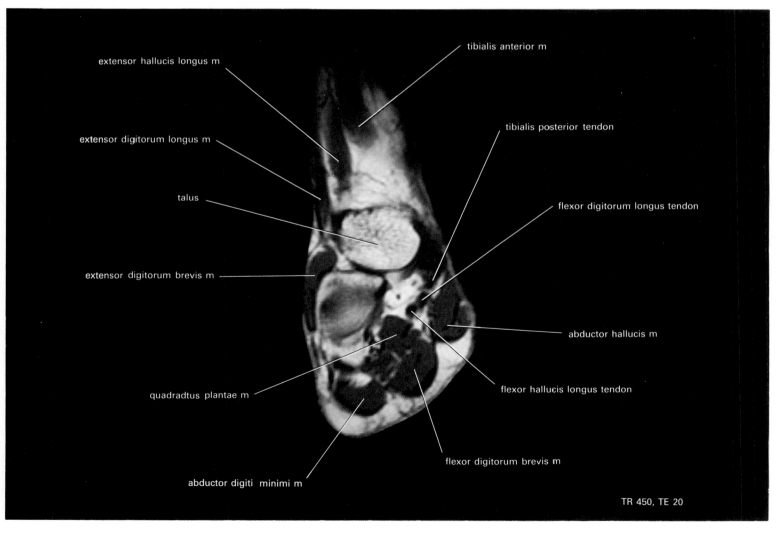

extensor hallucis longus m

tibialis anterior m

extensor digitorum longus m

tibialis posterior tendon

talus

flexor digitorum longus tendon

extensor digitorum brevis m

abductor hallucis m

quadradtus plantae m

flexor hallucis longus tendon

abductor digiti minimi m

flexor digitorum brevis m

TR 450, TE 20

Section 5F from behind.

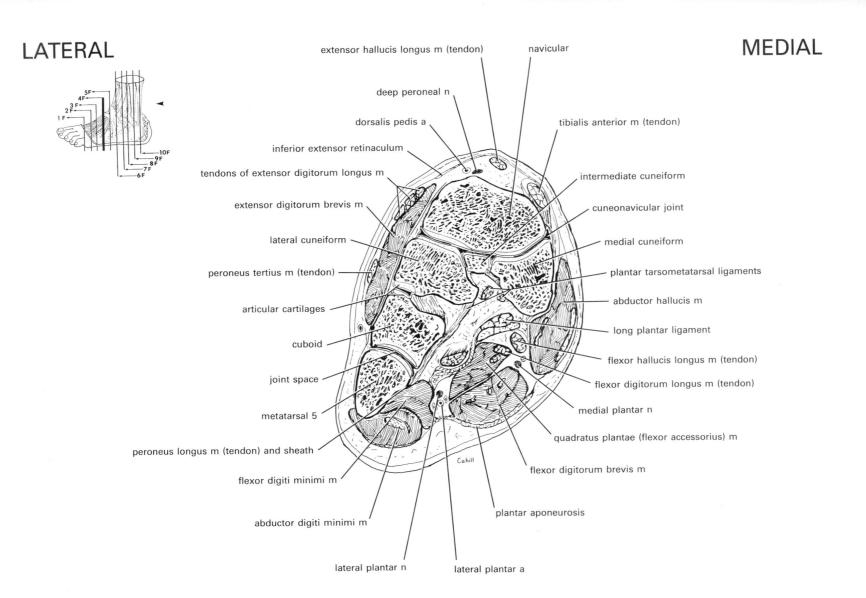

extensor hallucis longus m (tendon)

navicular

deep peroneal n

tibialis anterior m (tendon)

dorsalis pedis a

inferior extensor retinaculum

intermediate cuneiform

tendons of extensor digitorum longus m

cuneonavicular joint

extensor digitorum brevis m

medial cuneiform

lateral cuneiform

plantar tarsometatarsal ligaments

peroneus tertius m (tendon)

abductor hallucis m

articular cartilages

long plantar ligament

cuboid

flexor hallucis longus m (tendon)

joint space

flexor digitorum longus m (tendon)

metatarsal 5

medial plantar n

peroneus longus m (tendon) and sheath

quadratus plantae (flexor accessorius) m

flexor digiti minimi m

flexor digitorum brevis m

abductor digiti minimi m

plantar aponeurosis

lateral plantar n

lateral plantar a

Cahill

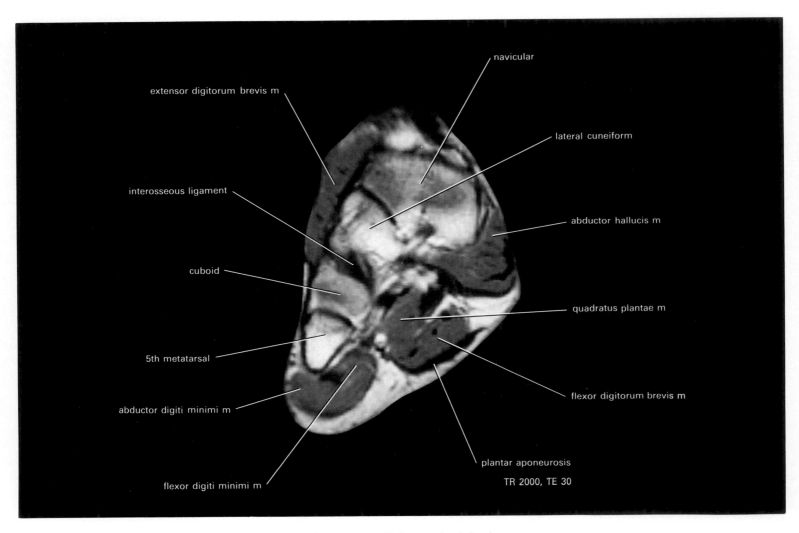

navicular

extensor digitorum brevis m

lateral cuneiform

interosseous ligament

abductor hallucis m

cuboid

quadratus plantae m

5th metatarsal

abductor digiti minimi m

flexor digitorum brevis m

plantar aponeurosis

flexor digiti minimi m

TR 2000, TE 30

Section 4F from behind.

deep peroneal n

extensor hallucis longus m (tendon)

dorsalis pedis a

intermediate cuneiform

medial cuneiform

extensor hallucis brevis m

extensor digitorum longus m (tendon)

great saphenous v

lateral cuneiform

tibialis anterior m (tendon)

peroneus tertius m (tendon)

plantar tarsometatarsal ligaments

metatarsal 2

peroneus longus m (tendon)

extensor digitorum brevis m

metatarsal 1

metatarsal 3

abductor hallucis m

metatarsal 4

plantar aponeurosis

perforating a

flexor hallucis longus m (tendon)

metatarsal 5

medial plantar n and a

abductor digiti minimi m

flexor digitorum longus and quadratus plantae mm

flexor digiti minimi brevis m

flexor digitorum brevis m

third plantar interosseous m

plantar arch

oblique head of adductor hallucis m

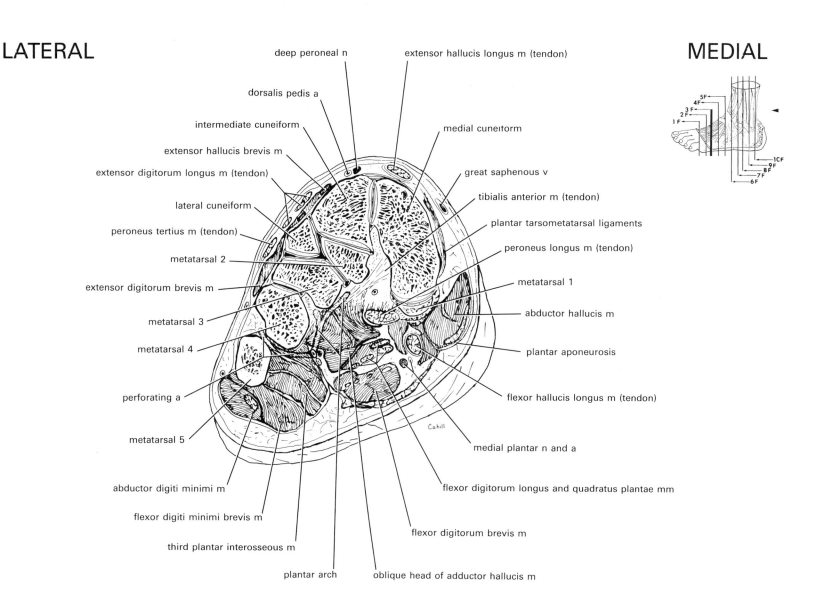

Cahill

peroneus longus tendon

medial cunieform

intermediate cunieform

abductor hallucis m

3rd metatarsal

flexor hallucis longus tendon

4th metatarsal

5th metatarsal

plantar aponeurosis

flexor digitorum brevis m

TR 450, TE 20

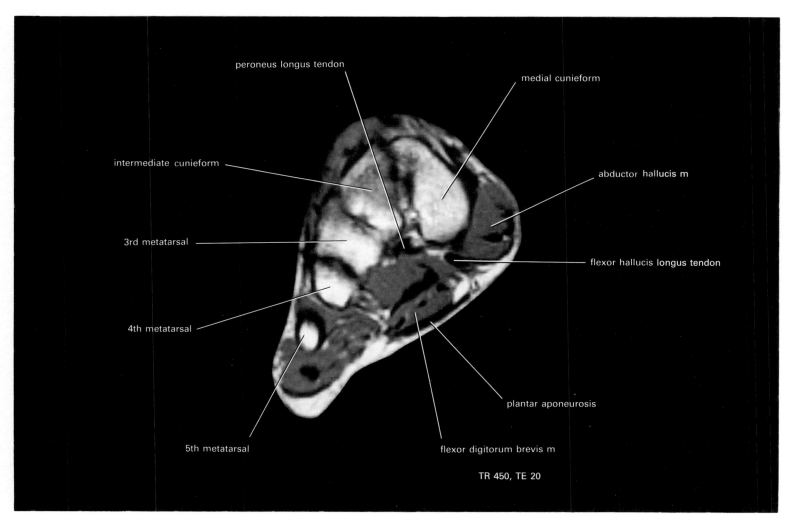

Section 3F from behind.

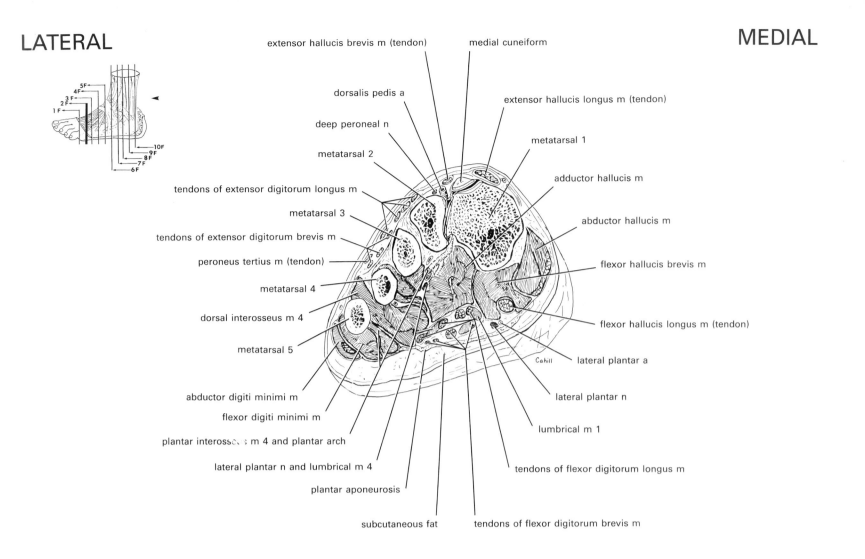

extensor hallucis brevis m (tendon)

medial cuneiform

dorsalis pedis a

extensor hallucis longus m (tendon)

deep peroneal n

metatarsal 1

metatarsal 2

adductor hallucis m

tendons of extensor digitorum longus m

metatarsal 3

abductor hallucis m

tendons of extensor digitorum brevis m

peroneus tertius m (tendon)

flexor hallucis brevis m

metatarsal 4

dorsal interosseus m 4

flexor hallucis longus m (tendon)

metatarsal 5

Cahill

lateral plantar a

abductor digiti minimi m

lateral plantar n

flexor digiti minimi m

lumbrical m 1

plantar interosseus m 4 and plantar arch

lateral plantar n and lumbrical m 4

tendons of flexor digitorum longus m

plantar aponeurosis

subcutaneous fat

tendons of flexor digitorum brevis m

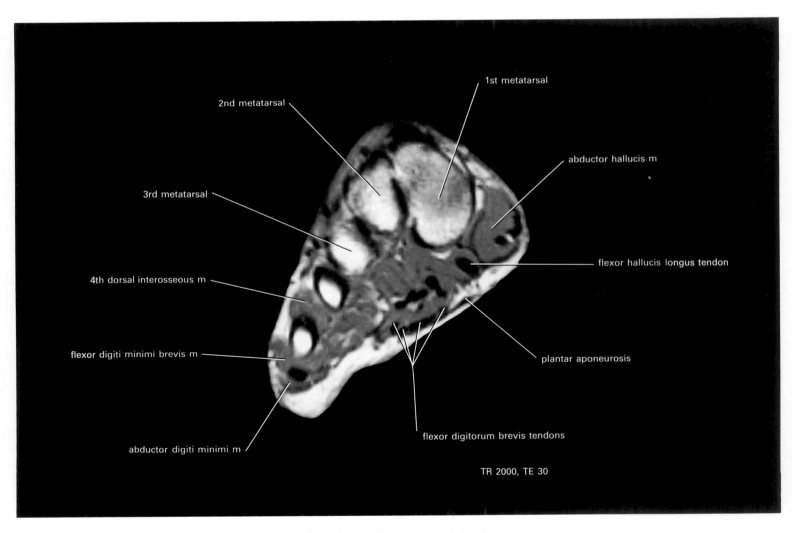

1st metatarsal

2nd metatarsal

abductor hallucis m

3rd metatarsal

flexor hallucis longus tendon

4th dorsal interosseous m

flexor digiti minimi brevis m

plantar aponeurosis

abductor digiti minimi m

flexor digitorum brevis tendons

TR 2000, TE 30

Section 2F from behind.

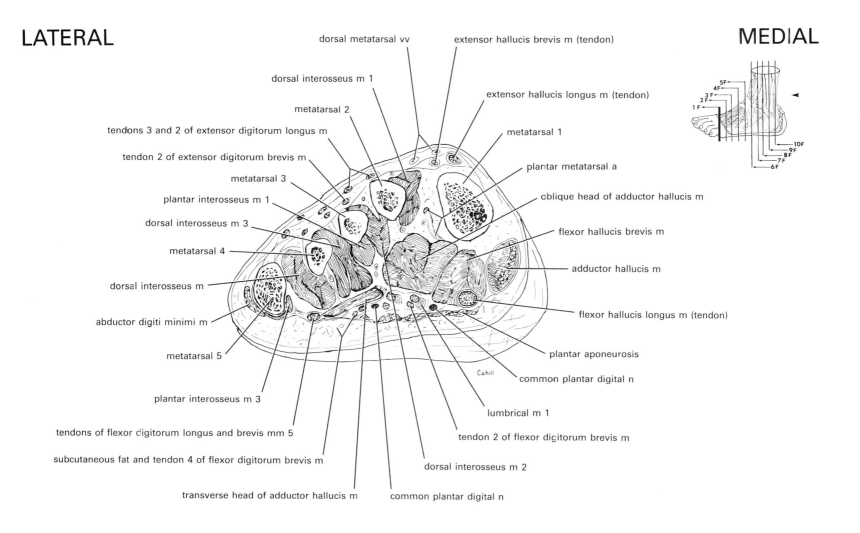

dorsal metatarsal vv

extensor hallucis brevis m (tendon)

dorsal interosseus m 1

extensor hallucis longus m (tendon)

metatarsal 2

tendons 3 and 2 of extensor digitorum longus m

metatarsal 1

tendon 2 of extensor digitorum brevis m

plantar metatarsal a

metatarsal 3

oblique head of adductor hallucis m

plantar interosseus m 1

dorsal interosseus m 3

flexor hallucis brevis m

metatarsal 4

adductor hallucis m

dorsal interosseus m

flexor hallucis longus m (tendon)

abductor digiti minimi m

metatarsal 5

plantar aponeurosis

common plantar digital n

plantar interosseus m 3

lumbrical m 1

tendons of flexor digitorum longus and brevis mm 5

tendon 2 of flexor digitorum brevis m

subcutaneous fat and tendon 4 of flexor digitorum brevis m

dorsal interosseus m 2

transverse head of adductor hallucis m

common plantar digital n

Cahill

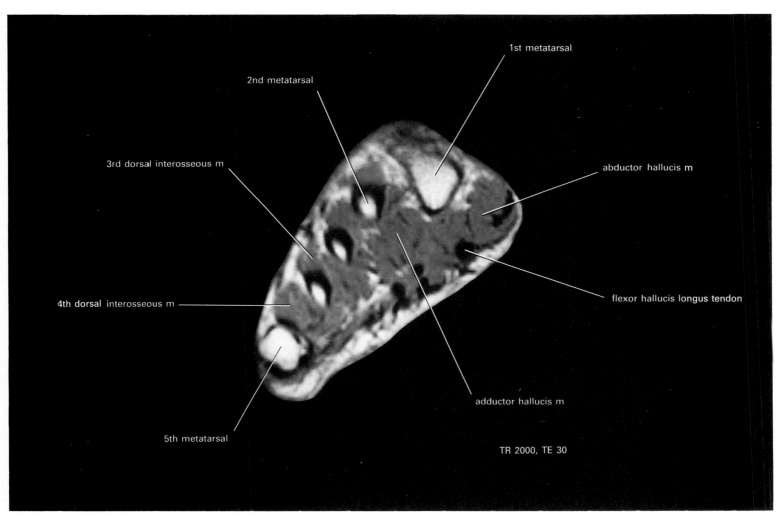

1st metatarsal

2nd metatarsal

3rd dorsal interosseous m

abductor hallucis m

4th dorsal interosseous m

flexor hallucis longus tendon

adductor hallucis m

5th metatarsal

TR 2000, TE 30

Section 1F from behind.

The Left Knee in Sagittal Planes

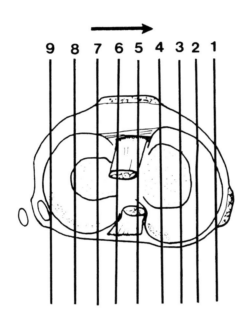

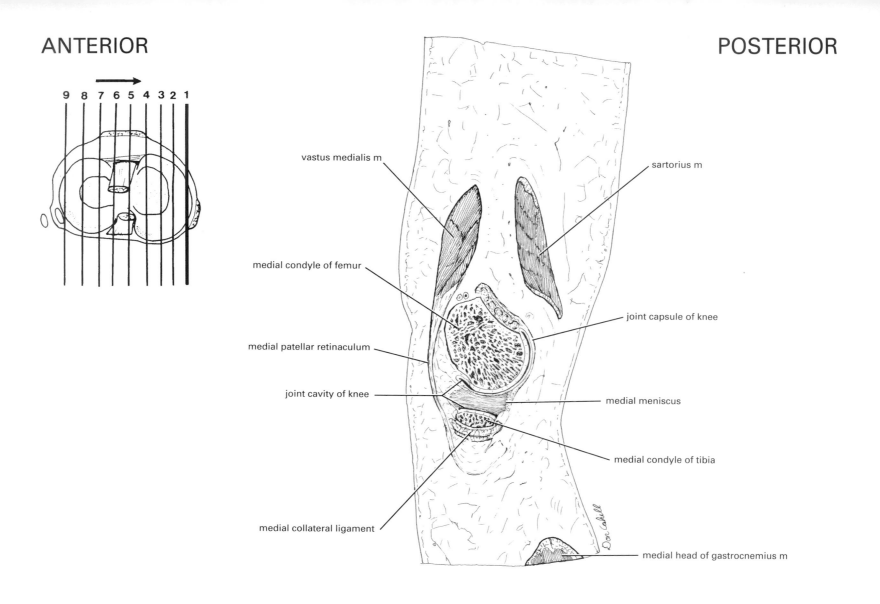

9 8 7 6 5 4 3 2 1

vastus medialis m

sartorius m

medial condyle of femur

joint capsule of knee

medial patellar retinaculum

joint cavity of knee

medial meniscus

medial condyle of tibia

medial collateral ligament

medial head of gastrocnemius m

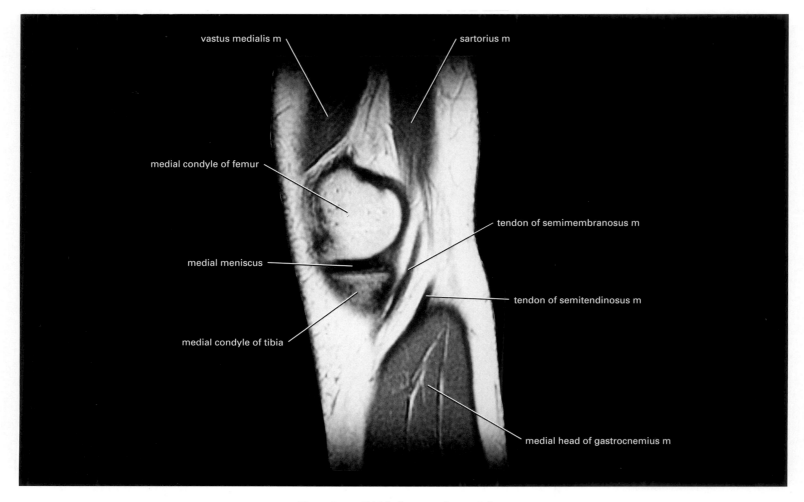

vastus medialis m

sartorius m

medial condyle of femur

tendon of semimembranosus m

medial meniscus

tendon of semitendinosus m

medial condyle of tibia

medial head of gastrocnemius m

Section SK1 from the side.

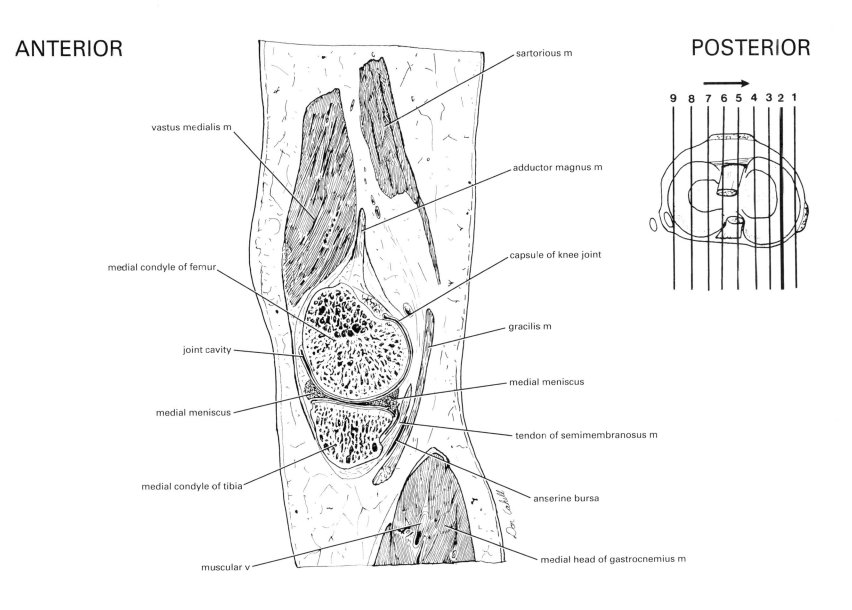

sartorious m

vastus medialis m

adductor magnus m

medial condyle of femur

capsule of knee joint

gracilis m

joint cavity

medial meniscus

medial meniscus

tendon of semimembranosus m

medial condyle of tibia

anserine bursa

muscular v

medial head of gastrocnemius m

9 8 7 6 5 4 3 2 1

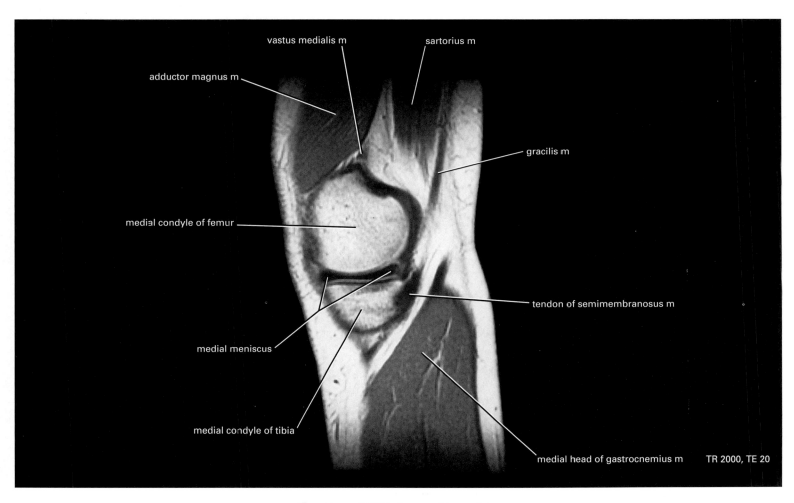

vastus medialis m

sartorius m

adductor magnus m

gracilis m

medial condyle of femur

tendon of semimembranosus m

medial meniscus

medial condyle of tibia

medial head of gastrocnemius m

TR 2000, TE 20

Section SK2 from the side.

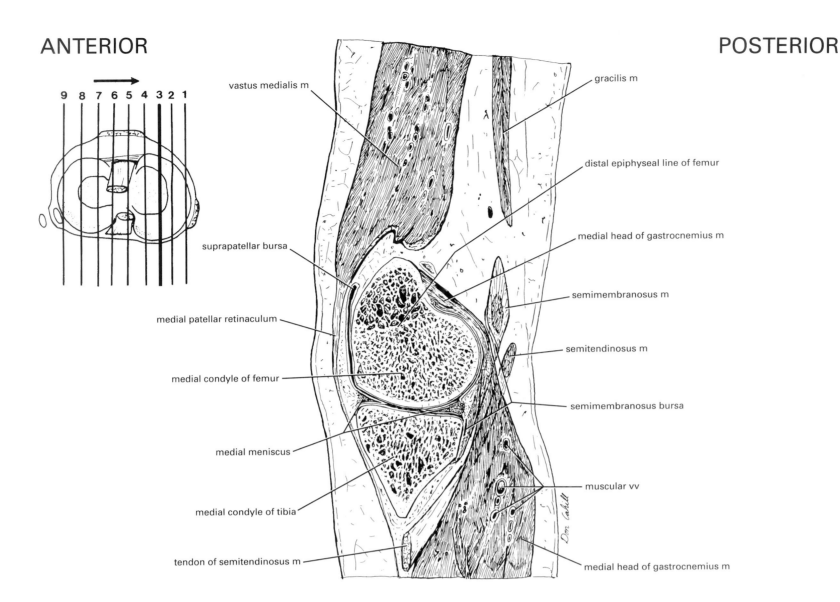

vastus medialis m

gracilis m

distal epiphyseal line of femur

medial head of gastrocnemius m

suprapatellar bursa

semimembranosus m

medial patellar retinaculum

semitendinosus m

medial condyle of femur

semimembranosus bursa

medial meniscus

muscular vv

medial condyle of tibia

tendon of semitendinosus m

medial head of gastrocnemius m

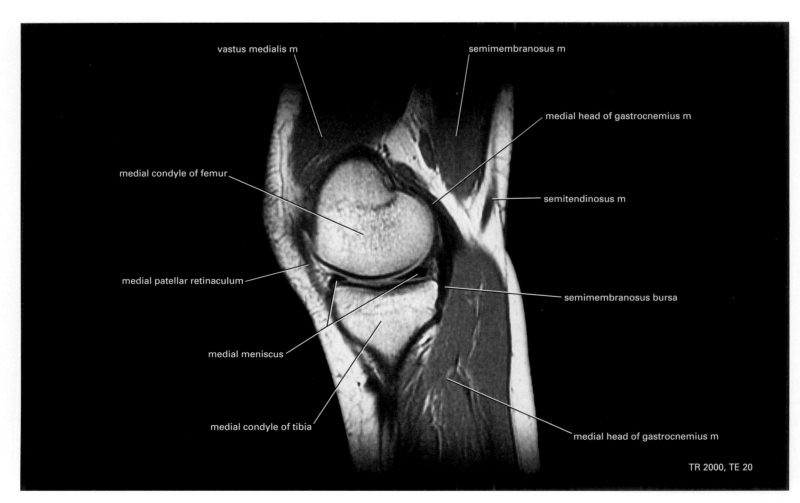

vastus medialis m

semimembranosus m

medial head of gastrocnemius m

medial condyle of femur

semitendinosus m

medial patellar retinaculum

semimembranosus bursa

medial meniscus

medial condyle of tibia

medial head of gastrocnemius m

TR 2000, TE 20

Section SK3 from the side.

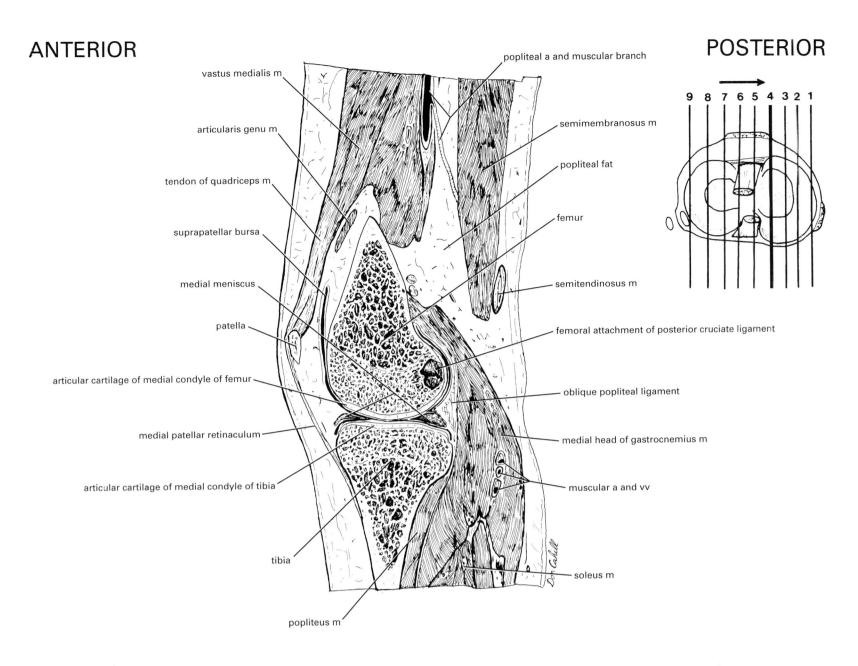

vastus medialis m

popliteal a and muscular branch

articularis genu m

semimembranosus m

tendon of quadriceps m

popliteal fat

suprapatellar bursa

femur

medial meniscus

semitendinosus m

patella

femoral attachment of posterior cruciate ligament

articular cartilage of medial condyle of femur

oblique popliteal ligament

medial patellar retinaculum

medial head of gastrocnemius m

articular cartilage of medial condyle of tibia

muscular a and vv

tibia

soleus m

popliteus m

9 8 7 6 5 4 3 2 1

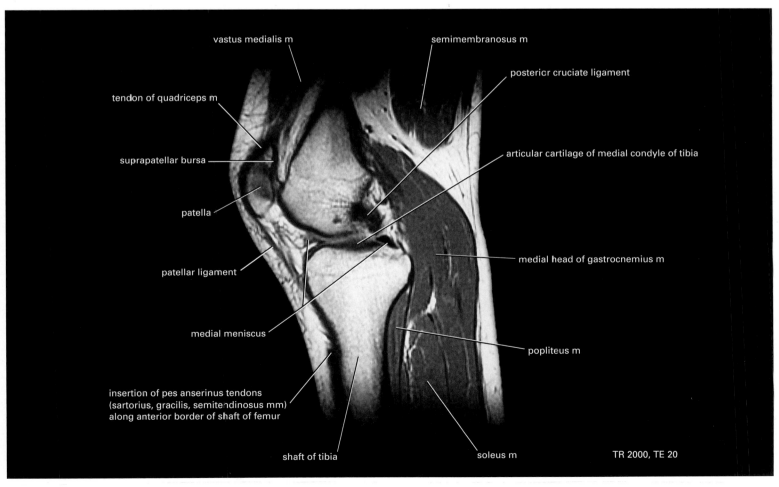

vastus medialis m

semimembranosus m

posterior cruciate ligament

tendon of quadriceps m

suprapatellar bursa

articular cartilage of medial condyle of tibia

patella

medial head of gastrocnemius m

patellar ligament

medial meniscus

popliteus m

insertion of pes anserinus tendons
(sartorius, gracilis, semitendinosus mm)
along anterior border of shaft of femur

shaft of tibia

soleus m

TR 2000, TE 20

Section SK4 from the side.

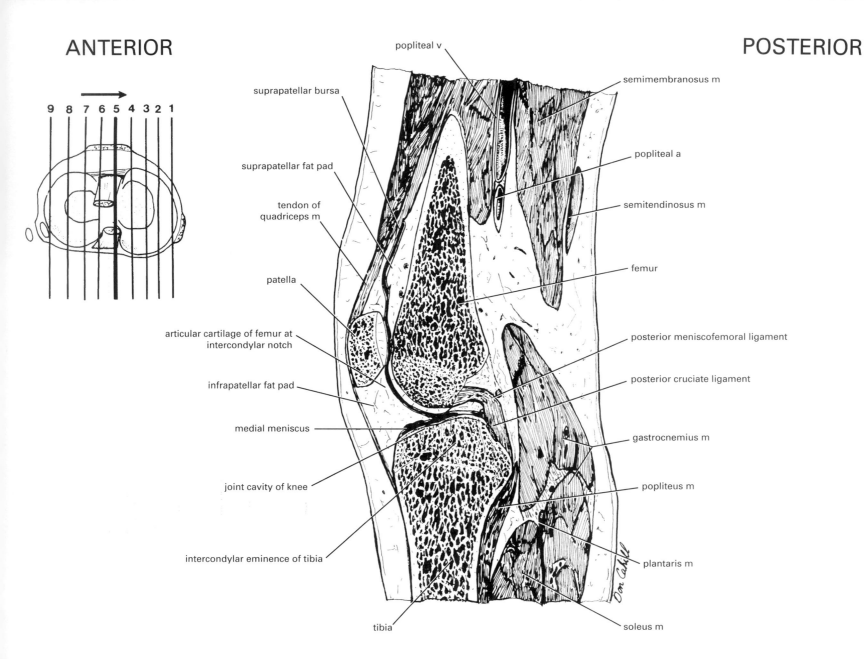

9 8 7 6 5 4 3 2 1

popliteal v

suprapatellar bursa

semimembranosus m

suprapatellar fat pad

popliteal a

tendon of
quadriceps m

semitendinosus m

patella

femur

articular cartilage of femur at
intercondylar notch

posterior meniscofemoral ligament

infrapatellar fat pad

posterior cruciate ligament

medial meniscus

gastrocnemius m

joint cavity of knee

popliteus m

intercondylar eminence of tibia

plantaris m

tibia

soleus m

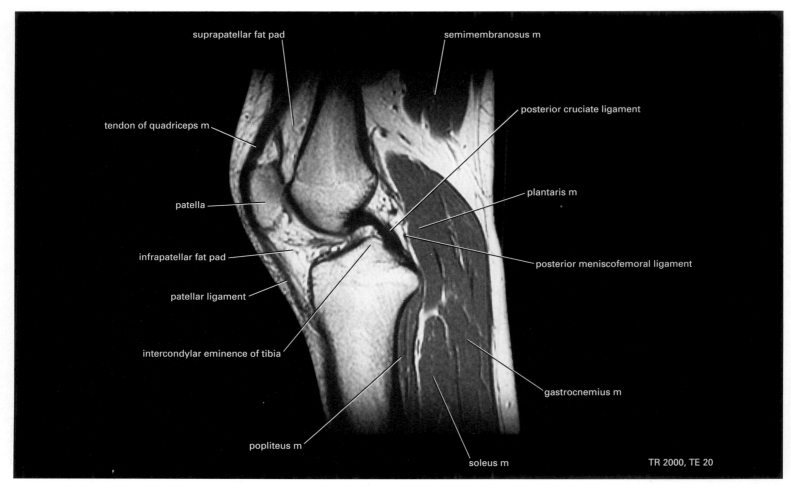

suprapatellar fat pad

semimembranosus m

tendon of quadriceps m

posterior cruciate ligament

patella

plantaris m

infrapatellar fat pad

posterior meniscofemoral ligament

patellar ligament

intercondylar eminence of tibia

gastrocnemius m

popliteus m

soleus m

TR 2000, TE 20

Section SK5 from the side.

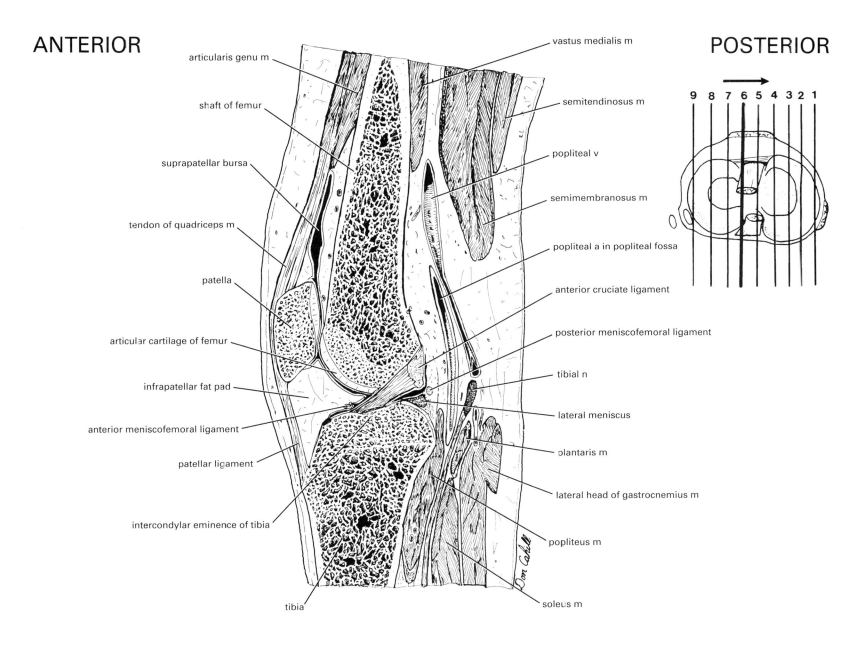

articularis genu m

shaft of femur

suprapatellar bursa

tendon of quadriceps m

patella

articular cartilage of femur

infrapatellar fat pad

anterior meniscofemoral ligament

patellar ligament

intercondylar eminence of tibia

tibia

vastus medialis m

semitendinosus m

popliteal v

semimembranosus m

popliteal a in popliteal fossa

anterior cruciate ligament

posterior meniscofemoral ligament

tibial n

lateral meniscus

plantaris m

lateral head of gastrocnemius m

popliteus m

soleus m

9 8 7 6 5 4 3 2 1

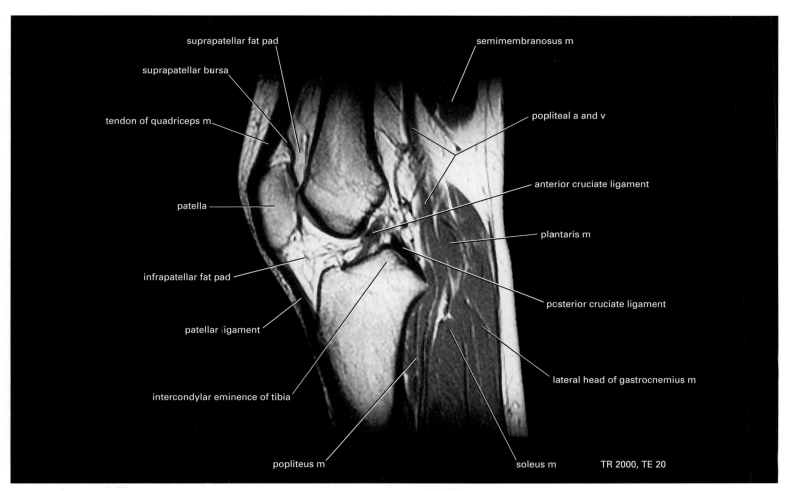

suprapatellar fat pad

suprapatellar bursa

tendon of quadriceps m

patella

infrapatellar fat pad

patellar ligament

intercondylar eminence of tibia

popliteus m

semimembranosus m

popliteal a and v

anterior cruciate ligament

plantaris m

posterior cruciate ligament

lateral head of gastrocnemius m

soleus m

TR 2000, TE 20

Section SK6 from the side.

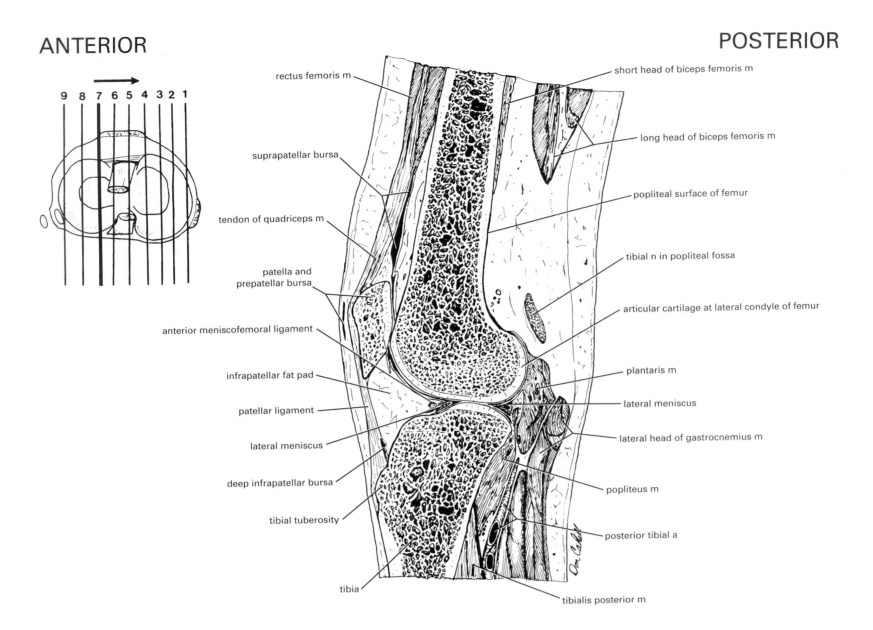

rectus femoris m

short head of biceps femoris m

suprapatellar bursa

long head of biceps femoris m

tendon of quadriceps m

popliteal surface of femur

patella and
prepatellar bursa

tibial n in popliteal fossa

anterior meniscofemoral ligament

articular cartilage at lateral condyle of femur

infrapatellar fat pad

plantaris m

patellar ligament

lateral meniscus

lateral meniscus

lateral head of gastrocnemius m

deep infrapatellar bursa

popliteus m

tibial tuberosity

posterior tibial a

tibia

tibialis posterior m

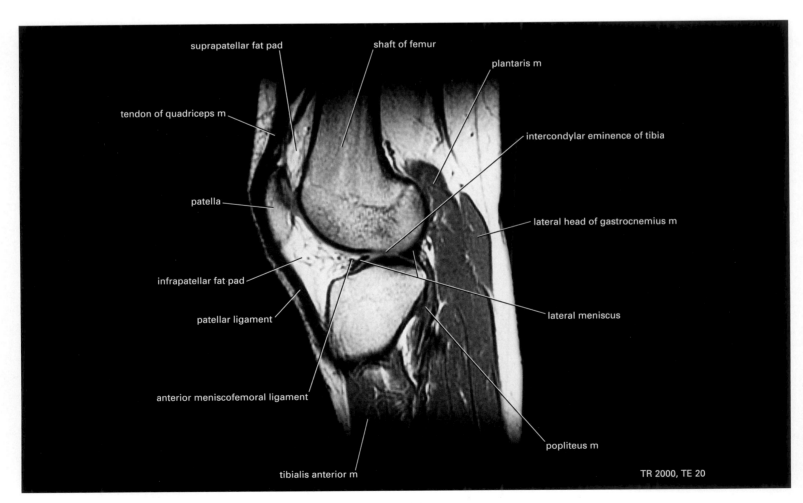

suprapatellar fat pad

shaft of femur

plantaris m

tendon of quadriceps m

intercondylar eminence of tibia

patella

lateral head of gastrocnemius m

infrapatellar fat pad

patellar ligament

lateral meniscus

anterior meniscofemoral ligament

popliteus m

tibialis anterior m

TR 2000, TE 20

Section SK7 from the side.

ANTERIOR

POSTERIOR

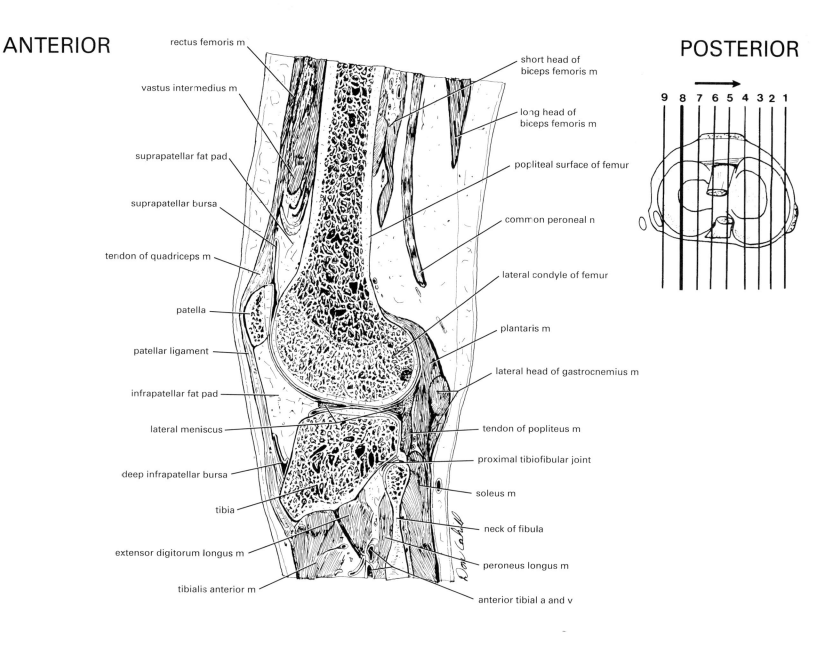

rectus femoris m

vastus intermedius m

suprapatellar fat pad

suprapatellar bursa

tendon of quadriceps m

patella

patellar ligament

infrapatellar fat pad

lateral meniscus

deep infrapatellar bursa

tibia

extensor digitorum longus m

tibialis anterior m

short head of biceps femoris m

long head of biceps femoris m

popliteal surface of femur

common peroneal n

lateral condyle of femur

plantaris m

lateral head of gastrocnemius m

tendon of popliteus m

proximal tibiofibular joint

soleus m

neck of fibula

peroneus longus m

anterior tibial a and v

9 8 7 6 5 4 3 2 1

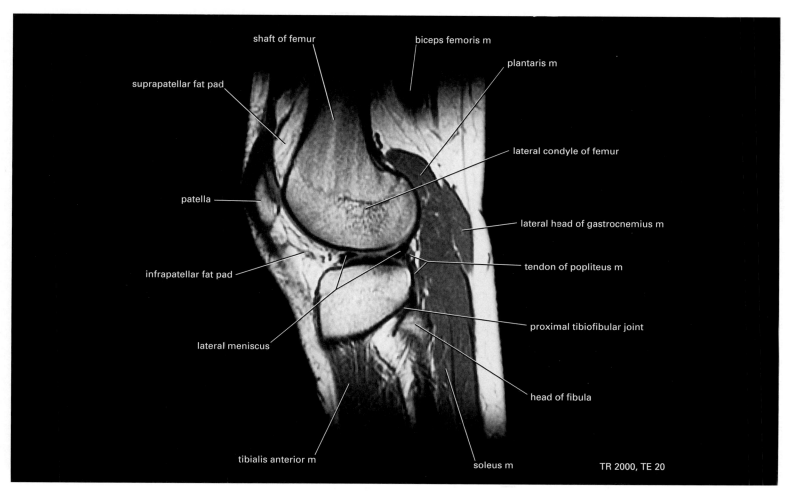

shaft of femur

suprapatellar fat pad

patella

infrapatellar fat pad

lateral meniscus

tibialis anterior m

biceps femoris m

plantaris m

lateral condyle of femur

lateral head of gastrocnemius m

tendon of popliteus m

proximal tibiofibular joint

head of fibula

soleus m

TR 2000, TE 20

Section SK8 from the side.

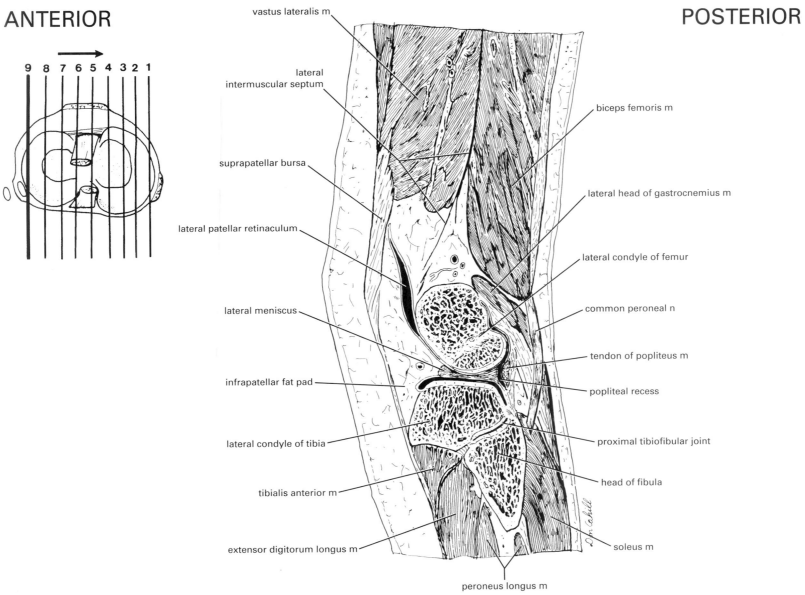

vastus lateralis m

lateral intermuscular septum

suprapatellar bursa

lateral patellar retinaculum

lateral meniscus

infrapatellar fat pad

lateral condyle of tibia

tibialis anterior m

extensor digitorum longus m

peroneus longus m

biceps femoris m

lateral head of gastrocnemius m

lateral condyle of femur

common peroneal n

tendon of popliteus m

popliteal recess

proximal tibiofibular joint

head of fibula

soleus m

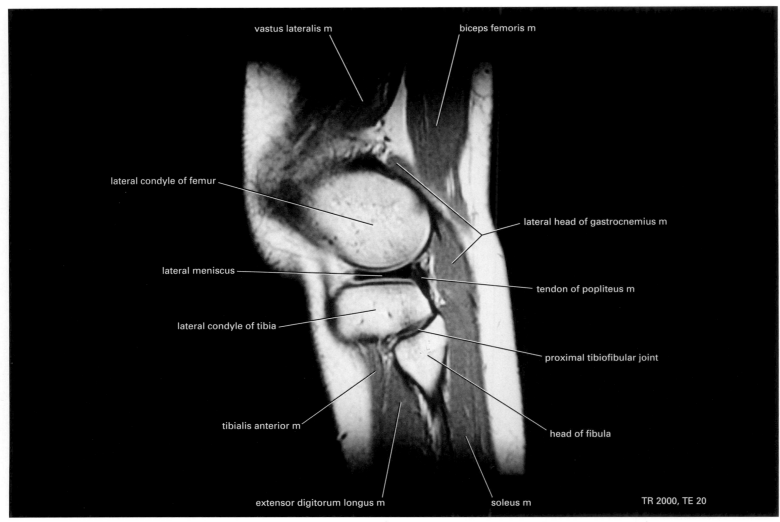

vastus lateralis m

biceps femoris m

lateral condyle of femur

lateral head of gastrocnemius m

lateral meniscus

tendon of popliteus m

lateral condyle of tibia

proximal tibiofibular joint

tibialis anterior m

head of fibula

extensor digitorum longus m

soleus m

TR 2000, TE 20

Section SK9 from the side.

The Left Knee in Coronal Planes

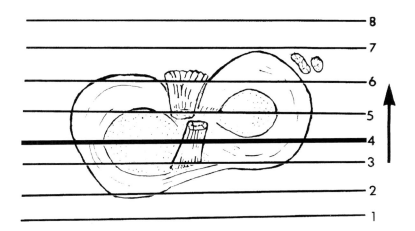

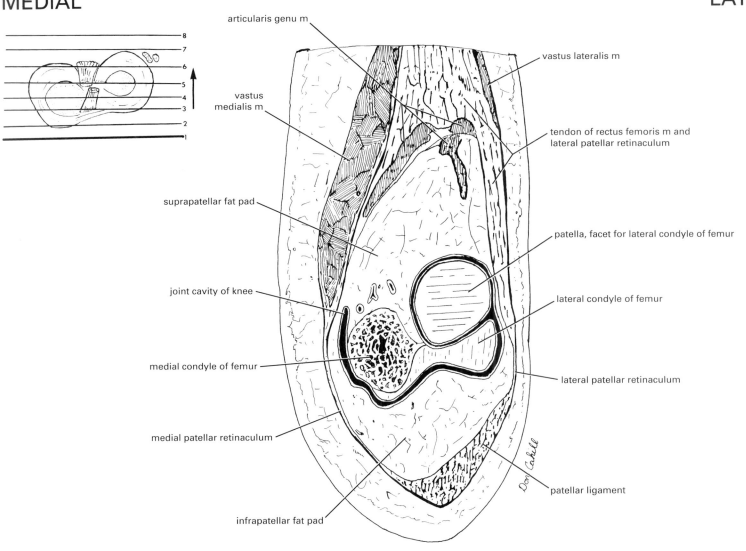

articularis genu m

vastus lateralis m

vastus medialis m

tendon of rectus femoris m and lateral patellar retinaculum

suprapatellar fat pad

patella, facet for lateral condyle of femur

joint cavity of knee

lateral condyle of femur

medial condyle of femur

lateral patellar retinaculum

medial patellar retinaculum

patellar ligament

infrapatellar fat pad

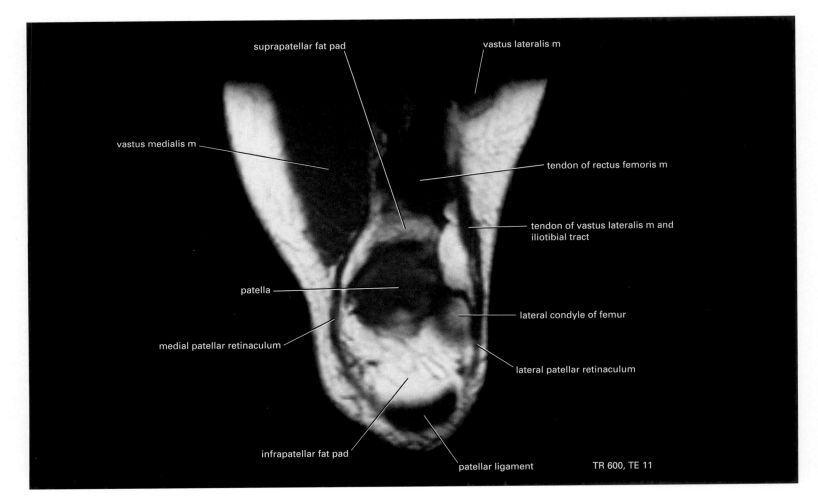

suprapatellar fat pad

vastus lateralis m

vastus medialis m

tendon of rectus femoris m

tendon of vastus lateralis m and iliotibial tract

patella

lateral condyle of femur

medial patellar retinaculum

lateral patellar retinaculum

infrapatellar fat pad

patellar ligament

TR 600, TE 11

Section CK1 from the front.

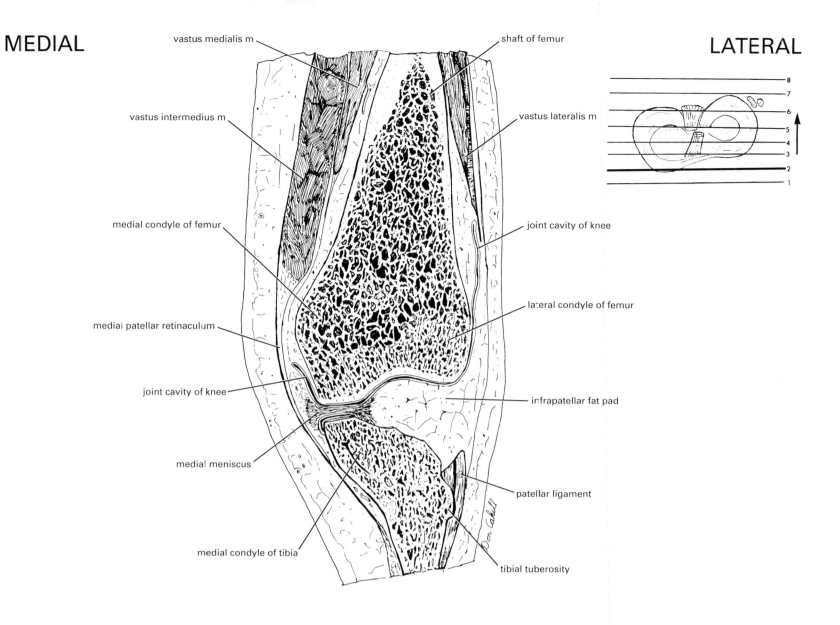

- vastus medialis m
- shaft of femur
- vastus intermedius m
- vastus lateralis m
- medial condyle of femur
- joint cavity of knee
- lateral condyle of femur
- medial patellar retinaculum
- joint cavity of knee
- infrapatellar fat pad
- medial meniscus
- patellar ligament
- medial condyle of tibia
- tibial tuberosity

Don Cahill

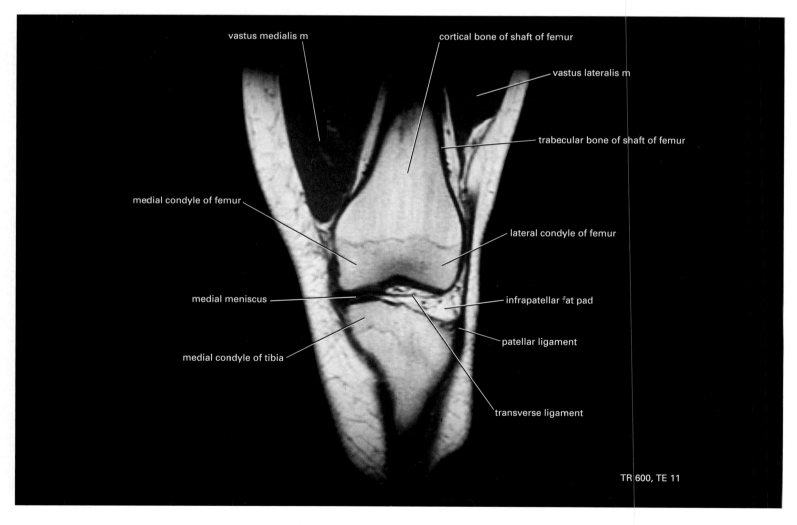

- vastus medialis m
- cortical bone of shaft of femur
- vastus lateralis m
- trabecular bone of shaft of femur
- medial condyle of femur
- lateral condyle of femur
- medial meniscus
- infrapatellar fat pad
- medial condyle of tibia
- patellar ligament
- transverse ligament

TR 600, TE 11

Section CK2 from the front.

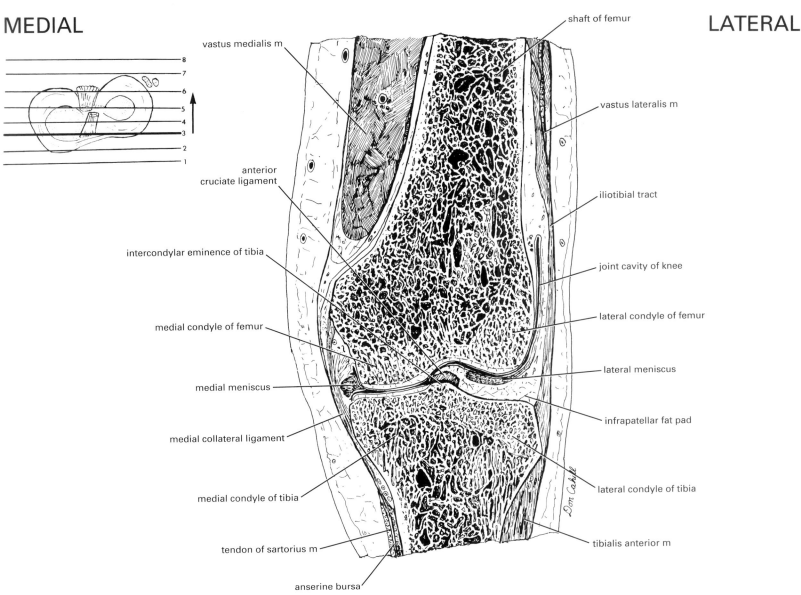

- shaft of femur
- vastus medialis m
- vastus lateralis m
- anterior cruciate ligament
- iliotibial tract
- intercondylar eminence of tibia
- joint cavity of knee
- medial condyle of femur
- lateral condyle of femur
- medial meniscus
- lateral meniscus
- medial collateral ligament
- infrapatellar fat pad
- medial condyle of tibia
- lateral condyle of tibia
- tendon of sartorius m
- tibialis anterior m
- anserine bursa

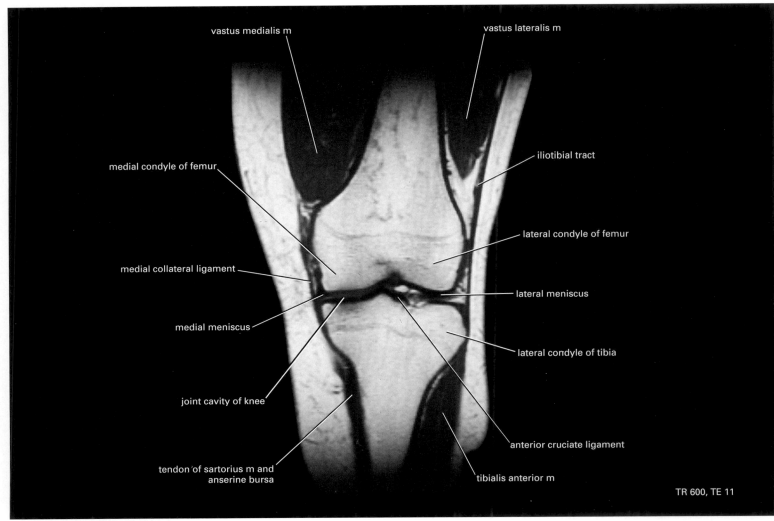

- vastus medialis m
- vastus lateralis m
- medial condyle of femur
- iliotibial tract
- lateral condyle of femur
- medial collateral ligament
- lateral meniscus
- medial meniscus
- lateral condyle of tibia
- joint cavity of knee
- anterior cruciate ligament
- tendon of sartorius m and anserine bursa
- tibialis anterior m

TR 600, TE 11

Section CK3 from the front.

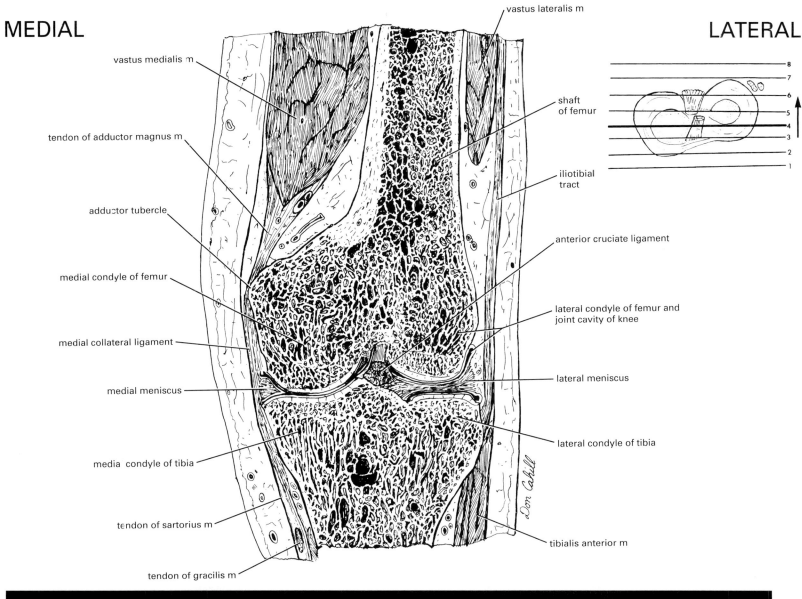

vastus lateralis m

vastus medialis m

tendon of adductor magnus m

shaft
of femur

adductor tubercle

iliotibial
tract

medial condyle of femur

anterior cruciate ligament

medial collateral ligament

lateral condyle of femur and
joint cavity of knee

medial meniscus

lateral meniscus

media condyle of tibia

lateral condyle of tibia

tendon of sartorius m

tibialis anterior m

tendon of gracilis m

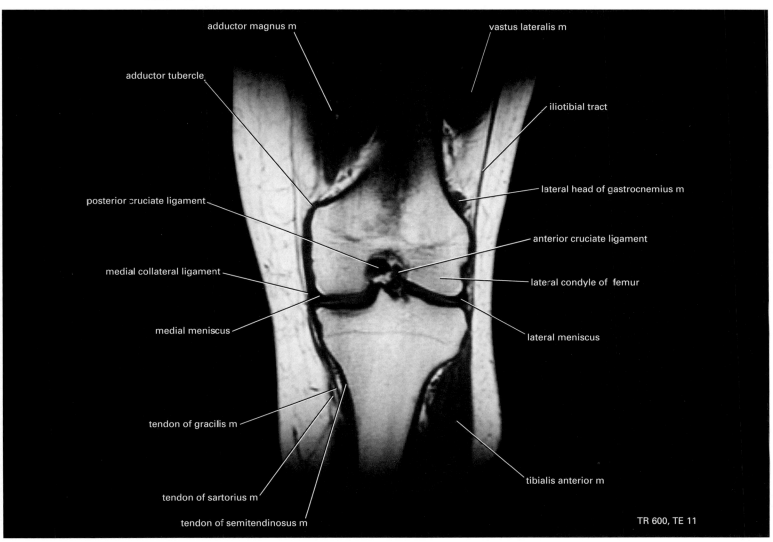

adductor magnus m

vastus lateralis m

adductor tubercle

iliotibial tract

posterior cruciate ligament

lateral head of gastrocnemius m

medial collateral ligament

anterior cruciate ligament

medial meniscus

lateral condyle of femur

lateral meniscus

tendon of gracilis m

tibialis anterior m

tendon of sartorius m

tendon of semitendinosus m

TR 600, TE 11

Section CK4 from the front.

MEDIAL

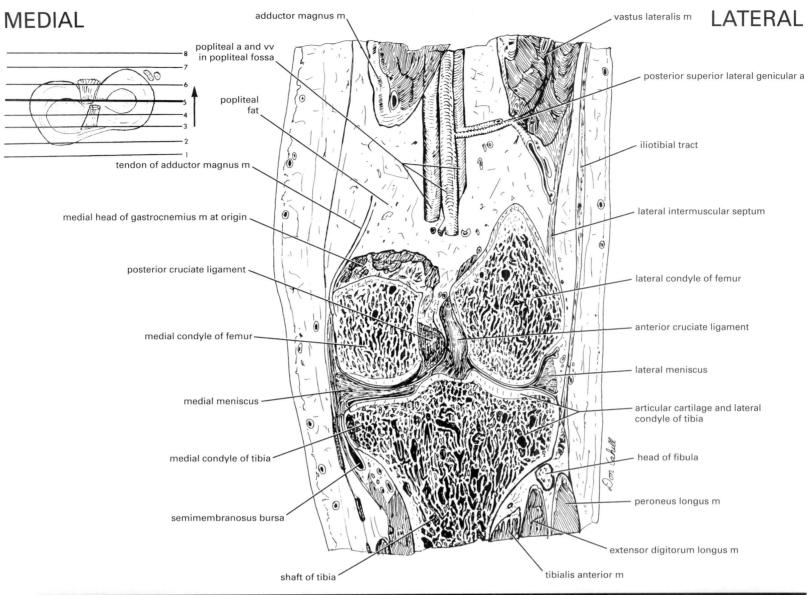

LATERAL

- adductor magnus m
- popliteal a and vv in popliteal fossa
- popliteal fat
- tendon of adductor magnus m
- medial head of gastrocnemius m at origin
- posterior cruciate ligament
- medial condyle of femur
- medial meniscus
- medial condyle of tibia
- semimembranosus bursa
- shaft of tibia

- vastus lateralis m
- posterior superior lateral genicular a
- iliotibial tract
- lateral intermuscular septum
- lateral condyle of femur
- anterior cruciate ligament
- lateral meniscus
- articular cartilage and lateral condyle of tibia
- head of fibula
- peroneus longus m
- extensor digitorum longus m
- tibialis anterior m

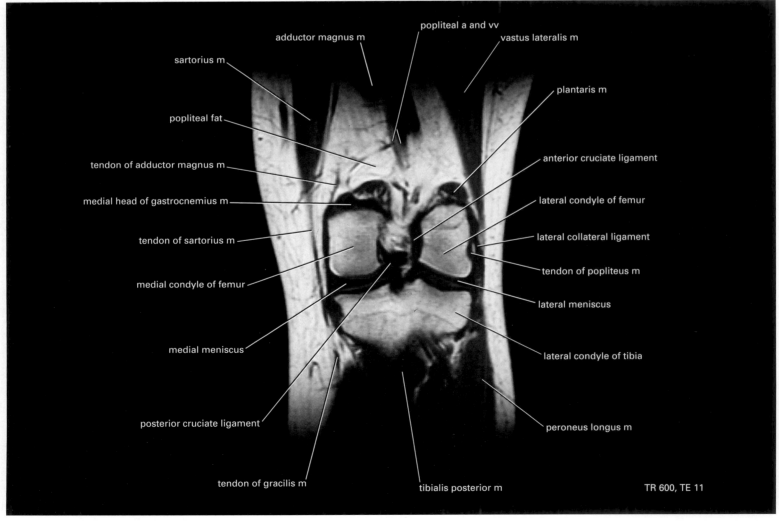

- adductor magnus m
- popliteal a and vv
- vastus lateralis m
- sartorius m
- plantaris m
- popliteal fat
- anterior cruciate ligament
- tendon of adductor magnus m
- lateral condyle of femur
- medial head of gastrocnemius m
- lateral collateral ligament
- tendon of sartorius m
- tendon of popliteus m
- medial condyle of femur
- lateral meniscus
- medial meniscus
- lateral condyle of tibia
- posterior cruciate ligament
- peroneus longus m
- tendon of gracilis m
- tibialis posterior m

TR 600, TE 11

Section CK5 from the front.

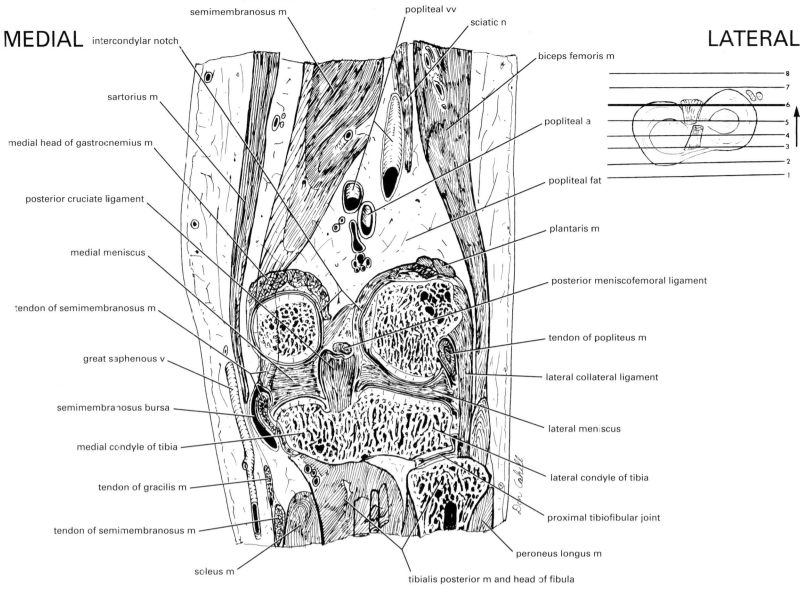

MEDIAL   intercondylar notch
LATERAL

- semimembranosus m
- popliteal vv
- sciatic n
- sartorius m
- biceps femoris m
- medial head of gastrocnemius m
- popliteal a
- posterior cruciate ligament
- popliteal fat
- medial meniscus
- plantaris m
- tendon of semimembranosus m
- posterior meniscofemoral ligament
- great saphenous v
- tendon of popliteus m
- semimembranosus bursa
- lateral collateral ligament
- medial condyle of tibia
- lateral meniscus
- tendon of gracilis m
- lateral condyle of tibia
- tendon of semimembranosus m
- proximal tibiofibular joint
- soleus m
- peroneus longus m
- tibialis posterior m and head of fibula

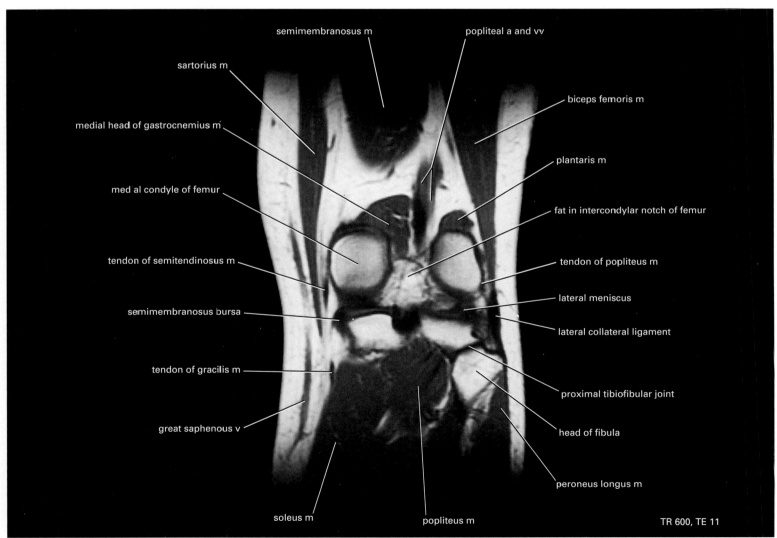

- semimembranosus m
- popliteal a and vv
- sartorius m
- biceps femoris m
- medial head of gastrocnemius m
- plantaris m
- medial condyle of femur
- fat in intercondylar notch of femur
- tendon of semitendinosus m
- tendon of popliteus m
- lateral meniscus
- semimembranosus bursa
- lateral collateral ligament
- tendon of gracilis m
- proximal tibiofibular joint
- great saphenous v
- head of fibula
- peroneus longus m
- soleus m
- popliteus m

TR 600, TE 11

Section CK6 from the front.

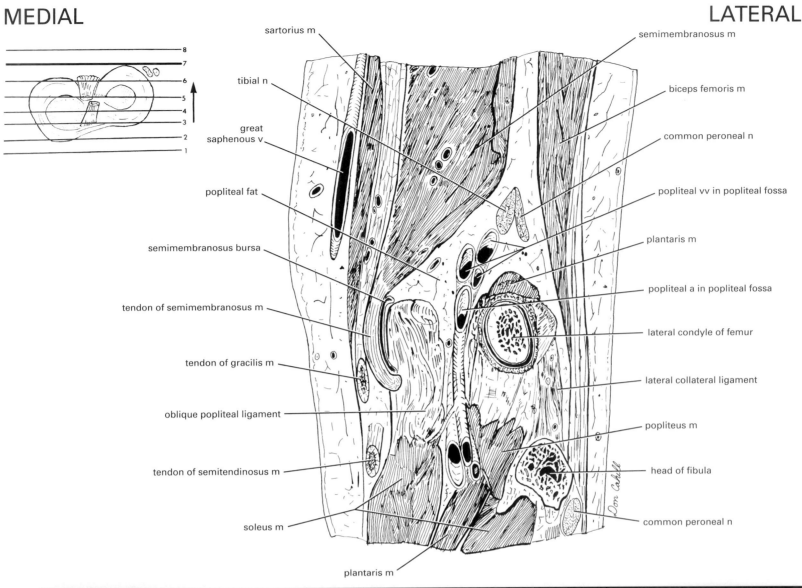

sartorius m

tibial n

great
saphenous v

popliteal fat

semimembranosus bursa

tendon of semimembranosus m

tendon of gracilis m

oblique popliteal ligament

tendon of semitendinosus m

soleus m

plantaris m

semimembranosus m

biceps femoris m

common peroneal n

popliteal vv in popliteal fossa

plantaris m

popliteal a in popliteal fossa

lateral condyle of femur

lateral collateral ligament

popliteus m

head of fibula

common peroneal n

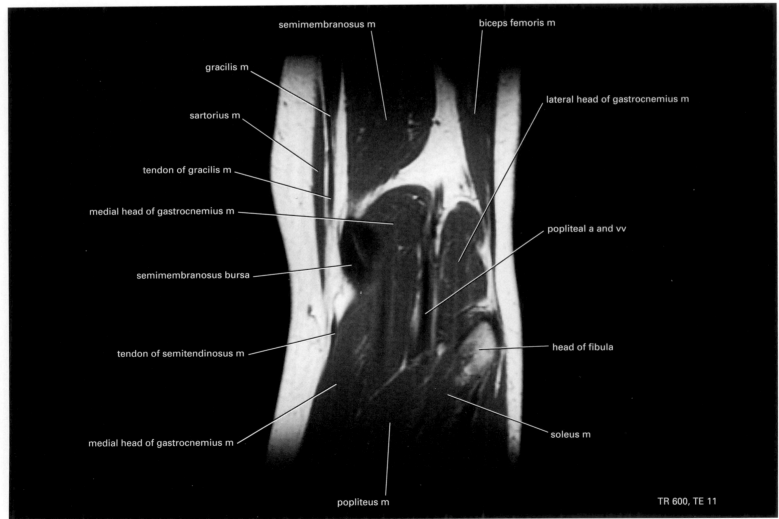

semimembranosus m

biceps femoris m

gracilis m

sartorius m

tendon of gracilis m

medial head of gastrocnemius m

semimembranosus bursa

tendon of semitendinosus m

medial head of gastrocnemius m

lateral head of gastrocnemius m

popliteal a and vv

head of fibula

soleus m

popliteus m

TR 600, TE 11

Section CK7 from the front.

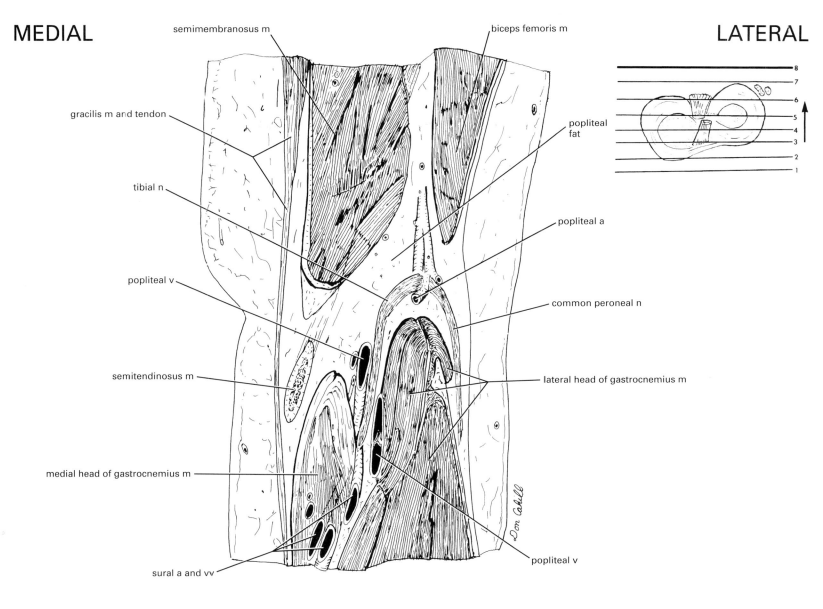

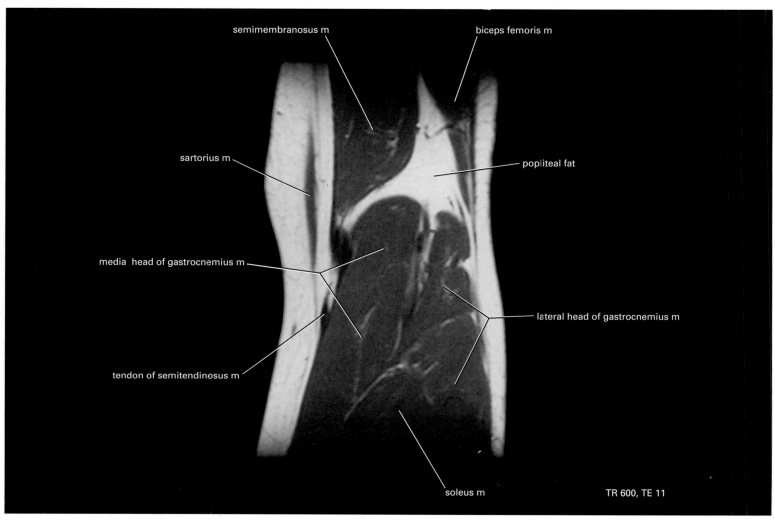

Section CK8 from the front.

The Right Upper Limb With Hand
in Pronation

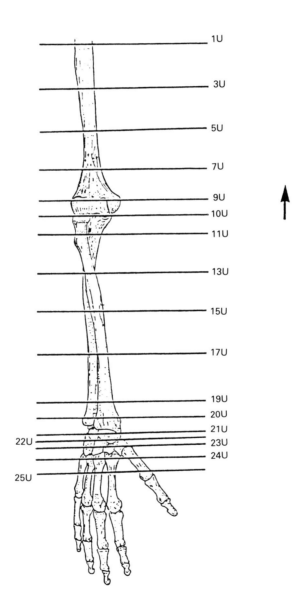

1U

3U

5U

7U

9U
10U
11U

13U

15U

17U

19U
20U
21U
22U
23U
24U

25U

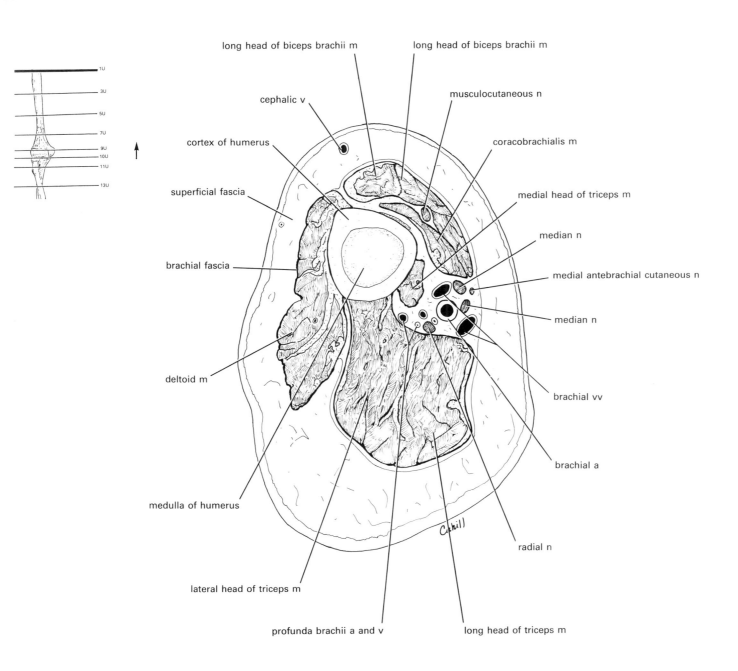

long head of biceps brachii m

long head of biceps brachii m

cephalic v

musculocutaneous n

cortex of humerus

coracobrachialis m

superficial fascia

medial head of triceps m

median n

brachial fascia

medial antebrachial cutaneous n

median n

deltoid m

brachial vv

brachial a

medulla of humerus

Cahill

radial n

lateral head of triceps m

profunda brachii a and v

long head of triceps m

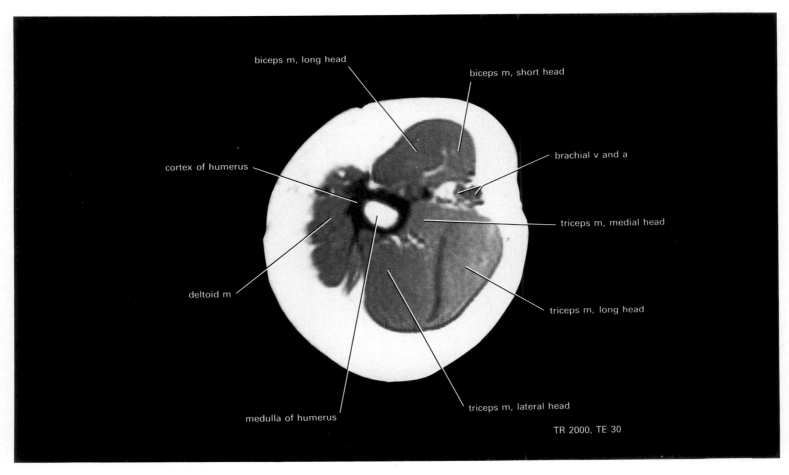

biceps m, long head

biceps m, short head

cortex of humerus

brachial v and a

triceps m, medial head

deltoid m

triceps m, long head

medulla of humerus

triceps m, lateral head

TR 2000, TE 30

Section 1U from below.

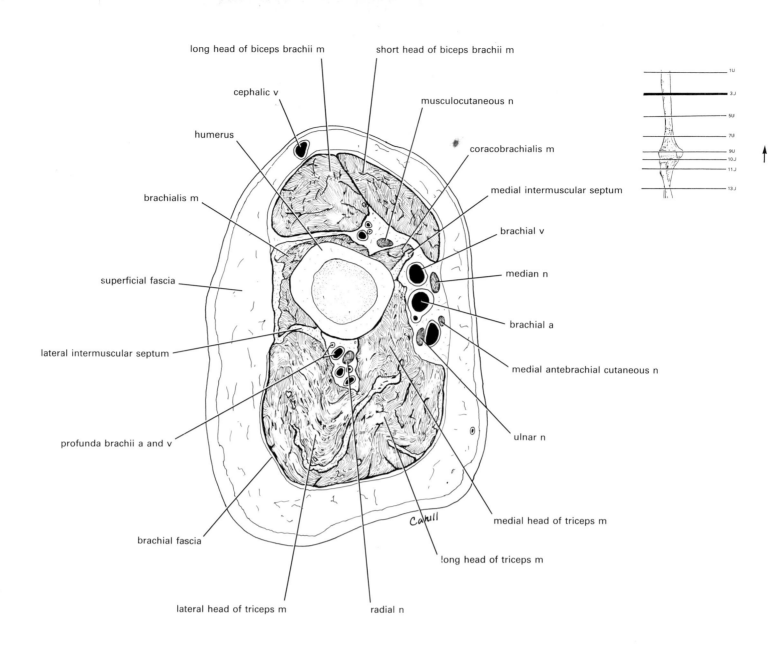

long head of biceps brachii m

short head of biceps brachii m

cephalic v

musculocutaneous n

humerus

coracobrachialis m

brachialis m

medial intermuscular septum

brachial v

superficial fascia

median n

brachial a

lateral intermuscular septum

medial antebrachial cutaneous n

profunda brachii a and v

ulnar n

medial head of triceps m

brachial fascia

long head of triceps m

lateral head of triceps m

radial n

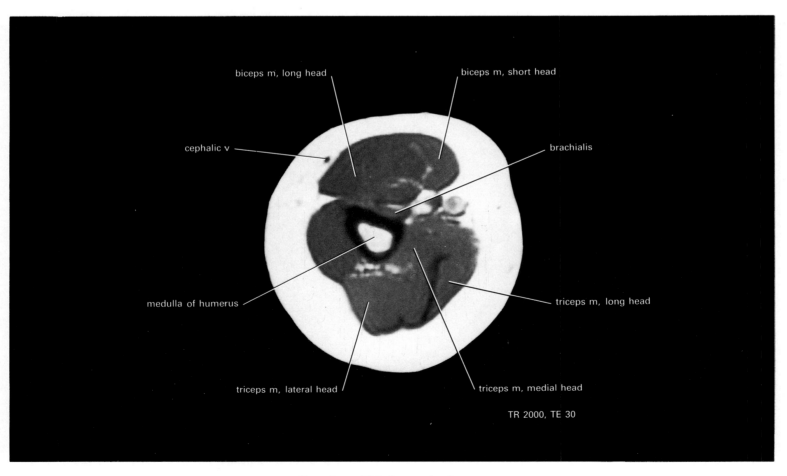

biceps m, long head

biceps m, short head

cephalic v

brachialis

medulla of humerus

triceps m, long head

triceps m, lateral head

triceps m, medial head

TR 2000, TE 30

Section 3U from below.

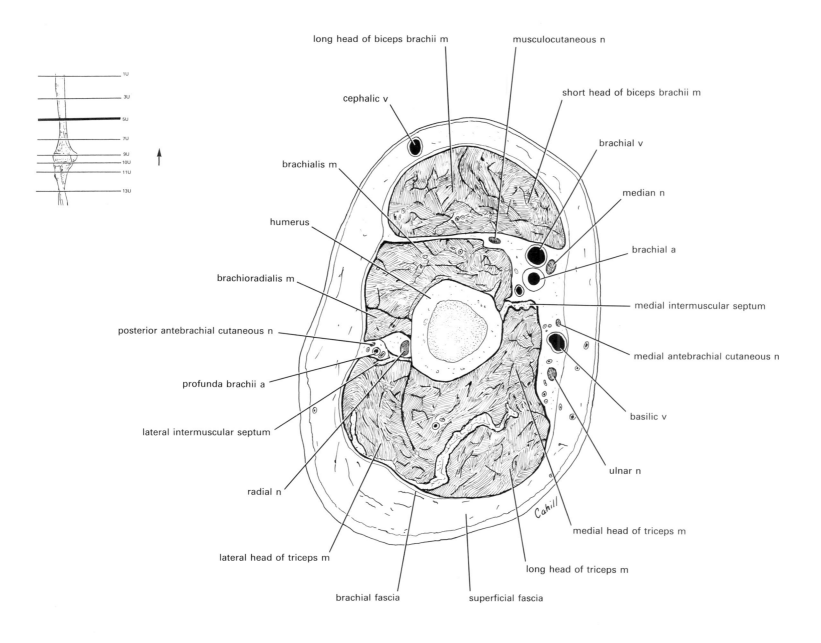

long head of biceps brachii m

musculocutaneous n

cephalic v

short head of biceps brachii m

brachialis m

brachial v

median n

humerus

brachial a

brachioradialis m

medial intermuscular septum

posterior antebrachial cutaneous n

medial antebrachial cutaneous n

profunda brachii a

basilic v

lateral intermuscular septum

ulnar n

radial n

medial head of triceps m

lateral head of triceps m

long head of triceps m

brachial fascia

superficial fascia

Cahill

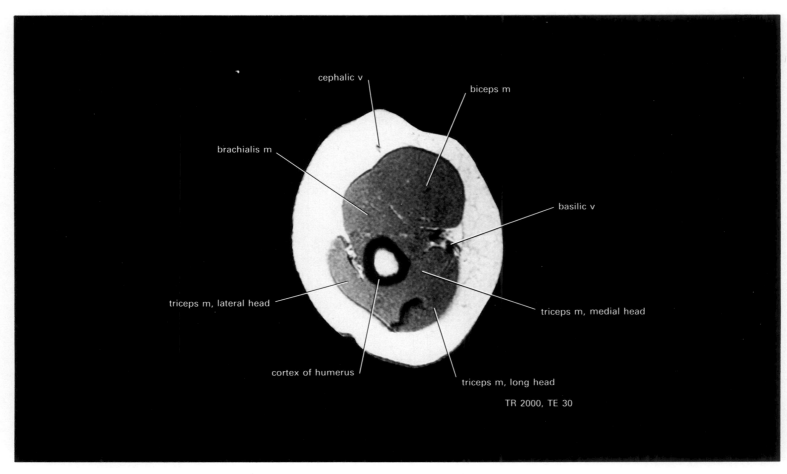

cephalic v

biceps m

brachialis m

basilic v

triceps m, lateral head

triceps m, medial head

cortex of humerus

triceps m, long head

TR 2000, TE 30

Section 5U from below.

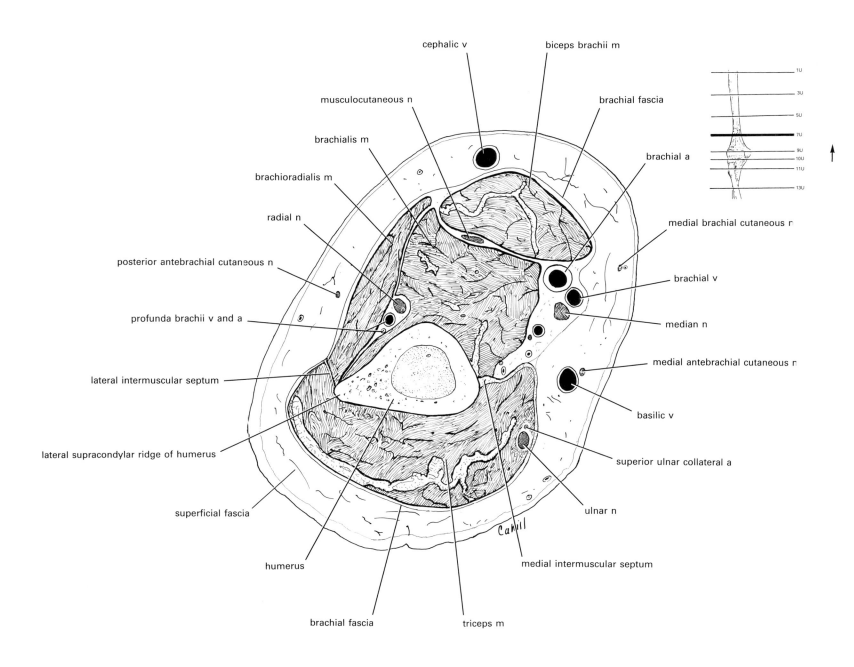

cephalic v — biceps brachii m

musculocutaneous n — brachial fascia

brachialis m

brachioradialis m — brachial a

radial n — medial brachial cutaneous n

posterior antebrachial cutaneous n — brachial v

profunda brachii v and a — median n

lateral intermuscular septum — medial antebrachial cutaneous n

— basilic v

lateral supracondylar ridge of humerus — superior ulnar collateral a

superficial fascia — ulnar n

humerus — medial intermuscular septum

brachial fascia — triceps m

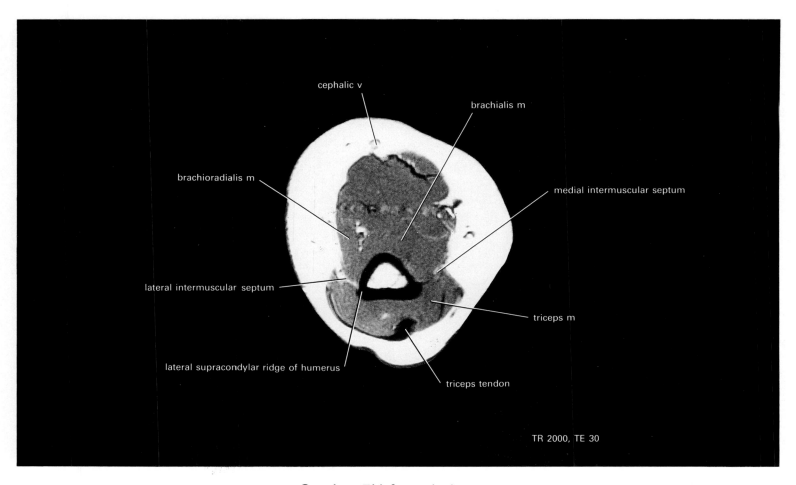

cephalic v — brachialis m

brachioradialis m — medial intermuscular septum

lateral intermuscular septum — triceps m

lateral supracondylar ridge of humerus — triceps tendon

TR 2000, TE 30

Section 7U from below.

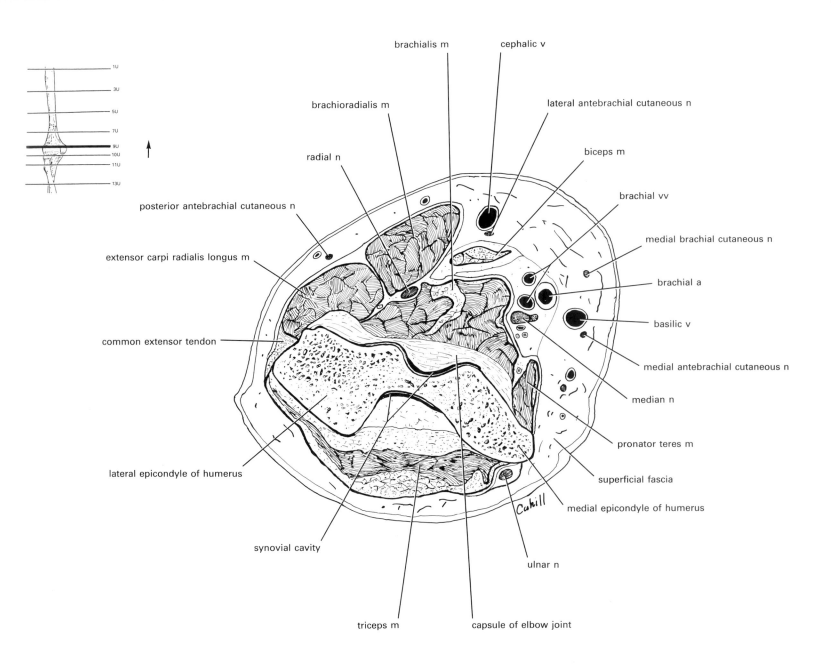

brachialis m

cephalic v

brachioradialis m

lateral antebrachial cutaneous n

radial n

biceps m

posterior antebrachial cutaneous n

brachial vv

extensor carpi radialis longus m

medial brachial cutaneous n

brachial a

common extensor tendon

basilic v

medial antebrachial cutaneous n

median n

lateral epicondyle of humerus

pronator teres m

superficial fascia

medial epicondyle of humerus

synovial cavity

ulnar n

triceps m

capsule of elbow joint

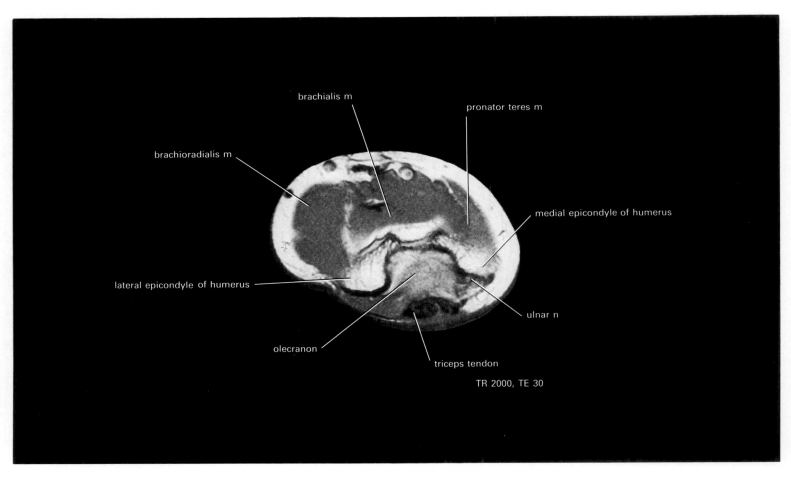

brachialis m

pronator teres m

brachioradialis m

medial epicondyle of humerus

lateral epicondyle of humerus

ulnar n

olecranon

triceps tendon

TR 2000, TE 30

Section 9U from below.

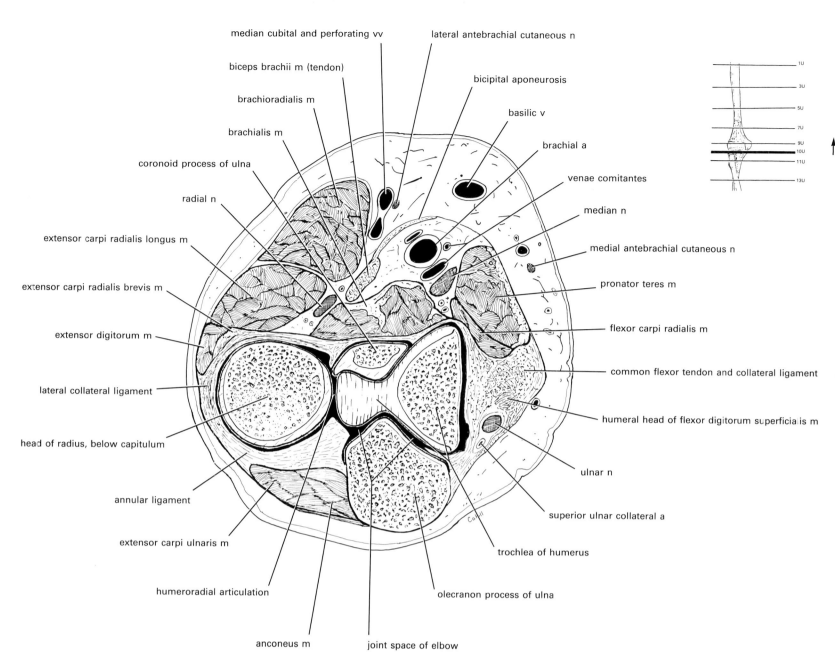

median cubital and perforating vv

biceps brachii m (tendon)

brachioradialis m

brachialis m

coronoid process of ulna

radial n

extensor carpi radialis longus m

extensor carpi radialis brevis m

extensor digitorum m

lateral collateral ligament

head of radius, below capitulum

annular ligament

extensor carpi ulnaris m

humeroradial articulation

anconeus m

lateral antebrachial cutaneous n

bicipital aponeurosis

basilic v

brachial a

venae comitantes

median n

medial antebrachial cutaneous n

pronator teres m

flexor carpi radialis m

common flexor tendon and collateral ligament

humeral head of flexor digitorum superficialis m

ulnar n

superior ulnar collateral a

trochlea of humerus

olecranon process of ulna

joint space of elbow

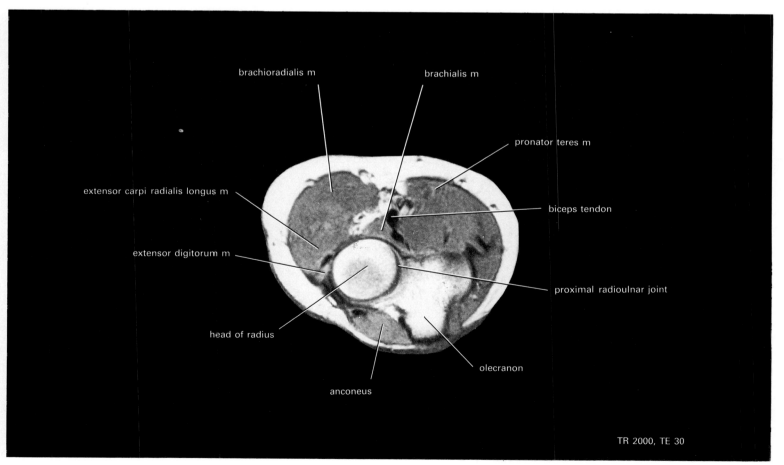

brachioradialis m

brachialis m

extensor carpi radialis longus m

pronator teres m

extensor digitorum m

biceps tendon

head of radius

proximal radioulnar joint

anconeus

olecranon

TR 2000, TE 30

Section 10U from below.

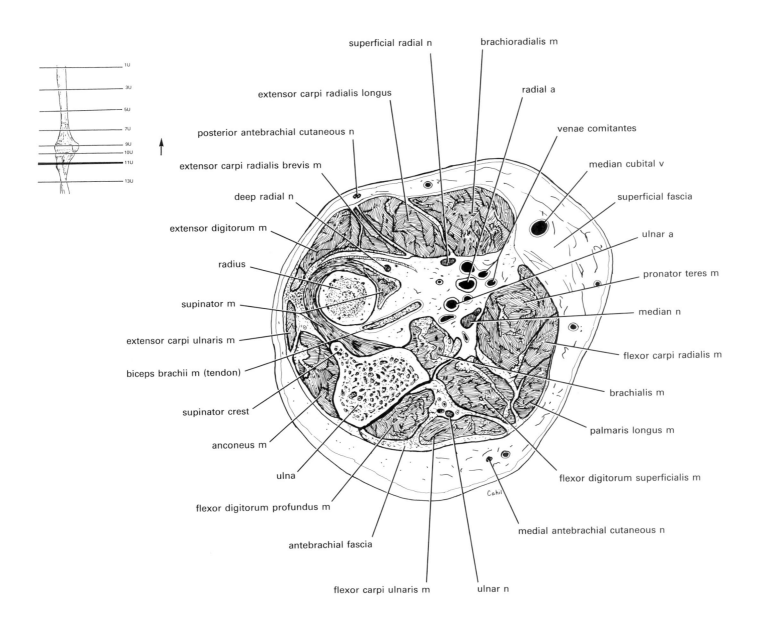

superficial radial n

brachioradialis m

extensor carpi radialis longus

radial a

posterior antebrachial cutaneous n

venae comitantes

extensor carpi radialis brevis m

median cubital v

deep radial n

superficial fascia

extensor digitorum m

ulnar a

radius

pronator teres m

supinator m

median n

extensor carpi ulnaris m

flexor carpi radialis m

biceps brachii m (tendon)

brachialis m

supinator crest

palmaris longus m

anconeus m

ulna

flexor digitorum superficialis m

flexor digitorum profundus m

medial antebrachial cutaneous n

antebrachial fascia

flexor carpi ulnaris m

ulnar n

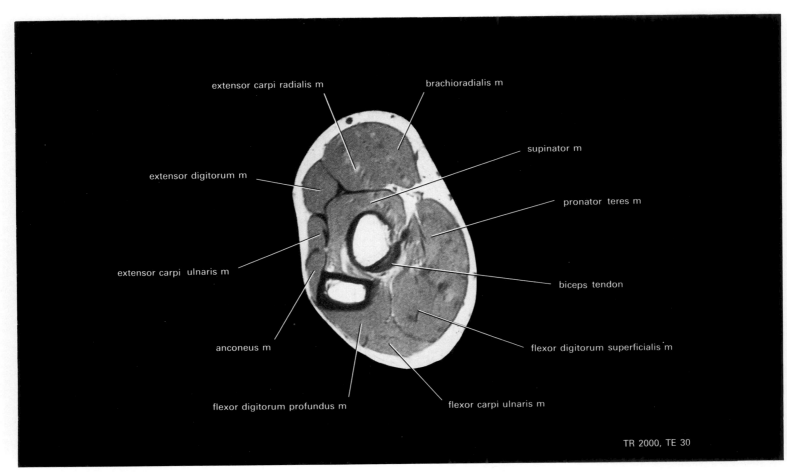

extensor carpi radialis m

brachioradialis m

supinator m

extensor digitorum m

pronator teres m

extensor carpi ulnaris m

biceps tendon

anconeus m

flexor digitorum superficialis m

flexor digitorum profundus m

flexor carpi ulnaris m

TR 2000, TE 30

Section 11U from below.

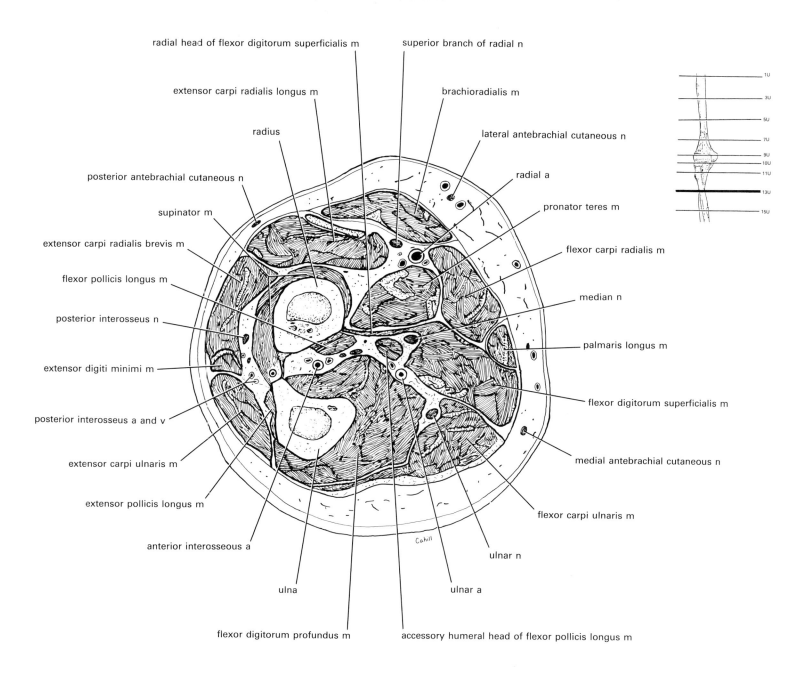

radial head of flexor digitorum superficialis m

extensor carpi radialis longus m

radius

posterior antebrachial cutaneous n

supinator m

extensor carpi radialis brevis m

flexor pollicis longus m

posterior interosseus n

extensor digiti minimi m

posterior interosseus a and v

extensor carpi ulnaris m

extensor pollicis longus m

anterior interosseous a

ulna

flexor digitorum profundus m

superior branch of radial n

brachioradialis m

lateral antebrachial cutaneous n

radial a

pronator teres m

flexor carpi radialis m

median n

palmaris longus m

flexor digitorum superficialis m

medial antebrachial cutaneous n

flexor carpi ulnaris m

ulnar n

ulnar a

accessory humeral head of flexor pollicis longus m

Cahill

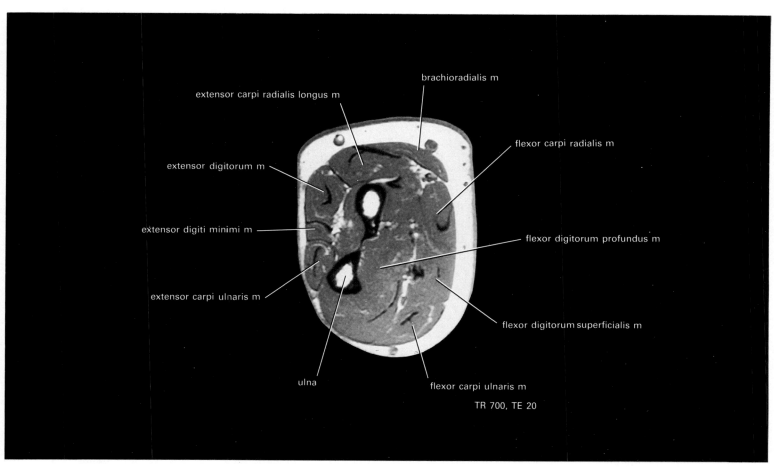

extensor carpi radialis longus m

brachioradialis m

extensor digitorum m

flexor carpi radialis m

extensor digiti minimi m

flexor digitorum profundus m

extensor carpi ulnaris m

flexor digitorum superficialis m

ulna

flexor carpi ulnaris m

TR 700, TE 20

Section 13U from below.

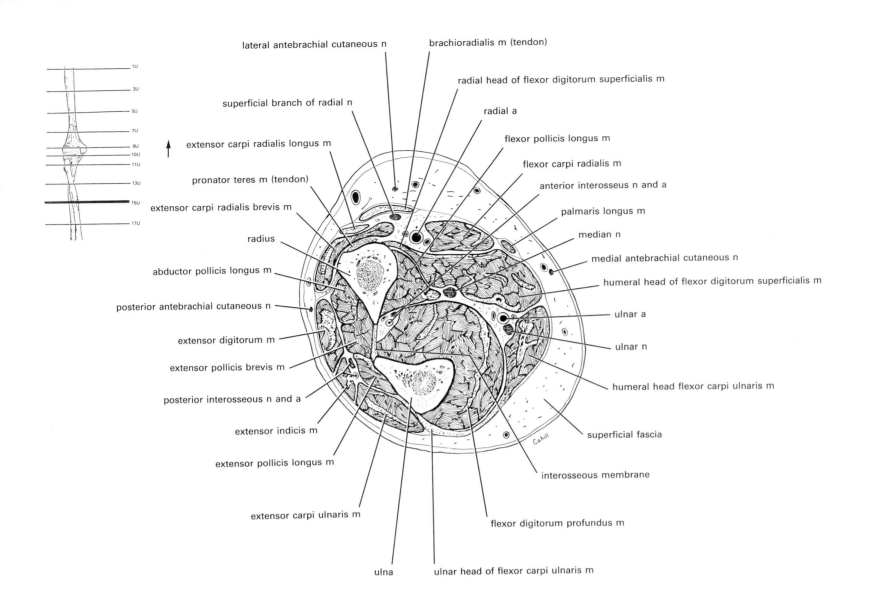

lateral antebrachial cutaneous n
brachioradialis m (tendon)
radial head of flexor digitorum superficialis m
superficial branch of radial n
radial a
extensor carpi radialis longus m
flexor pollicis longus m
flexor carpi radialis m
pronator teres m (tendon)
anterior interosseus n and a
extensor carpi radialis brevis m
palmaris longus m
radius
median n
abductor pollicis longus m
medial antebrachial cutaneous n
humeral head of flexor digitorum superficialis m
posterior antebrachial cutaneous n
ulnar a
extensor digitorum m
ulnar n
extensor pollicis brevis m
humeral head flexor carpi ulnaris m
posterior interosseous n and a
superficial fascia
extensor indicis m
interosseous membrane
extensor pollicis longus m
extensor carpi ulnaris m
flexor digitorum profundus m
ulna
ulnar head of flexor carpi ulnaris m

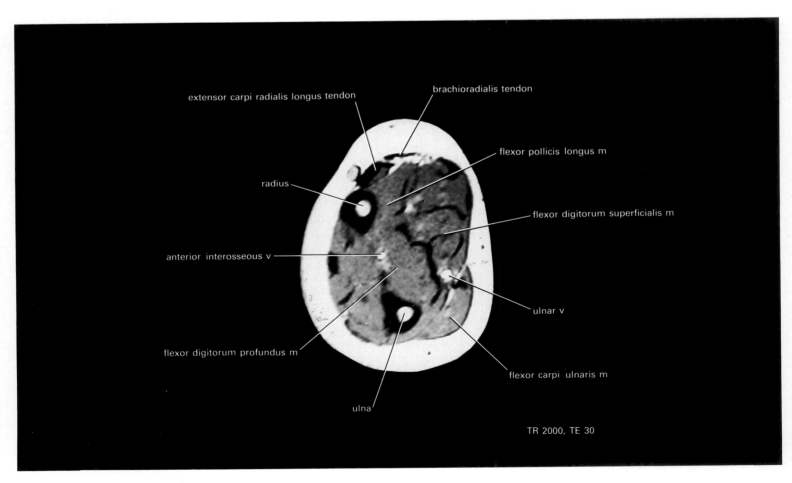

extensor carpi radialis longus tendon
brachioradialis tendon
flexor pollicis longus m
radius
flexor digitorum superficialis m
anterior interosseous v
ulnar v
flexor digitorum profundus m
flexor carpi ulnaris m
ulna
TR 2000, TE 30

Section 15U from below.

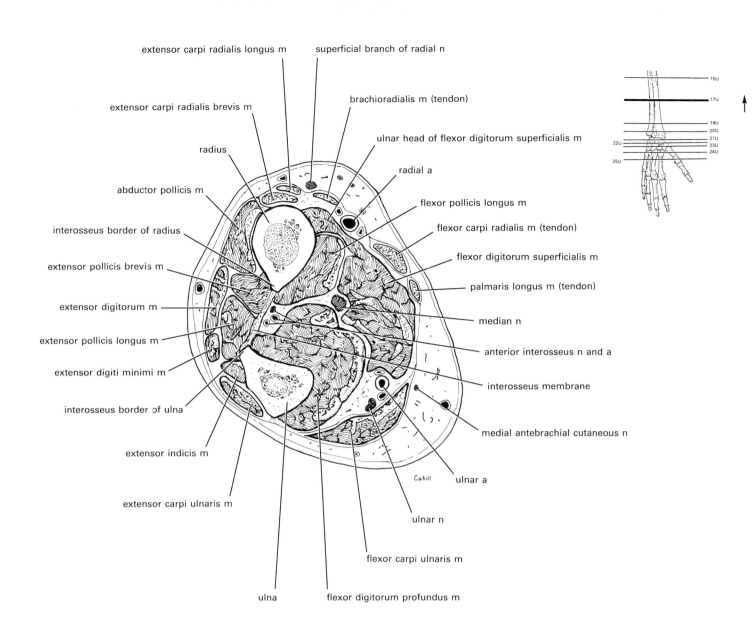

extensor carpi radialis longus m

superficial branch of radial n

extensor carpi radialis brevis m

brachioradialis m (tendon)

radius

ulnar head of flexor digitorum superficialis m

abductor pollicis m

radial a

interosseus border of radius

flexor pollicis longus m

extensor pollicis brevis m

flexor carpi radialis m (tendon)

extensor digitorum m

flexor digitorum superficialis m

extensor pollicis longus m

palmaris longus m (tendon)

extensor digiti minimi m

median n

interosseus border of ulna

anterior interosseus n and a

interosseus membrane

extensor indicis m

medial antebrachial cutaneous n

extensor carpi ulnaris m

ulnar a

ulnar n

flexor carpi ulnaris m

ulna

flexor digitorum profundus m

Cahill

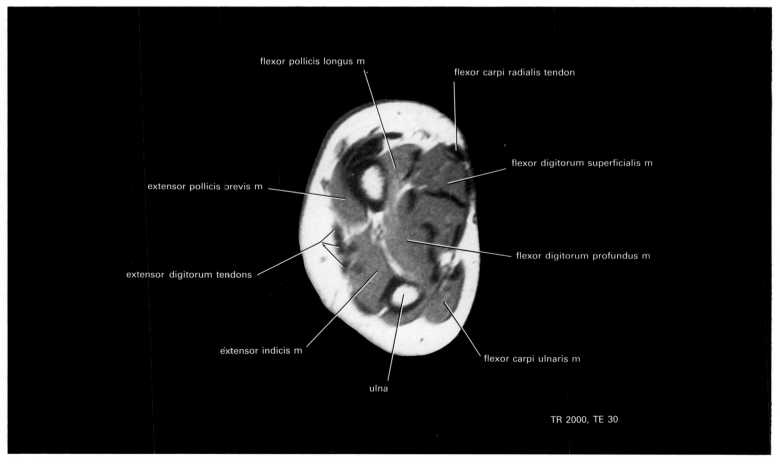

flexor pollicis longus m

flexor carpi radialis tendon

extensor pollicis brevis m

flexor digitorum superficialis m

extensor digitorum tendons

flexor digitorum profundus m

extensor indicis m

flexor carpi ulnaris m

ulna

TR 2000, TE 30

Section 17U from below.

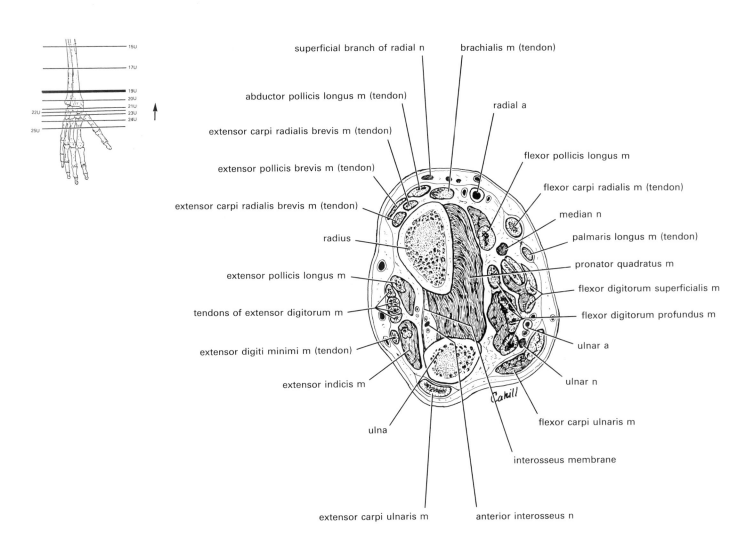

superficial branch of radial n

brachialis m (tendon)

abductor pollicis longus m (tendon)

radial a

extensor carpi radialis brevis m (tendon)

flexor pollicis longus m

extensor pollicis brevis m (tendon)

flexor carpi radialis m (tendon)

extensor carpi radialis brevis m (tendon)

median n

radius

palmaris longus m (tendon)

pronator quadratus m

extensor pollicis longus m

flexor digitorum superficialis m

tendons of extensor digitorum m

flexor digitorum profundus m

ulnar a

extensor digiti minimi m (tendon)

ulnar n

extensor indicis m

flexor carpi ulnaris m

ulna

interosseus membrane

extensor carpi ulnaris m

anterior interosseus n

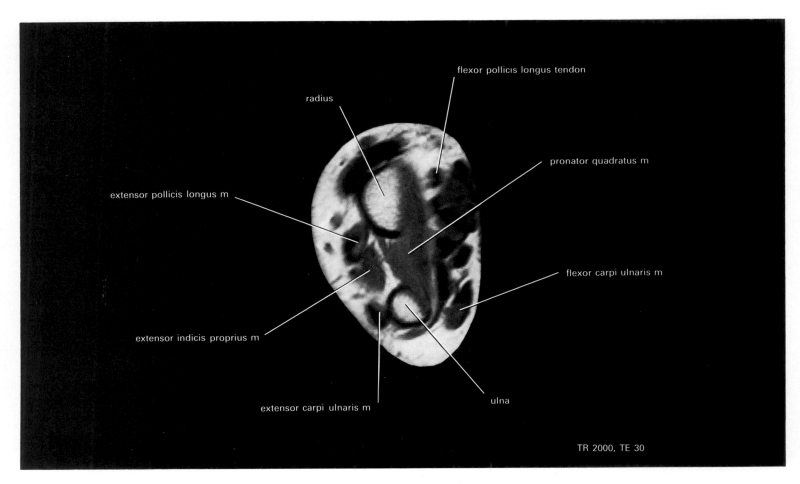

flexor pollicis longus tendon

radius

pronator quadratus m

extensor pollicis longus m

flexor carpi ulnaris m

extensor indicis proprius m

ulna

extensor carpi ulnaris m

TR 2000, TE 30

Section 19U from below.

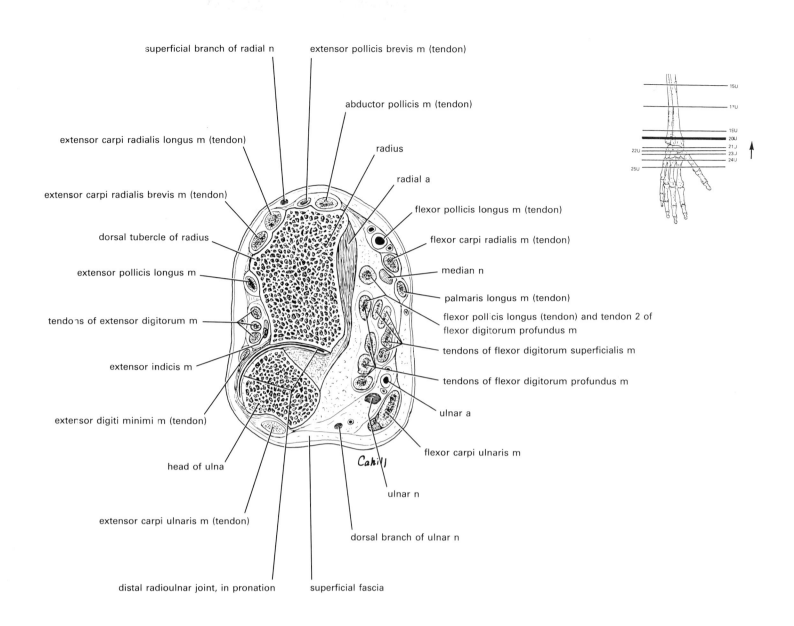

superficial branch of radial n
extensor pollicis brevis m (tendon)
abductor pollicis m (tendon)
extensor carpi radialis longus m (tendon)
radius
extensor carpi radialis brevis m (tendon)
radial a
dorsal tubercle of radius
flexor pollicis longus m (tendon)
extensor pollicis longus m
flexor carpi radialis m (tendon)
median n
palmaris longus m (tendon)
tendons of extensor digitorum m
flexor pollicis longus (tendon) and tendon 2 of flexor digitorum profundus m
extensor indicis m
tendons of flexor digitorum superficialis m
tendons of flexor digitorum profundus m
extensor digiti minimi m (tendon)
ulnar a
head of ulna
flexor carpi ulnaris m
Cahill
ulnar n
extensor carpi ulnaris m (tendon)
dorsal branch of ulnar n
distal radioulnar joint, in pronation
superficial fascia

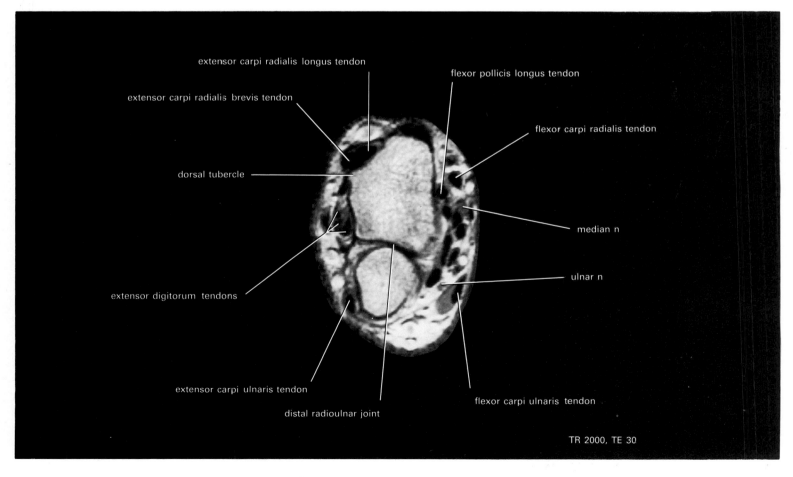

extensor carpi radialis longus tendon
flexor pollicis longus tendon
extensor carpi radialis brevis tendon
flexor carpi radialis tendon
dorsal tubercle
median n
ulnar n
extensor digitorum tendons
extensor carpi ulnaris tendon
flexor carpi ulnaris tendon
distal radioulnar joint

TR 2000, TE 30

Section 20U from below.

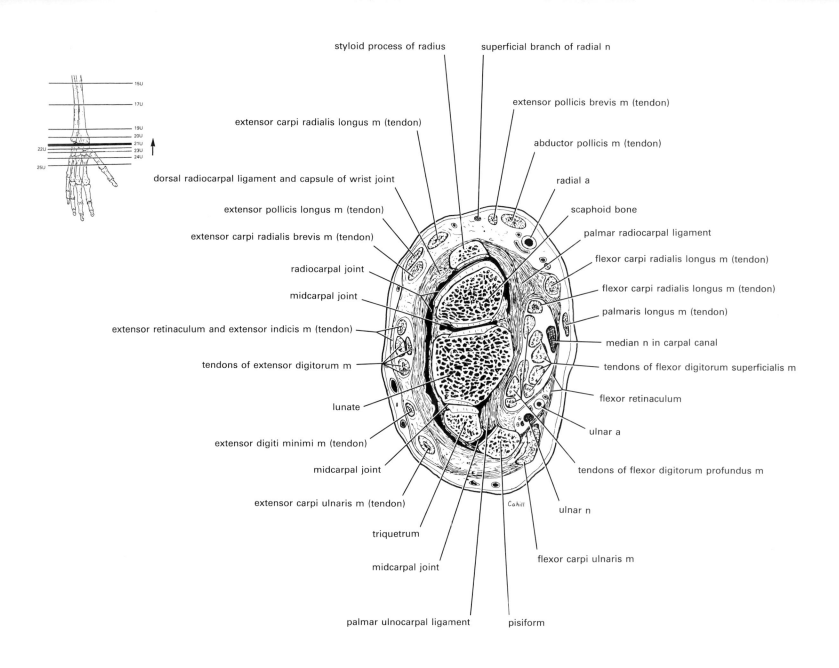

styloid process of radius

superficial branch of radial n

extensor carpi radialis longus m (tendon)

extensor pollicis brevis m (tendon)

abductor pollicis m (tendon)

dorsal radiocarpal ligament and capsule of wrist joint

radial a

scaphoid bone

extensor pollicis longus m (tendon)

palmar radiocarpal ligament

extensor carpi radialis brevis m (tendon)

flexor carpi radialis longus m (tendon)

radiocarpal joint

flexor carpi radialis longus m (tendon)

midcarpal joint

palmaris longus m (tendon)

extensor retinaculum and extensor indicis m (tendon)

median n in carpal canal

tendons of extensor digitorum m

tendons of flexor digitorum superficialis m

lunate

flexor retinaculum

ulnar a

extensor digiti minimi m (tendon)

tendons of flexor digitorum profundus m

midcarpal joint

ulnar n

extensor carpi ulnaris m (tendon)

flexor carpi ulnaris m

triquetrum

Cahill

midcarpal joint

palmar ulnocarpal ligament

pisiform

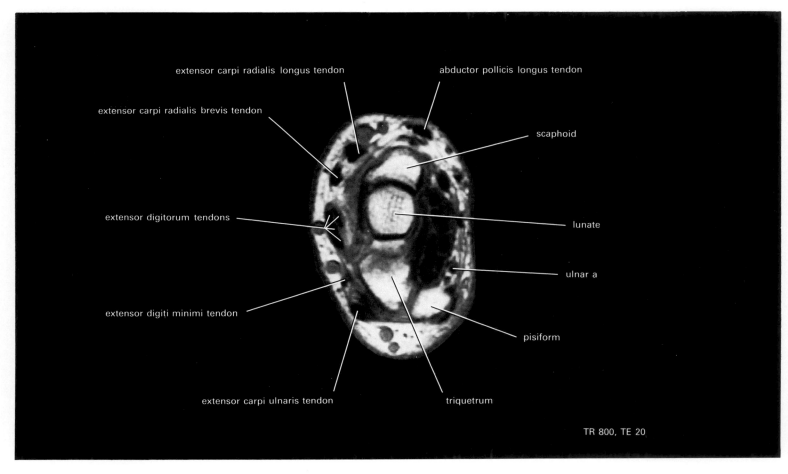

extensor carpi radialis longus tendon

abductor pollicis longus tendon

extensor carpi radialis brevis tendon

scaphoid

extensor digitorum tendons

lunate

ulnar a

extensor digiti minimi tendon

pisiform

extensor carpi ulnaris tendon

triquetrum

TR 800, TE 20

Section 21U from below.

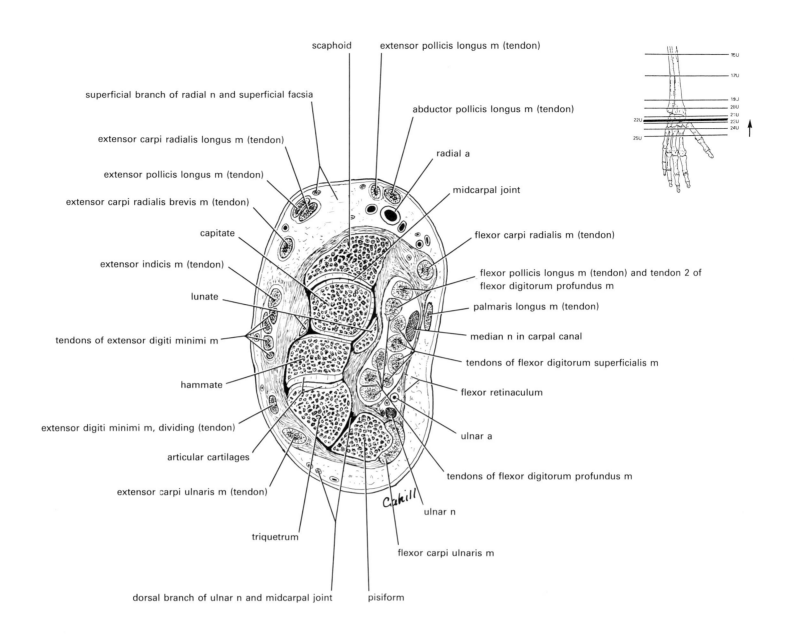

scaphoid

extensor pollicis longus m (tendon)

superficial branch of radial n and superficial facsia

abductor pollicis longus m (tendon)

extensor carpi radialis longus m (tendon)

radial a

extensor pollicis longus m (tendon)

midcarpal joint

extensor carpi radialis brevis m (tendon)

flexor carpi radialis m (tendon)

capitate

extensor indicis m (tendon)

flexor pollicis longus m (tendon) and tendon 2 of flexor digitorum profundus m

lunate

palmaris longus m (tendon)

tendons of extensor digiti minimi m

median n in carpal canal

tendons of flexor digitorum superficialis m

hammate

flexor retinaculum

extensor digiti minimi m, dividing (tendon)

ulnar a

articular cartilages

tendons of flexor digitorum profundus m

extensor carpi ulnaris m (tendon)

ulnar n

triquetrum

flexor carpi ulnaris m

dorsal branch of ulnar n and midcarpal joint

pisiform

Cahill

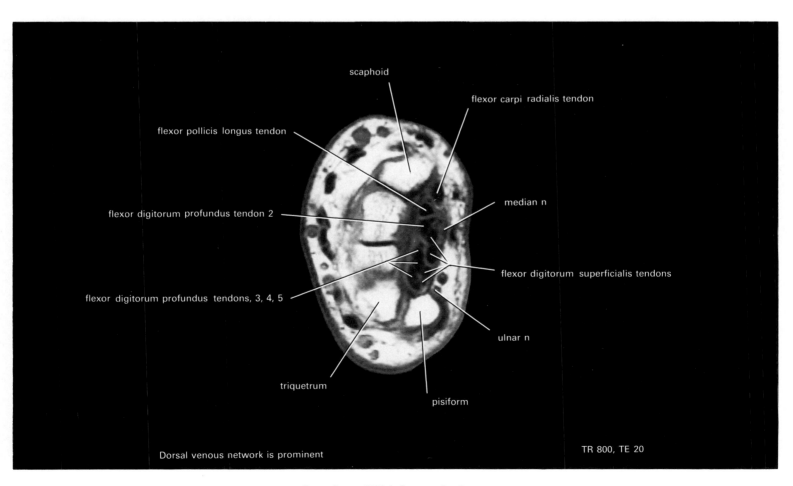

scaphoid

flexor carpi radialis tendon

flexor pollicis longus tendon

flexor digitorum profundus tendon 2

median n

flexor digitorum profundus tendons, 3, 4, 5

flexor digitorum superficialis tendons

triquetrum

ulnar n

pisiform

Dorsal venous network is prominent

TR 800, TE 20

Section 22U from below.

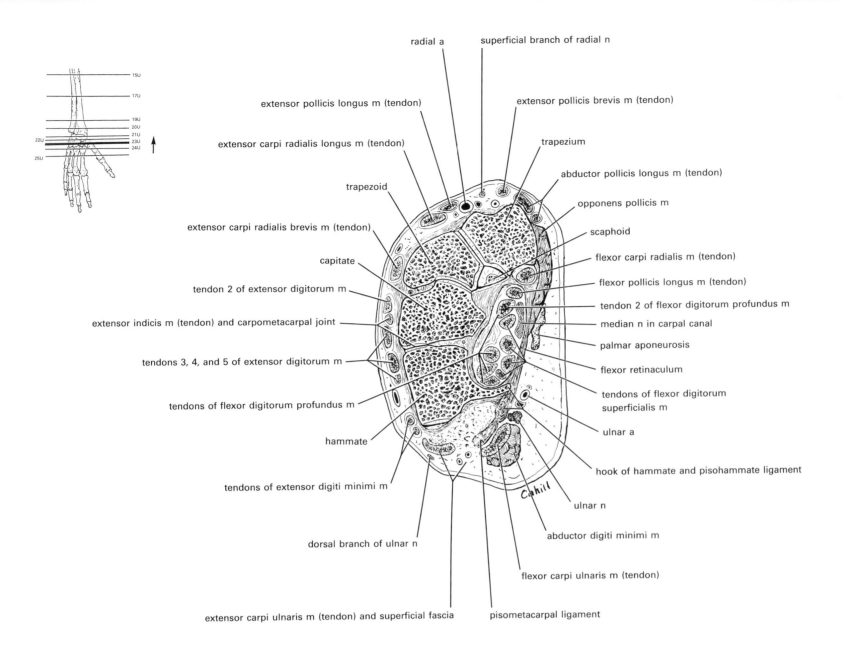

radial a

superficial branch of radial n

extensor pollicis longus m (tendon)

extensor pollicis brevis m (tendon)

extensor carpi radialis longus m (tendon)

trapezium

abductor pollicis longus m (tendon)

trapezoid

opponens pollicis m

extensor carpi radialis brevis m (tendon)

scaphoid

capitate

flexor carpi radialis m (tendon)

flexor pollicis longus m (tendon)

tendon 2 of extensor digitorum m

tendon 2 of flexor digitorum profundus m

extensor indicis m (tendon) and carpometacarpal joint

median n in carpal canal

palmar aponeurosis

tendons 3, 4, and 5 of extensor digitorum m

flexor retinaculum

tendons of flexor digitorum profundus m

tendons of flexor digitorum superficialis m

hammate

ulnar a

tendons of extensor digiti minimi m

hook of hammate and pisohammate ligament

ulnar n

dorsal branch of ulnar n

abductor digiti minimi m

flexor carpi ulnaris m (tendon)

extensor carpi ulnaris m (tendon) and superficial fascia

pisometacarpal ligament

Cahill

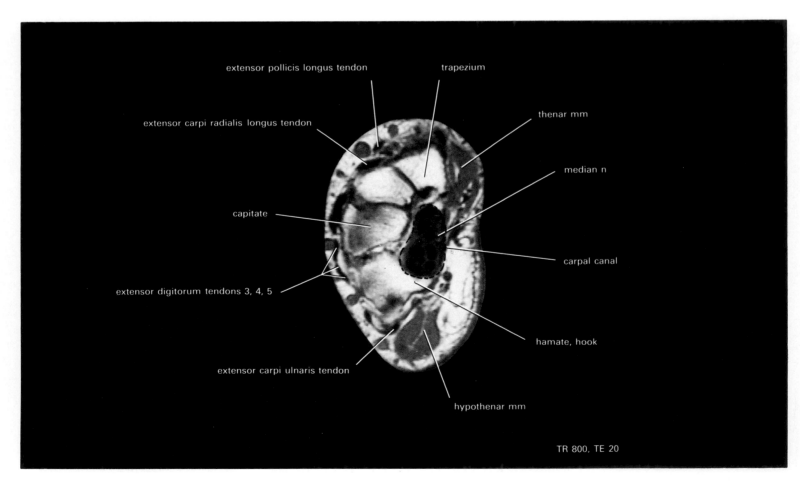

extensor pollicis longus tendon

trapezium

extensor carpi radialis longus tendon

thenar mm

capitate

median n

carpal canal

extensor digitorum tendons 3, 4, 5

hamate, hook

extensor carpi ulnaris tendon

hypothenar mm

TR 800, TE 20

Section 23U from below.

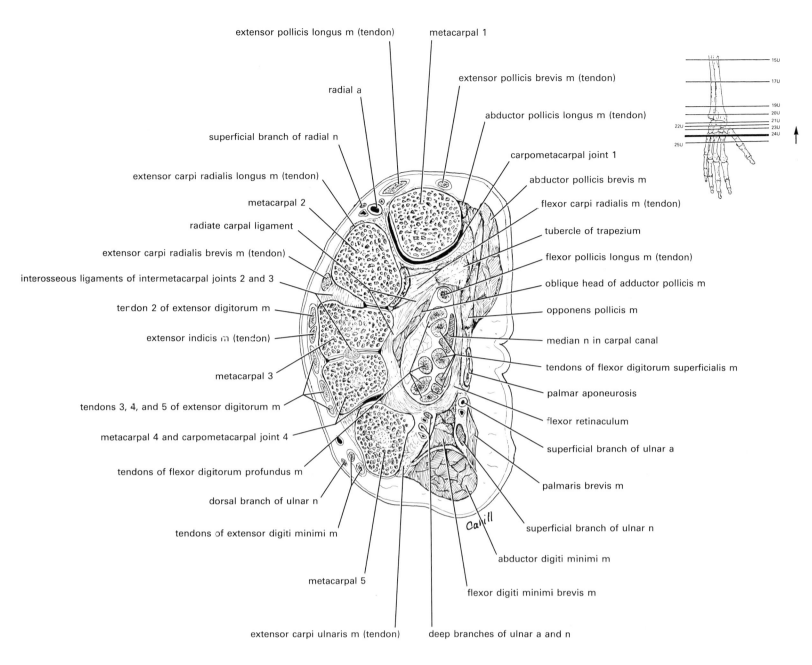

extensor pollicis longus m (tendon)

metacarpal 1

radial a

extensor pollicis brevis m (tendon)

abductor pollicis longus m (tendon)

superficial branch of radial n

carpometacarpal joint 1

extensor carpi radialis longus m (tendon)

abductor pollicis brevis m

metacarpal 2

flexor carpi radialis m (tendon)

radiate carpal ligament

tubercle of trapezium

extensor carpi radialis brevis m (tendon)

flexor pollicis longus m (tendon)

interosseous ligaments of intermetacarpal joints 2 and 3

oblique head of adductor pollicis m

tendon 2 of extensor digitorum m

opponens pollicis m

extensor indicis m (tendon)

median n in carpal canal

metacarpal 3

tendons of flexor digitorum superficialis m

tendons 3, 4, and 5 of extensor digitorum m

palmar aponeurosis

metacarpal 4 and carpometacarpal joint 4

flexor retinaculum

tendons of flexor digitorum profundus m

superficial branch of ulnar a

dorsal branch of ulnar n

palmaris brevis m

tendons of extensor digiti minimi m

superficial branch of ulnar n

abductor digiti minimi m

metacarpal 5

flexor digiti minimi brevis m

Cahill

extensor carpi ulnaris m (tendon)

deep branches of ulnar a and n

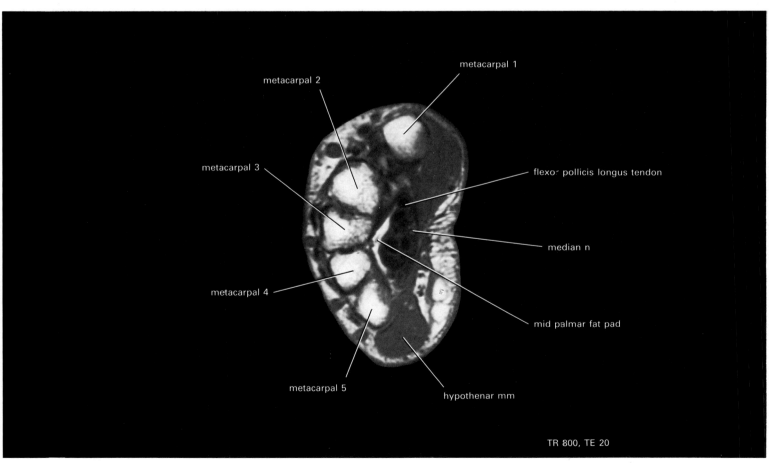

metacarpal 1

metacarpal 2

metacarpal 3

flexor pollicis longus tendon

median n

metacarpal 4

mid palmar fat pad

metacarpal 5

hypothenar mm

TR 800, TE 20

Section 24U from below.

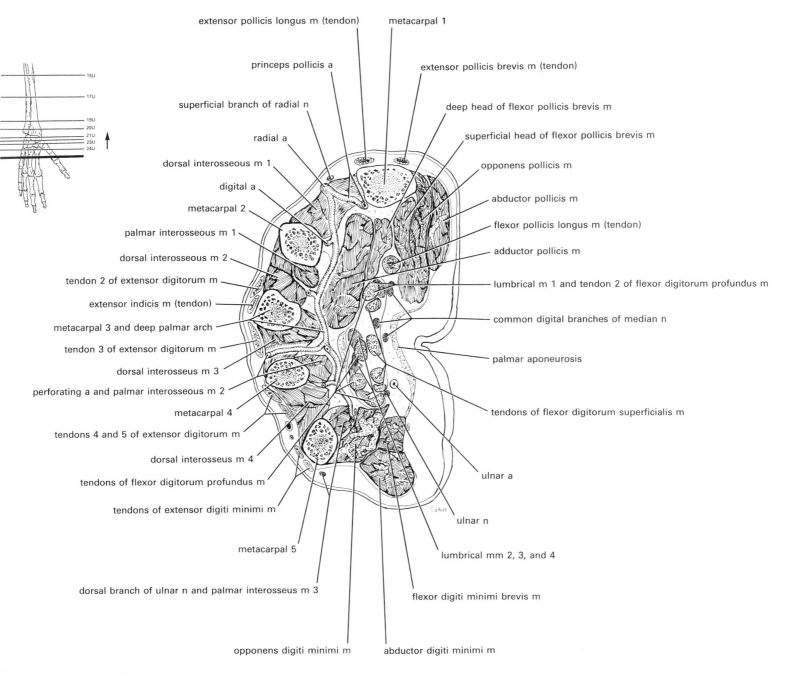

extensor pollicis longus m (tendon)

metacarpal 1

princeps pollicis a

extensor pollicis brevis m (tendon)

superficial branch of radial n

deep head of flexor pollicis brevis m

radial a

superficial head of flexor pollicis brevis m

dorsal interosseous m 1

opponens pollicis m

digital a

abductor pollicis m

metacarpal 2

flexor pollicis longus m (tendon)

palmar interosseous m 1

adductor pollicis m

dorsal interosseous m 2

tendon 2 of extensor digitorum m

lumbrical m 1 and tendon 2 of flexor digitorum profundus m

extensor indicis m (tendon)

metacarpal 3 and deep palmar arch

common digital branches of median n

tendon 3 of extensor digitorum m

dorsal interosseus m 3

palmar aponeurosis

perforating a and palmar interosseous m 2

metacarpal 4

tendons 4 and 5 of extensor digitorum m

tendons of flexor digitorum superficialis m

dorsal interosseus m 4

tendons of flexor digitorum profundus m

ulnar a

tendons of extensor digiti minimi m

ulnar n

metacarpal 5

lumbrical mm 2, 3, and 4

dorsal branch of ulnar n and palmar interosseus m 3

flexor digiti minimi brevis m

opponens digiti minimi m

abductor digiti minimi m

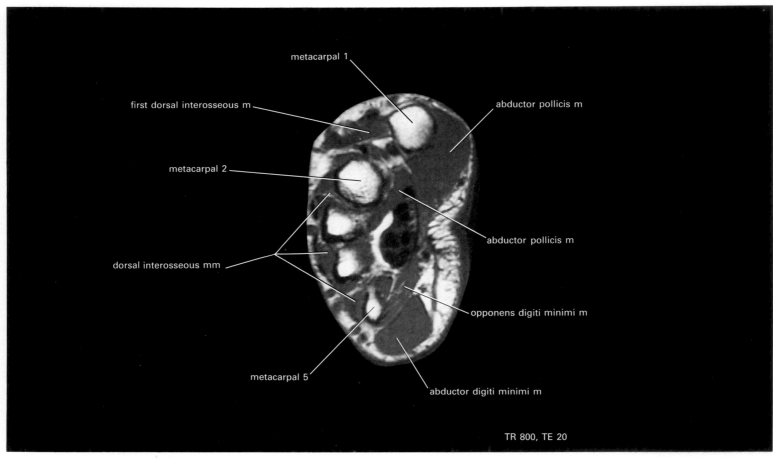

metacarpal 1

first dorsal interosseous m

abductor pollicis m

metacarpal 2

abductor pollicis m

dorsal interosseous mm

opponens digiti minimi m

metacarpal 5

abductor digiti minimi m

TR 800, TE 20

Section 25U from below.

The Right Shoulder in Sagittal Planes

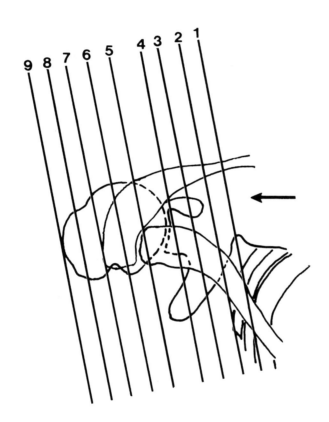

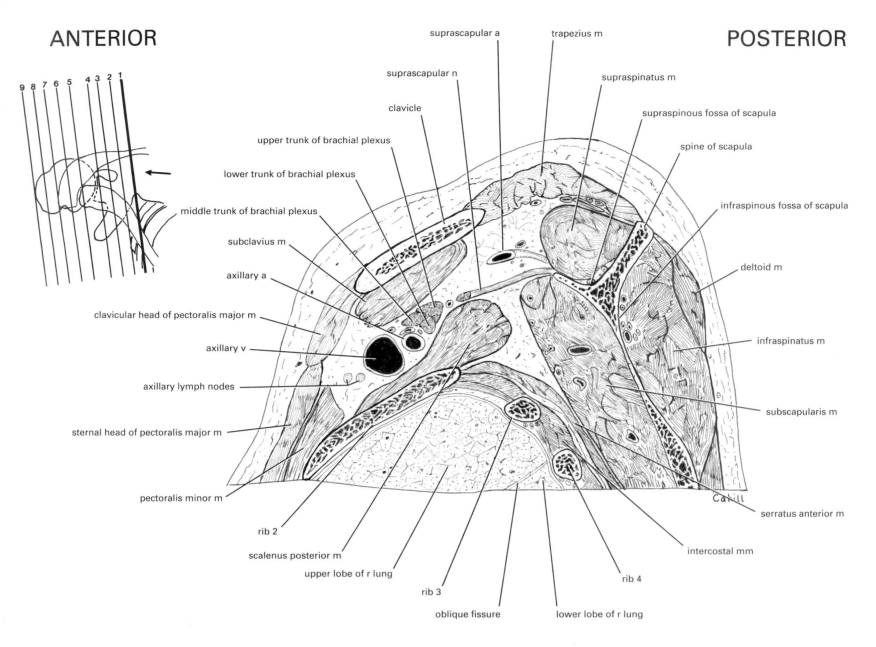

ANTERIOR

POSTERIOR

9 8 7 6 5 4 3 2 1

suprascapular a

trapezius m

suprascapular n

supraspinatus m

clavicle

supraspinous fossa of scapula

upper trunk of brachial plexus

spine of scapula

lower trunk of brachial plexus

infraspinous fossa of scapula

middle trunk of brachial plexus

subclavius m

deltoid m

axillary a

clavicular head of pectoralis major m

axillary v

infraspinatus m

axillary lymph nodes

subscapularis m

sternal head of pectoralis major m

pectoralis minor m

serratus anterior m

rib 2

intercostal mm

scalenus posterior m

upper lobe of r lung

rib 4

rib 3

oblique fissure

lower lobe of r lung

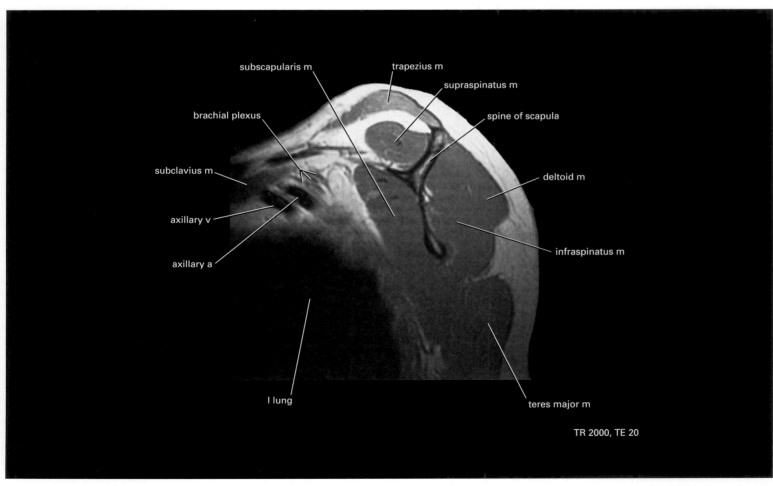

subscapularis m

trapezius m

supraspinatus m

brachial plexus

spine of scapula

subclavius m

deltoid m

axillary v

axillary a

infraspinatus m

l lung

teres major m

TR 2000, TE 20

Section SS1 from midline.

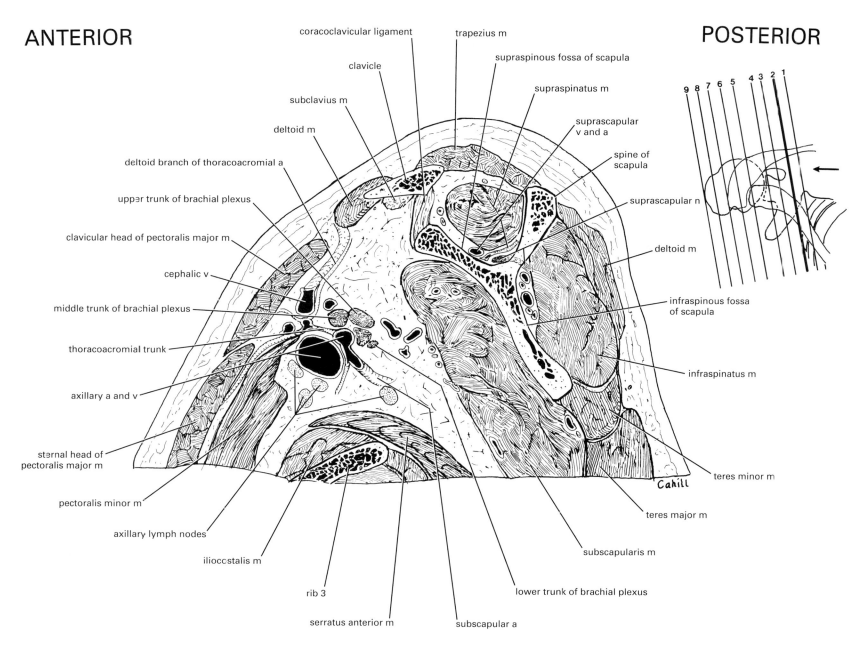

ANTERIOR

POSTERIOR

coracoclavicular ligament

trapezius m

clavicle

supraspinous fossa of scapula

subclavius m

supraspinatus m

deltoid m

suprascapular
v and a

deltoid branch of thoracoacromial a

spine of
scapula

upper trunk of brachial plexus

suprascapular n

clavicular head of pectoralis major m

deltoid m

cephalic v

middle trunk of brachial plexus

infraspinous fossa
of scapula

thoracoacromial trunk

infraspinatus m

axillary a and v

sternal head of
pectoralis major m

teres minor m

pectoralis minor m

teres major m

axillary lymph nodes

subscapularis m

iliocostalis m

lower trunk of brachial plexus

rib 3

subscapular a

serratus anterior m

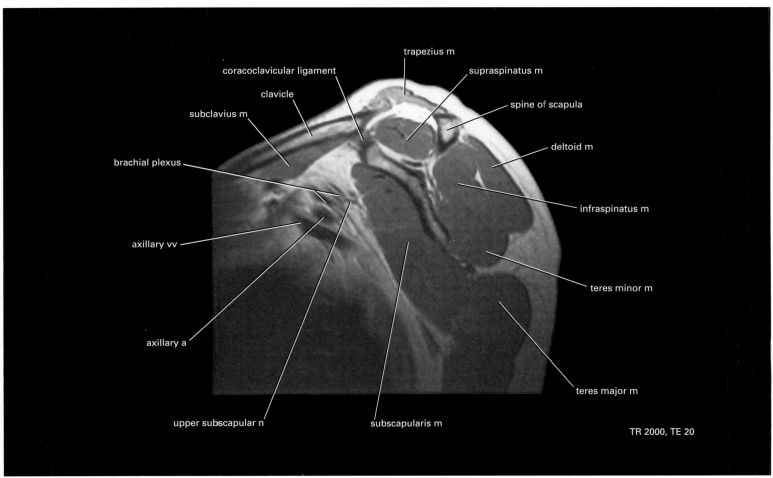

coracoclavicular ligament

trapezius m

clavicle

supraspinatus m

subclavius m

spine of scapula

brachial plexus

deltoid m

axillary vv

infraspinatus m

axillary a

teres minor m

teres major m

upper subscapular n

subscapularis m

TR 2000, TE 20

Section SS2 from midline.

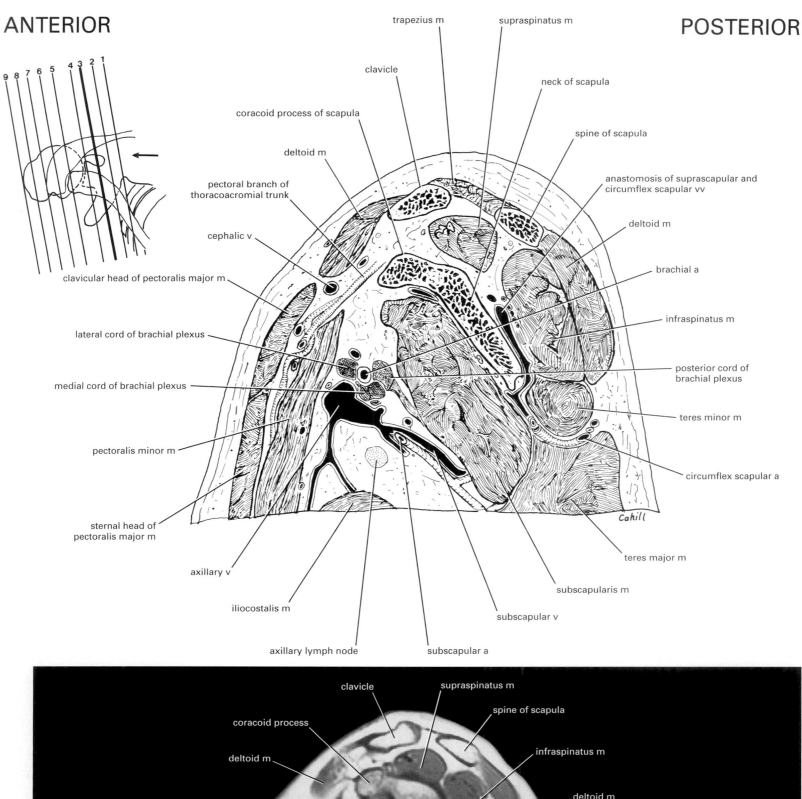

ANTERIOR

POSTERIOR

trapezius m

supraspinatus m

clavicle

neck of scapula

coracoid process of scapula

spine of scapula

deltoid m

anastomosis of suprascapular and
circumflex scapular vv

pectoral branch of
thoracoacromial trunk

deltoid m

cephalic v

brachial a

clavicular head of pectoralis major m

infraspinatus m

lateral cord of brachial plexus

posterior cord of
brachial plexus

medial cord of brachial plexus

teres minor m

pectoralis minor m

circumflex scapular a

sternal head of
pectoralis major m

teres major m

axillary v

subscapularis m

iliocostalis m

subscapular v

axillary lymph node

subscapular a

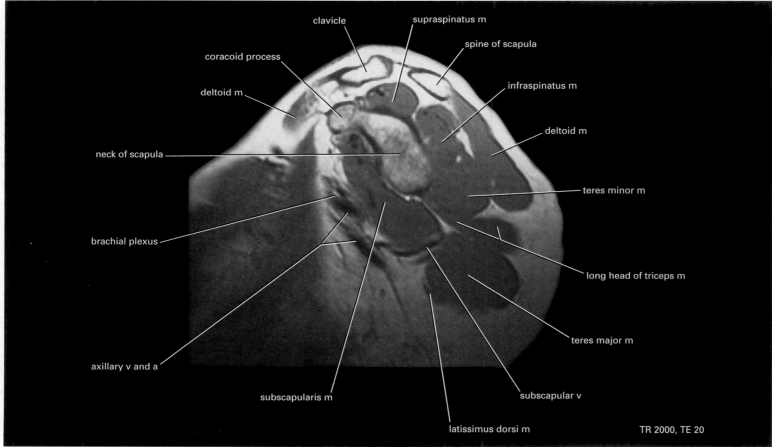

clavicle

supraspinatus m

coracoid process

spine of scapula

deltoid m

infraspinatus m

deltoid m

neck of scapula

teres minor m

brachial plexus

long head of triceps m

teres major m

axillary v and a

subscapularis m

subscapular v

latissimus dorsi m

TR 2000, TE 20

Section SS3 from midline.

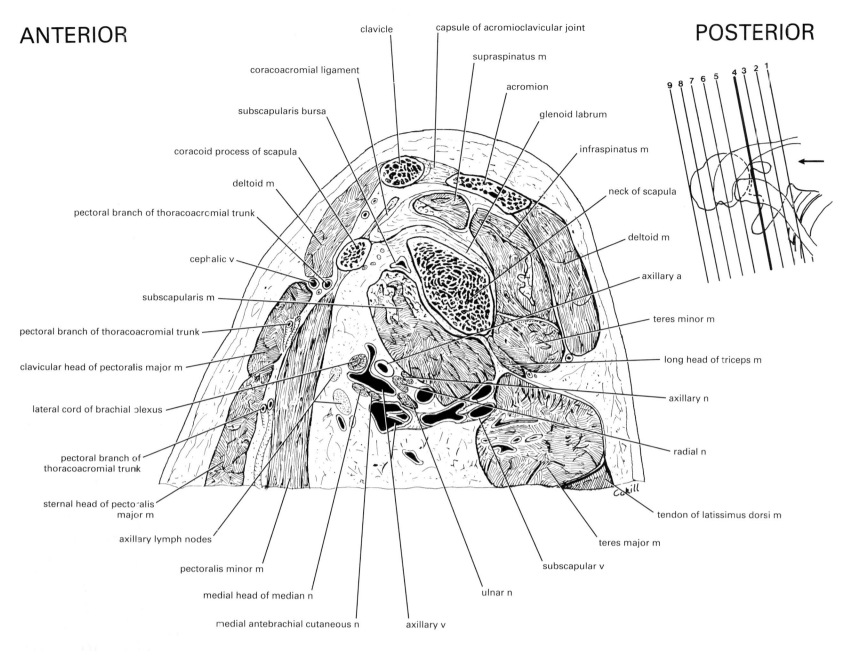

clavicle

capsule of acromioclavicular joint

supraspinatus m

coracoacromial ligament

acromion

subscapularis bursa

glenoid labrum

coracoid process of scapula

infraspinatus m

deltoid m

neck of scapula

pectoral branch of thoracoacromial trunk

deltoid m

cephalic v

axillary a

subscapularis m

teres minor m

pectoral branch of thoracoacromial trunk

long head of triceps m

clavicular head of pectoralis major m

axillary n

lateral cord of brachial plexus

radial n

pectoral branch of thoracoacromial trunk

tendon of latissimus dorsi m

sternal head of pectoralis major m

teres major m

axillary lymph nodes

subscapular v

pectoralis minor m

medial head of median n

ulnar n

medial antebrachial cutaneous n

axillary v

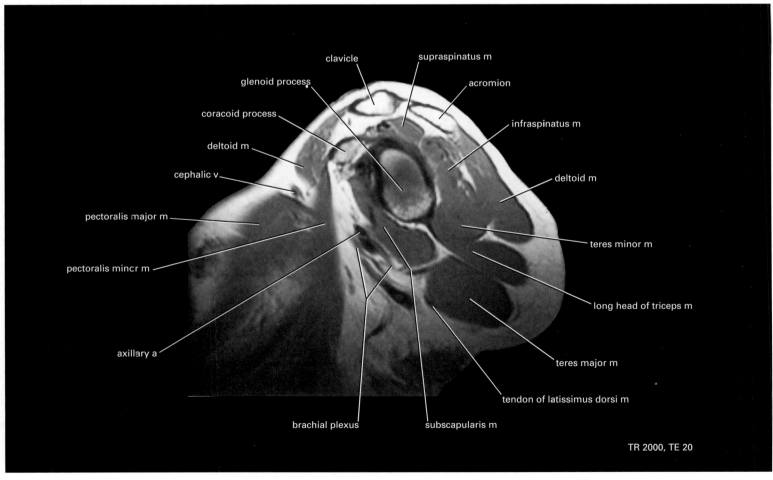

clavicle

supraspinatus m

glenoid process

acromion

coracoid process

infraspinatus m

deltoid m

deltoid m

cephalic v

pectoralis major m

teres minor m

pectoralis minor m

long head of triceps m

axillary a

teres major m

tendon of latissimus dorsi m

brachial plexus

subscapularis m

TR 2000, TE 20

Section SS4 from midline.

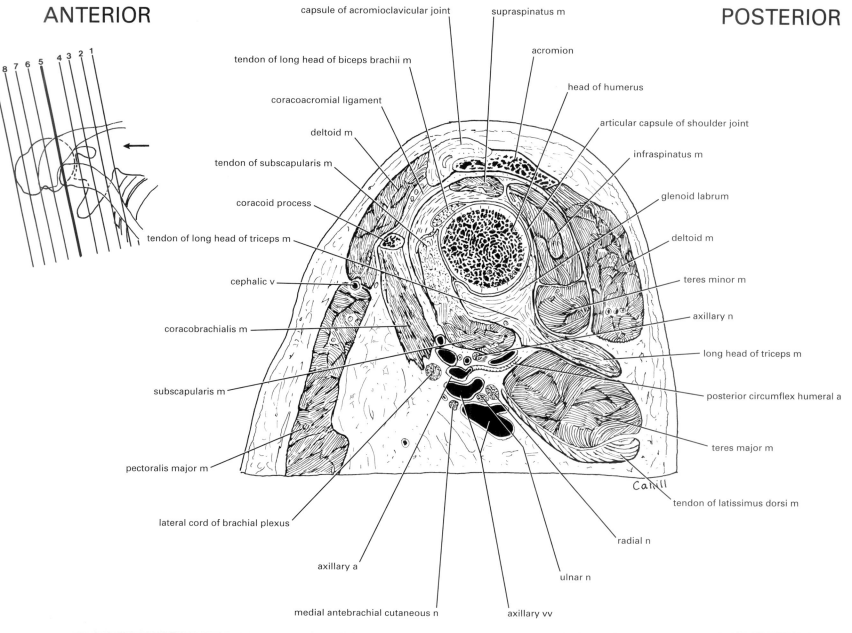

ANTERIOR

9 8 7 6 5 4 3 2 1

POSTERIOR

capsule of acromioclavicular joint

supraspinatus m

acromion

tendon of long head of biceps brachii m

head of humerus

coracoacromial ligament

articular capsule of shoulder joint

deltoid m

infraspinatus m

tendon of subscapularis m

glenoid labrum

coracoid process

deltoid m

tendon of long head of triceps m

teres minor m

cephalic v

axillary n

coracobrachialis m

long head of triceps m

posterior circumflex humeral a

subscapularis m

teres major m

pectoralis major m

tendon of latissimus dorsi m

lateral cord of brachial plexus

radial n

axillary a

ulnar n

medial antebrachial cutaneous n

axillary vv

Cahill

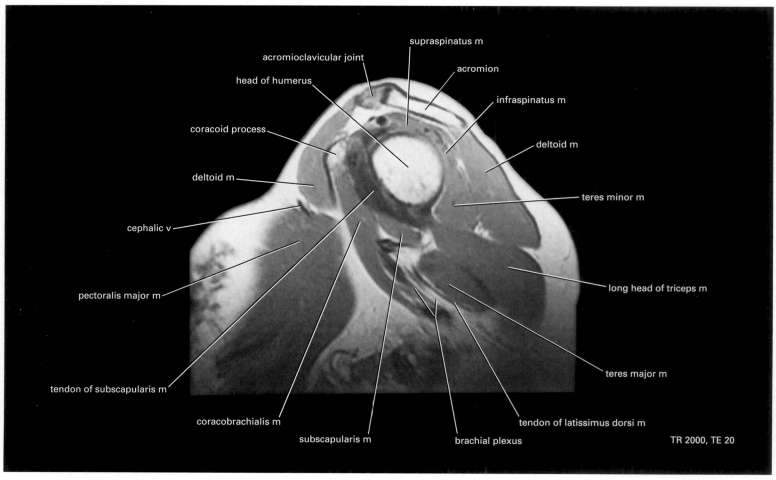

supraspinatus m

acromioclavicular joint

acromion

head of humerus

infraspinatus m

coracoid process

deltoid m

deltoid m

teres minor m

cephalic v

long head of triceps m

pectoralis major m

teres major m

tendon of subscapularis m

coracobrachialis m

tendon of latissimus dorsi m

subscapularis m

brachial plexus

TR 2000, TE 20

Section SS5 from midline.

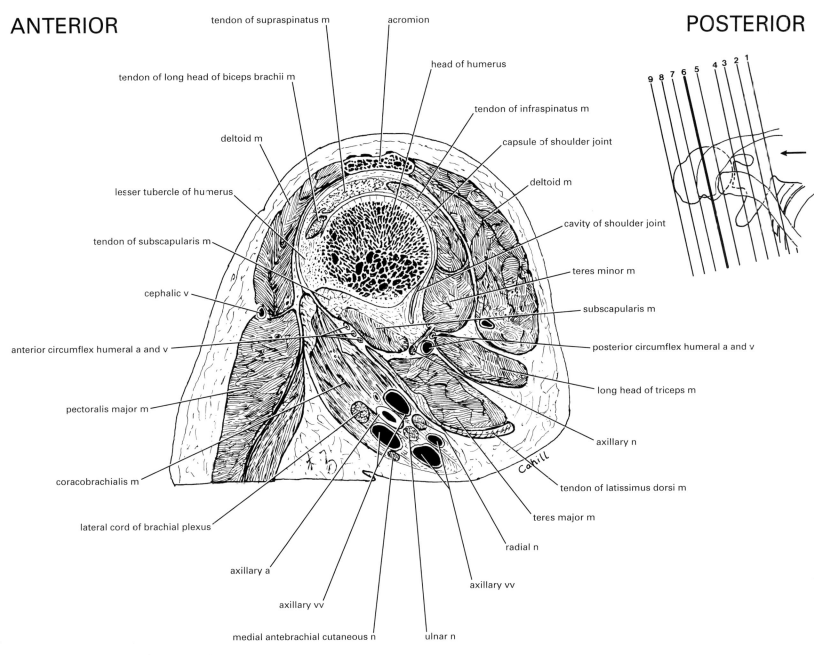

tendon of supraspinatus m

acromion

head of humerus

tendon of long head of biceps brachii m

tendon of infraspinatus m

deltoid m

capsule of shoulder joint

deltoid m

lesser tubercle of humerus

cavity of shoulder joint

tendon of subscapularis m

teres minor m

cephalic v

subscapularis m

anterior circumflex humeral a and v

posterior circumflex humeral a and v

pectoralis major m

long head of triceps m

coracobrachialis m

axillary n

tendon of latissimus dorsi m

lateral cord of brachial plexus

teres major m

radial n

axillary a

axillary vv

axillary vv

medial antebrachial cutaneous n

ulnar n

Cahill

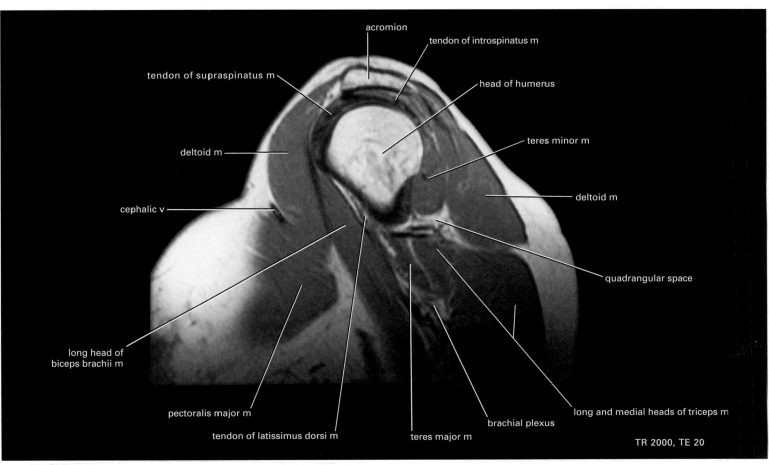

acromion

tendon of introspinatus m

tendon of supraspinatus m

head of humerus

deltoid m

teres minor m

cephalic v

deltoid m

quadrangular space

long head of
biceps brachii m

long and medial heads of triceps m

pectoralis major m

brachial plexus

tendon of latissimus dorsi m

teres major m

TR 2000, TE 20

Section SS6 from midline.

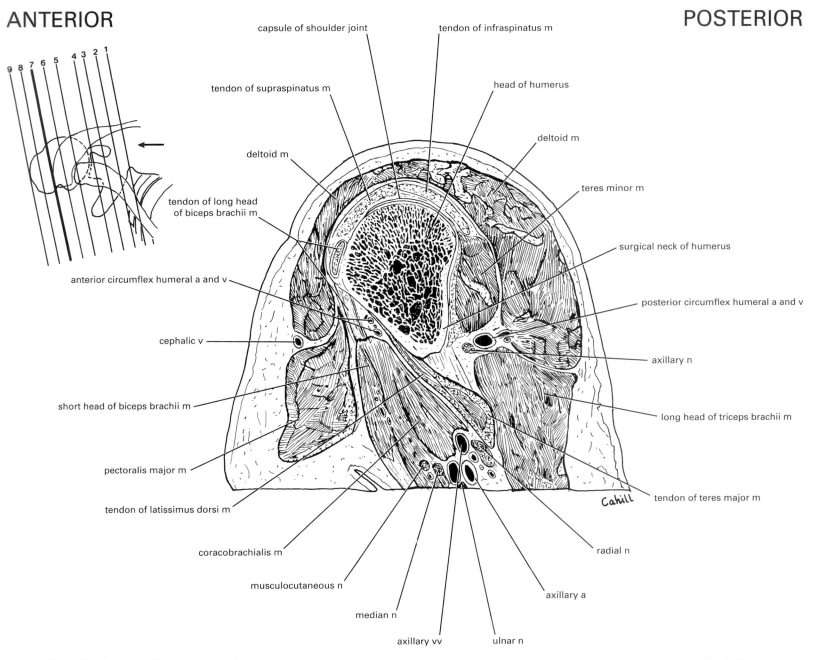

capsule of shoulder joint

tendon of infraspinatus m

tendon of supraspinatus m

head of humerus

deltoid m

deltoid m

teres minor m

tendon of long head of biceps brachii m

surgical neck of humerus

anterior circumflex humeral a and v

posterior circumflex humeral a and v

cephalic v

axillary n

short head of biceps brachii m

long head of triceps brachii m

pectoralis major m

tendon of teres major m

tendon of latissimus dorsi m

radial n

coracobrachialis m

musculocutaneous n

axillary a

median n

axillary vv

ulnar n

Cahill

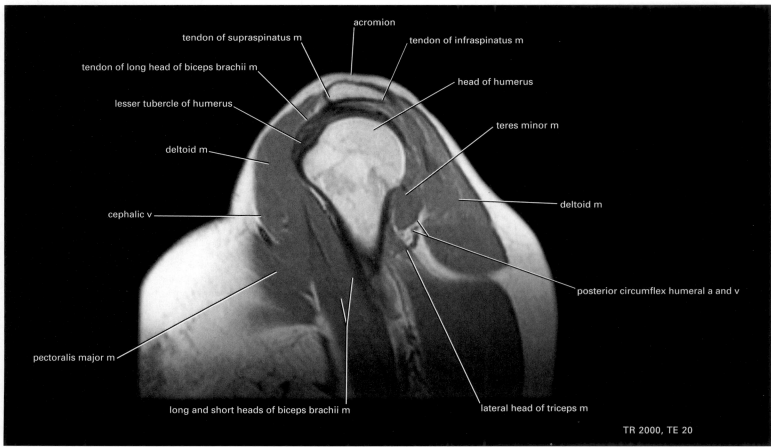

acromion

tendon of supraspinatus m

tendon of infraspinatus m

tendon of long head of biceps brachii m

head of humerus

lesser tubercle of humerus

teres minor m

deltoid m

deltoid m

cephalic v

posterior circumflex humeral a and v

pectoralis major m

long and short heads of biceps brachii m

lateral head of triceps m

TR 2000, TE 20

Section SS7 from midline.

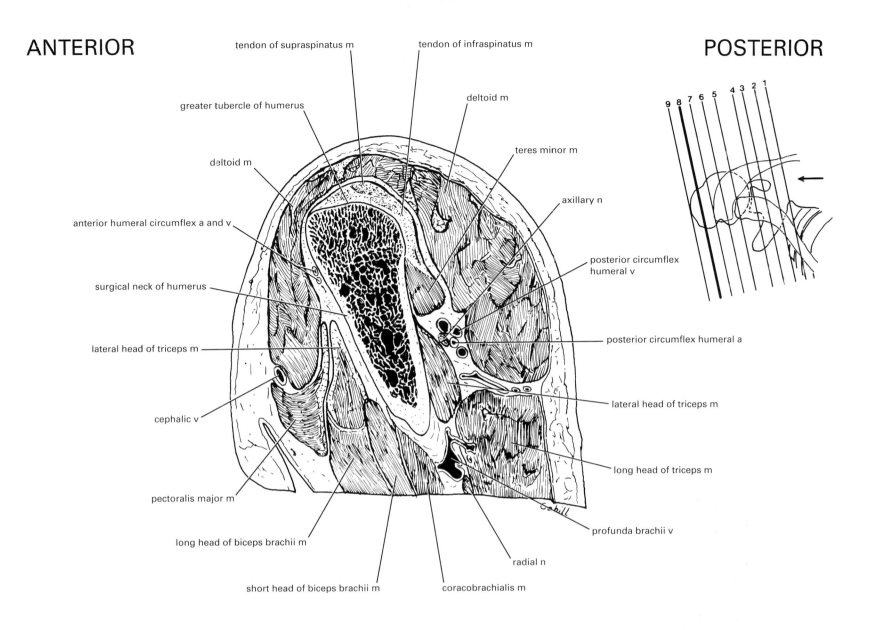

tendon of supraspinatus m

tendon of infraspinatus m

deltoid m

greater tubercle of humerus

teres minor m

deltoid m

axillary n

anterior humeral circumflex a and v

posterior circumflex humeral v

surgical neck of humerus

lateral head of triceps m

posterior circumflex humeral a

cephalic v

lateral head of triceps m

long head of triceps m

pectoralis major m

long head of biceps brachii m

profunda brachii v

short head of biceps brachii m

coracobrachialis m

radial n

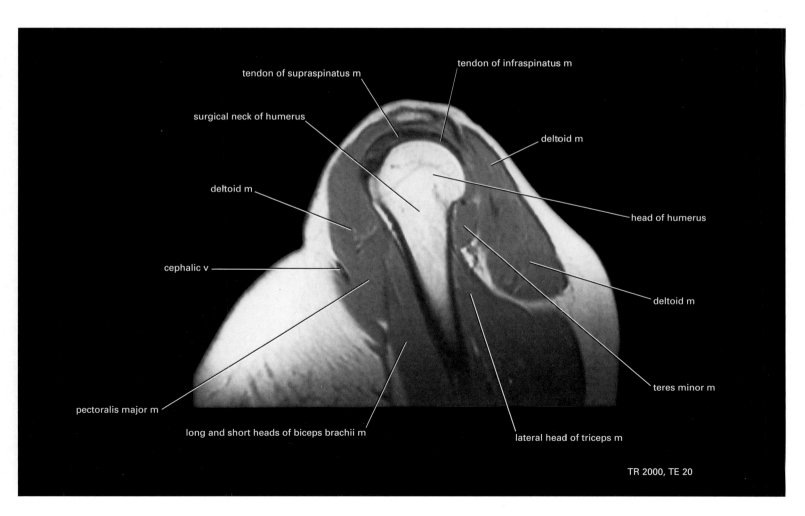

tendon of supraspinatus m

tendon of infraspinatus m

surgical neck of humerus

deltoid m

deltoid m

head of humerus

cephalic v

deltoid m

teres minor m

pectoralis major m

long and short heads of biceps brachii m

lateral head of triceps m

TR 2000, TE 20

Section SS8 from midline.

ANTERIOR   POSTERIOR

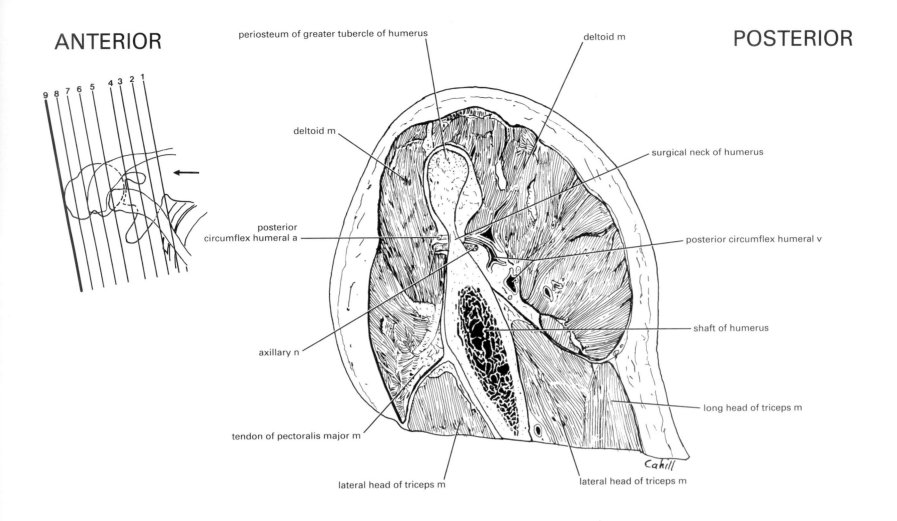

periosteum of greater tubercle of humerus

deltoid m

deltoid m

surgical neck of humerus

posterior circumflex humeral a

posterior circumflex humeral v

axillary n

shaft of humerus

tendon of pectoralis major m

long head of triceps m

lateral head of triceps m

lateral head of triceps m

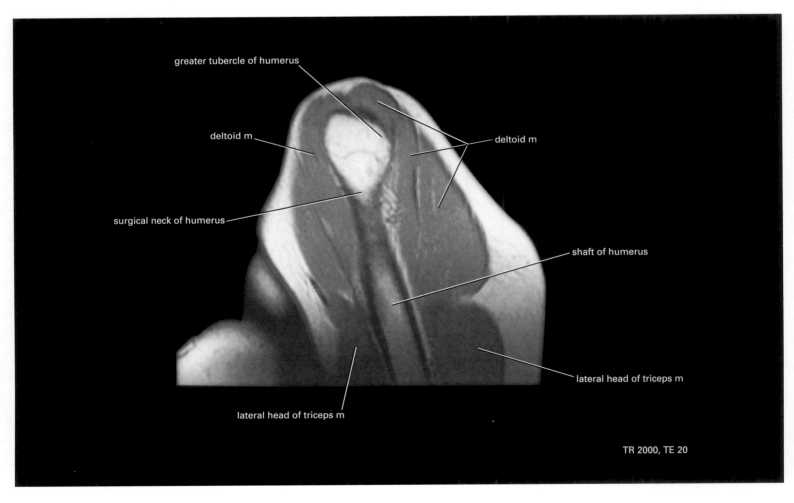

greater tubercle of humerus

deltoid m

deltoid m

surgical neck of humerus

shaft of humerus

lateral head of triceps m

lateral head of triceps m

TR 2000, TE 20

Section SS9 from midline.

The Left Shoulder in Coronal Planes

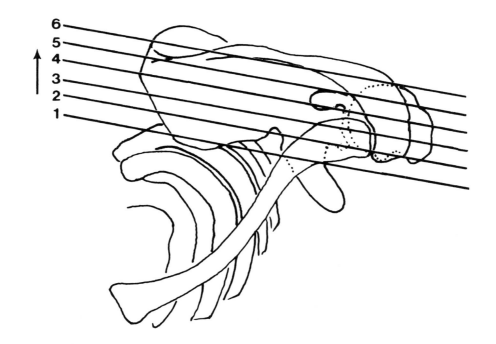

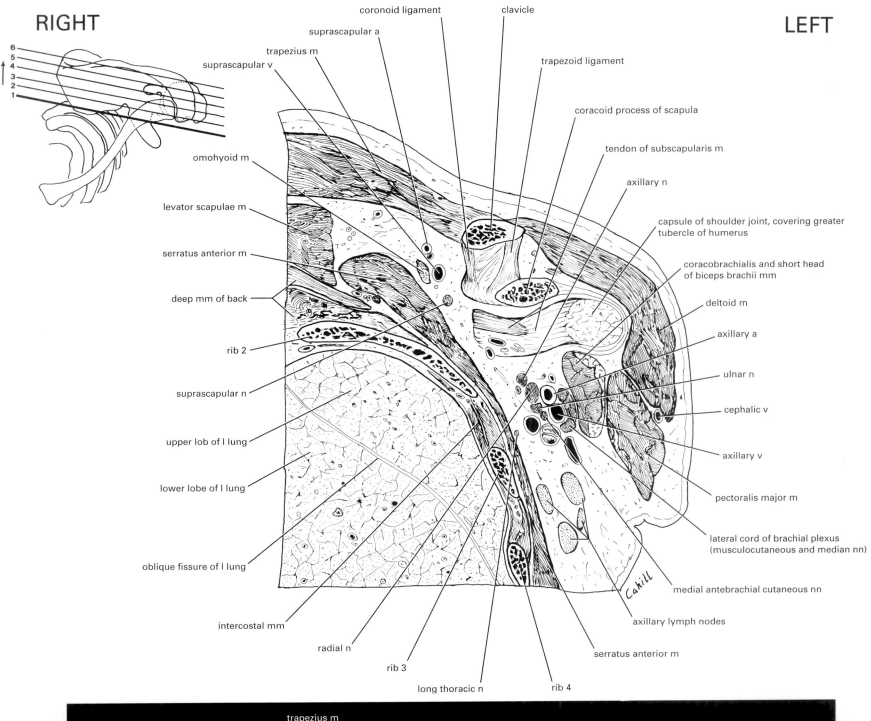

coronoid ligament

suprascapular a

clavicle

trapezius m

suprascapular v

trapezoid ligament

coracoid process of scapula

omohyoid m

tendon of subscapularis m

axillary n

levator scapulae m

capsule of shoulder joint, covering greater tubercle of humerus

serratus anterior m

coracobrachialis and short head of biceps brachii mm

deep mm of back

deltoid m

rib 2

axillary a

suprascapular n

ulnar n

cephalic v

upper lob of l lung

axillary v

lower lobe of l lung

pectoralis major m

oblique fissure of l lung

lateral cord of brachial plexus (musculocutaneous and median nn)

medial antebrachial cutaneous nn

intercostal mm

axillary lymph nodes

radial n

serratus anterior m

rib 3

long thoracic n

rib 4

Cahill

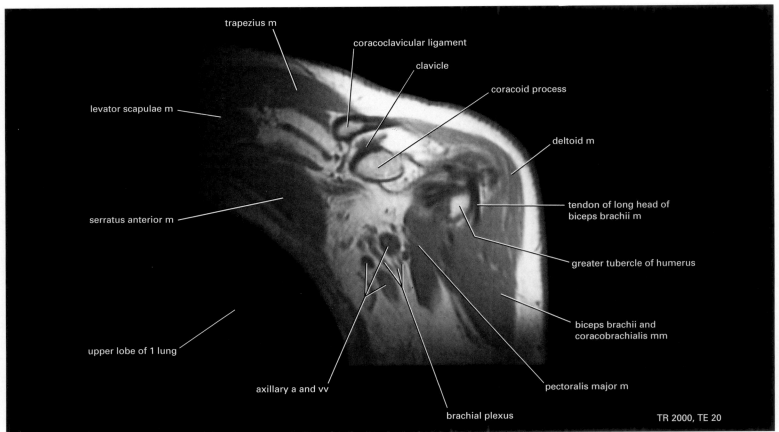

trapezius m

coracoclavicular ligament

clavicle

coracoid process

levator scapulae m

deltoid m

tendon of long head of biceps brachii m

serratus anterior m

greater tubercle of humerus

upper lobe of 1 lung

biceps brachii and coracobrachialis mm

axillary a and vv

pectoralis major m

brachial plexus

TR 2000, TE 20

Section CS1 from the front.

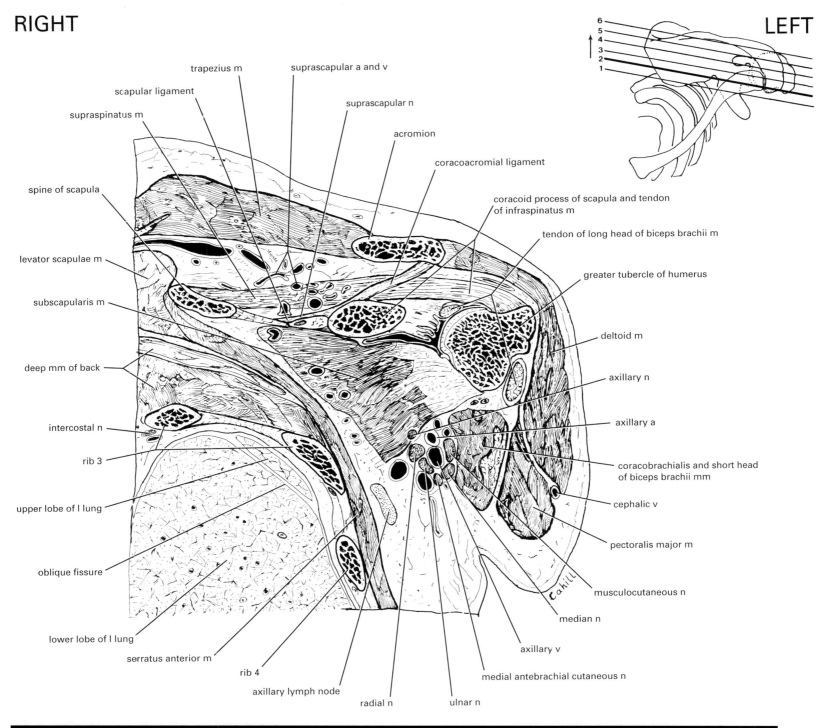

trapezius m
scapular ligament
suprascapular a and v
suprascapular n
supraspinatus m
acromion
coracoacromial ligament
spine of scapula
coracoid process of scapula and tendon of infraspinatus m
tendon of long head of biceps brachii m
levator scapulae m
greater tubercle of humerus
subscapularis m
deltoid m
deep mm of back
axillary n
axillary a
intercostal n
coracobrachialis and short head of biceps brachii mm
rib 3
cephalic v
upper lobe of l lung
pectoralis major m
oblique fissure
musculocutaneous n
median n
lower lobe of l lung
serratus anterior m
axillary v
rib 4
medial antebrachial cutaneous n
axillary lymph node
radial n
ulnar n

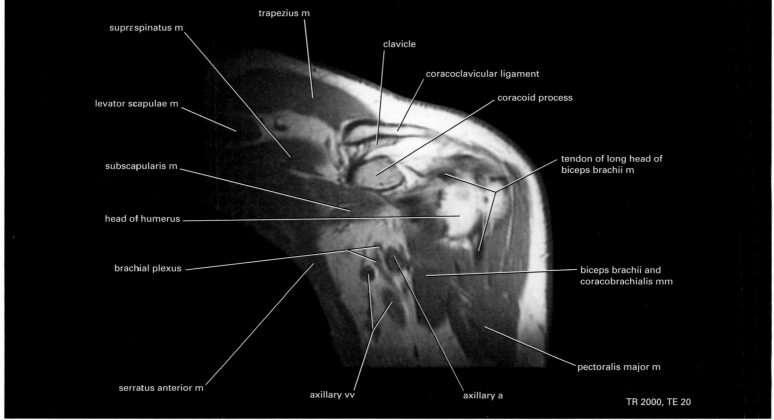

suprazspinatus m
trapezius m
clavicle
coracoclavicular ligament
levator scapulae m
coracoid process
subscapularis m
tendon of long head of biceps brachii m
head of humerus
brachial plexus
biceps brachii and coracobrachialis mm
pectoralis major m
serratus anterior m
axillary vv
axillary a
TR 2000, TE 20

Section CS2 from the front.

RIGHT   LEFT

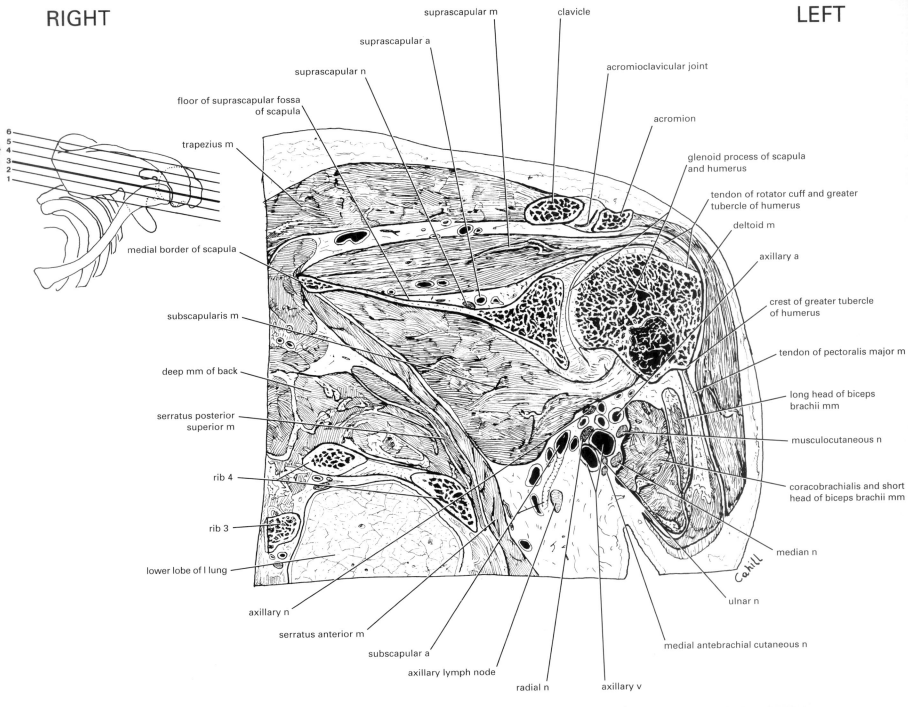

suprascapular m
clavicle
suprascapular a
suprascapular n
acromioclavicular joint
floor of suprascapular fossa
of scapula
acromion
trapezius m
glenoid process of scapula
and humerus
tendon of rotator cuff and greater
tubercle of humerus
deltoid m
medial border of scapula
axillary a
subscapularis m
crest of greater tubercle
of humerus
deep mm of back
tendon of pectoralis major m
serratus posterior
superior m
long head of biceps
brachii mm
rib 4
musculocutaneous n
rib 3
coracobrachialis and short
head of biceps brachii mm
lower lobe of l lung
median n
axillary n
ulnar n
serratus anterior m
subscapular a
medial antebrachial cutaneous n
axillary lymph node
radial n   axillary v

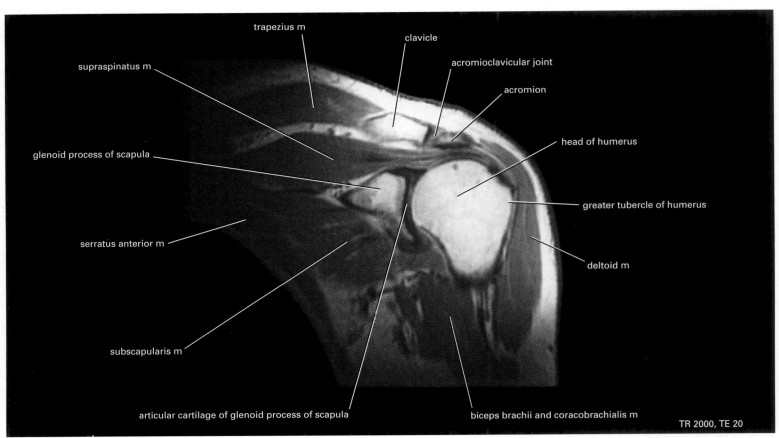

trapezius m
clavicle
supraspinatus m
acromioclavicular joint
acromion
glenoid process of scapula
head of humerus
serratus anterior m
greater tubercle of humerus
subscapularis m
deltoid m
articular cartilage of glenoid process of scapula
biceps brachii and coracobrachialis m
TR 2000, TE 20

Section CS3 from the front.

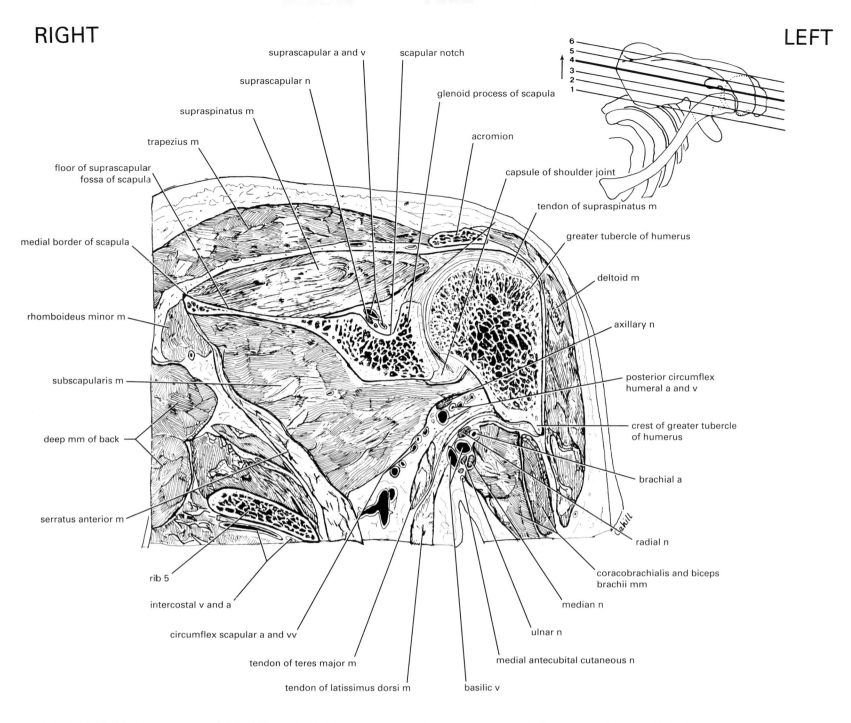

suprascapular a and v

scapular notch

suprascapular n

glenoid process of scapula

supraspinatus m

acromion

trapezius m

capsule of shoulder joint

floor of suprascapular
fossa of scapula

tendon of supraspinatus m

medial border of scapula

greater tubercle of humerus

deltoid m

rhomboideus minor m

axillary n

subscapularis m

posterior circumflex
humeral a and v

deep mm of back

crest of greater tubercle
of humerus

brachial a

serratus anterior m

radial n

rib 5

coracobrachialis and biceps
brachii mm

intercostal v and a

median n

circumflex scapular a and vv

ulnar n

tendon of teres major m

medial antecubital cutaneous n

tendon of latissimus dorsi m

basilic v

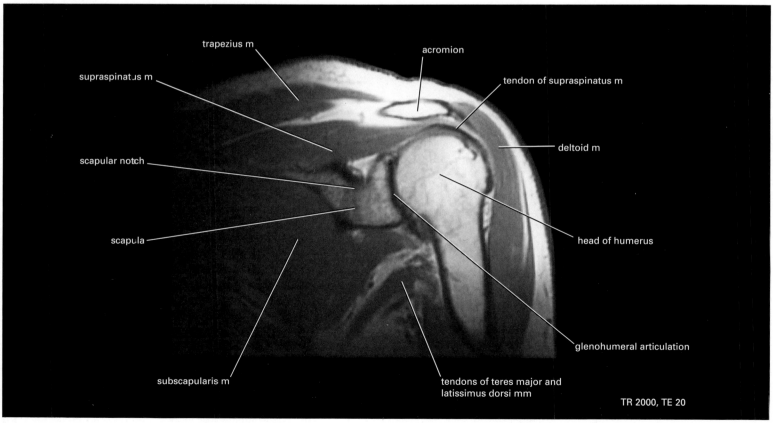

trapezius m

acromion

supraspinatus m

tendon of supraspinatus m

deltoid m

scapular notch

scapula

head of humerus

subscapularis m

glenohumeral articulation

tendons of teres major and
latissimus dorsi mm

TR 2000, TE 20

Section CS4 from the front.

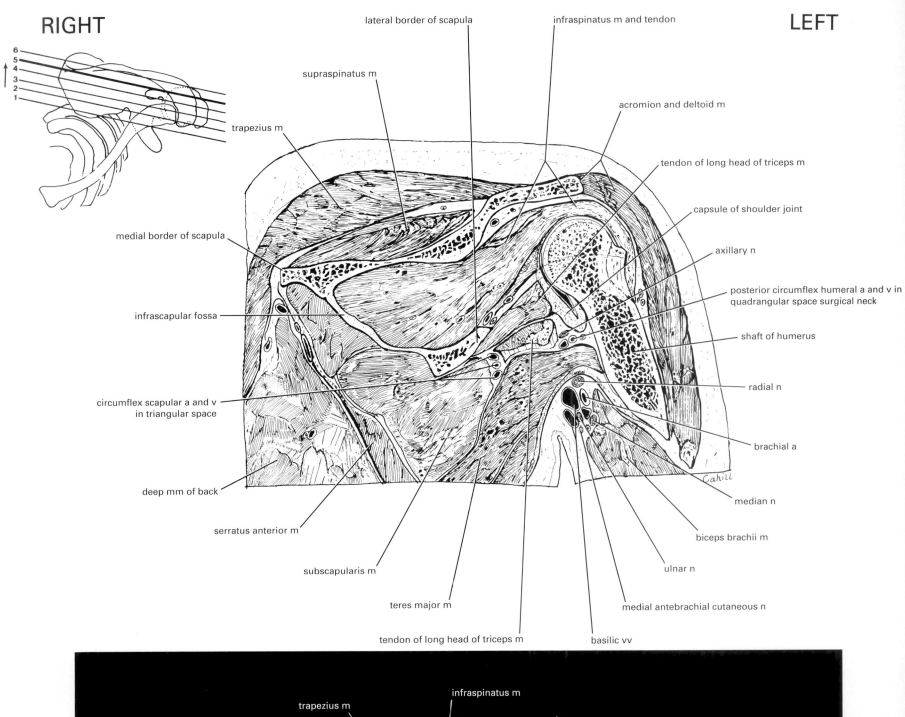

lateral border of scapula

infraspinatus m and tendon

supraspinatus m

acromion and deltoid m

trapezius m

tendon of long head of triceps m

capsule of shoulder joint

medial border of scapula

axillary n

posterior circumflex humeral a and v in
quadrangular space surgical neck

infrascapular fossa

shaft of humerus

radial n

circumflex scapular a and v
in triangular space

brachial a

deep mm of back

median n

biceps brachii m

serratus anterior m

ulnar n

subscapularis m

medial antebrachial cutaneous n

teres major m

basilic vv

tendon of long head of triceps m

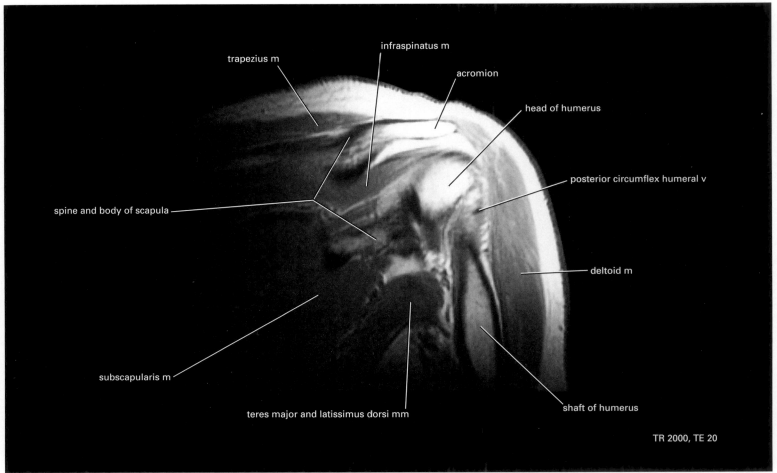

infraspinatus m

trapezius m

acromion

head of humerus

spine and body of scapula

posterior circumflex humeral v

deltoid m

subscapularis m

shaft of humerus

teres major and latissimus dorsi mm

TR 2000, TE 20

Section CS5 from the front.

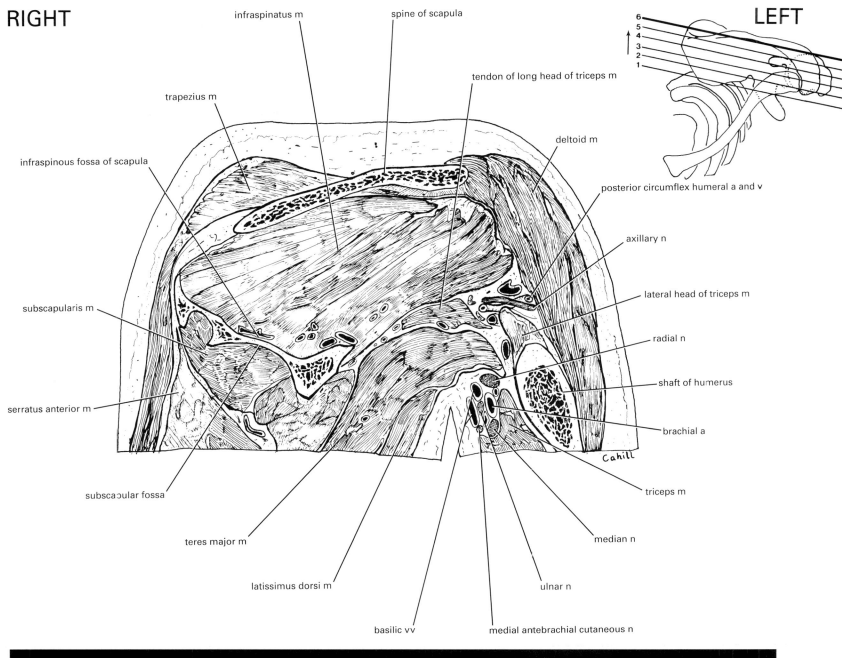

infraspinatus m

spine of scapula

tendon of long head of triceps m

trapezius m

deltoid m

infraspinous fossa of scapula

posterior circumflex humeral a and v

axillary n

lateral head of triceps m

subscapularis m

radial n

shaft of humerus

serratus anterior m

brachial a

triceps m

subscapular fossa

median n

teres major m

latissimus dorsi m

ulnar n

basilic vv

medial antebrachial cutaneous n

Cahill

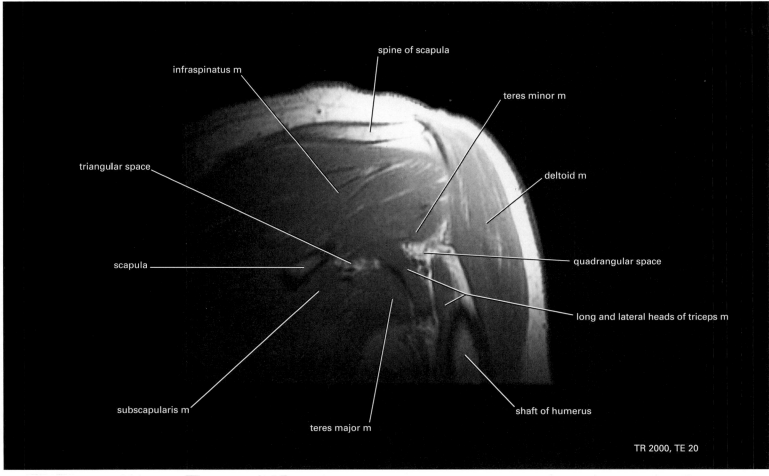

infraspinatus m

spine of scapula

teres minor m

triangular space

deltoid m

scapula

quadrangular space

long and lateral heads of triceps m

subscapularis m

teres major m

shaft of humerus

TR 2000, TE 20

Section CS6 from the front.

The Head 20° From Orbitomeatal Plane

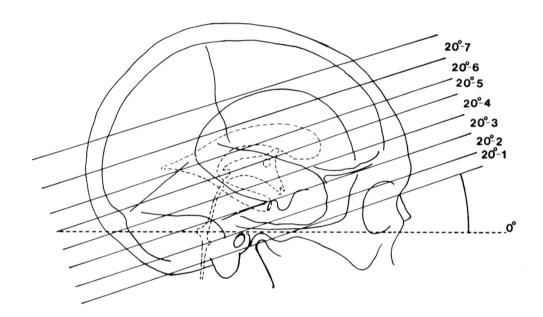

20°-7
20°-6
20°-5
20°-4
20°-3
20°-2
20°-1

0°

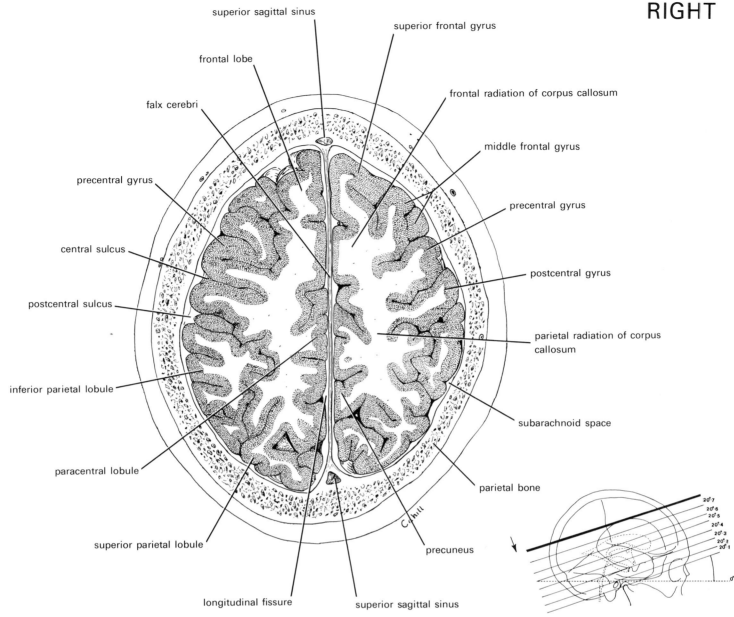

superior sagittal sinus

superior frontal gyrus

frontal lobe

falx cerebri

frontal radiation of corpus callosum

middle frontal gyrus

precentral gyrus

precentral gyrus

central sulcus

postcentral gyrus

postcentral sulcus

parietal radiation of corpus callosum

inferior parietal lobule

subarachnoid space

paracentral lobule

parietal bone

superior parietal lobule

precuneus

longitudinal fissure

superior sagittal sinus

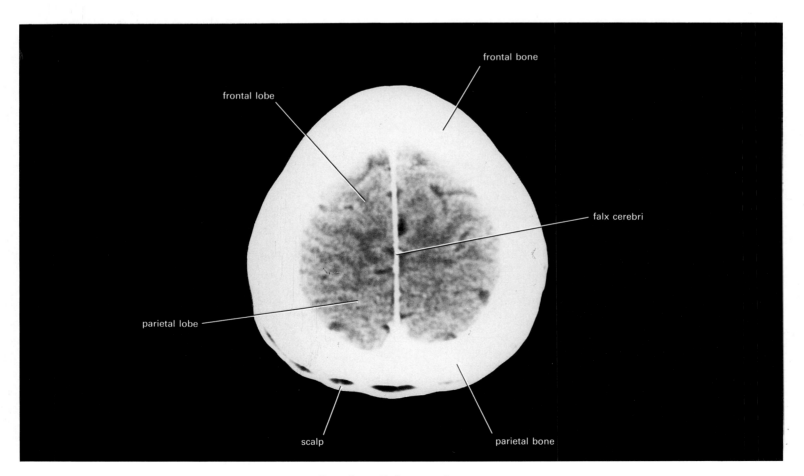

frontal bone

frontal lobe

falx cerebri

parietal lobe

scalp

parietal bone

Section 7 from above.

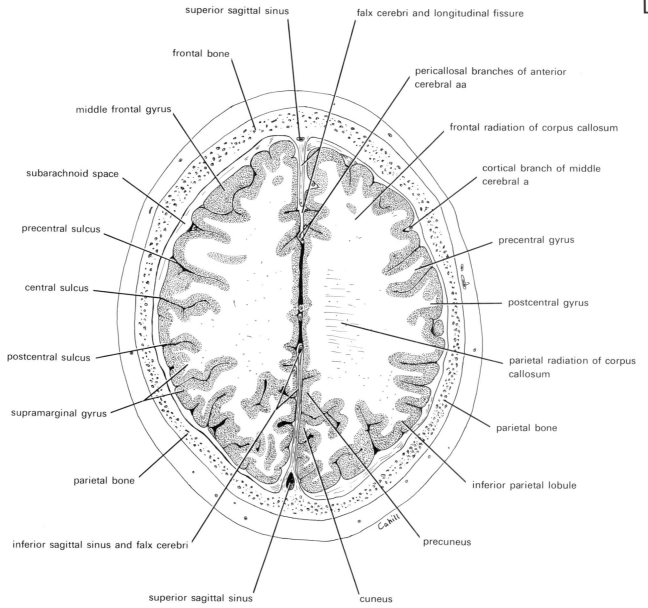

superior sagittal sinus

falx cerebri and longitudinal fissure

frontal bone

pericallosal branches of anterior cerebral aa

middle frontal gyrus

frontal radiation of corpus callosum

subarachnoid space

cortical branch of middle cerebral a

precentral sulcus

precentral gyrus

central sulcus

postcentral gyrus

postcentral sulcus

parietal radiation of corpus callosum

supramarginal gyrus

parietal bone

parietal bone

inferior parietal lobule

inferior sagittal sinus and falx cerebri

precuneus

superior sagittal sinus

cuneus

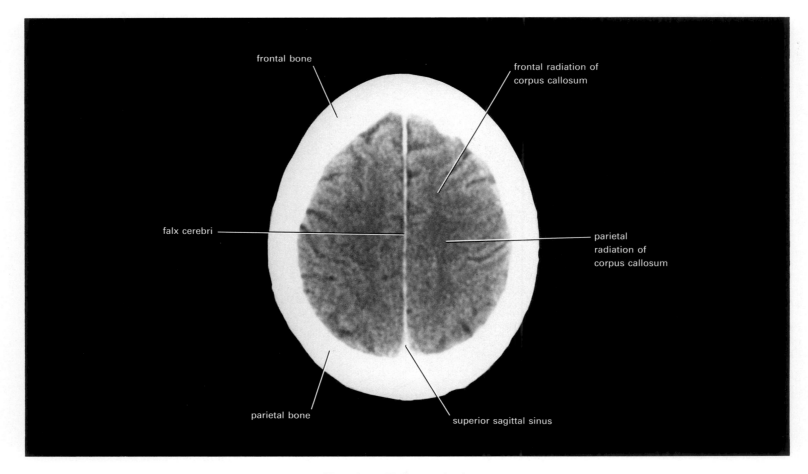

frontal bone

frontal radiation of corpus callosum

falx cerebri

parietal radiation of corpus callosum

parietal bone

superior sagittal sinus

Section 7 from below.

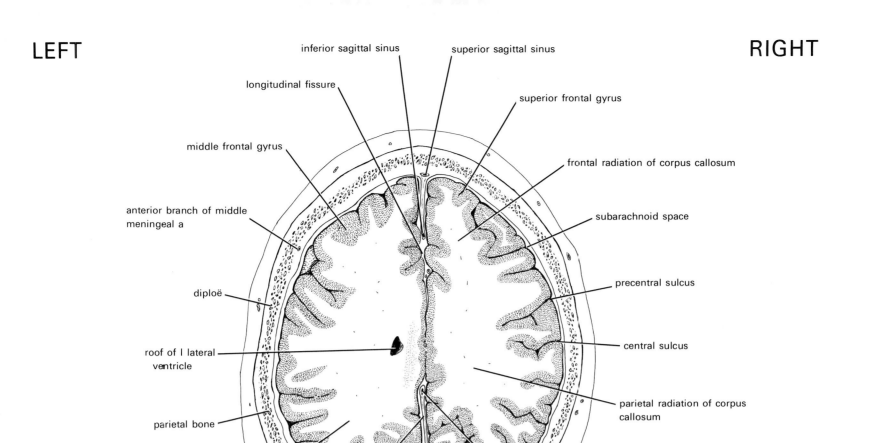

inferior sagittal sinus
superior sagittal sinus
longitudinal fissure
superior frontal gyrus
middle frontal gyrus
frontal radiation of corpus callosum
anterior branch of middle meningeal a
subarachnoid space
diploë
precentral sulcus
roof of l lateral ventricle
central sulcus
parietal bone
parietal radiation of corpus callosum
occipital raciation of corpus callosum
parietal bone
inferior sagittal sinus
falx cerebri
occipital lobe
parietooccipital sulcus
superior sagittal sinus
longitudinal fissure

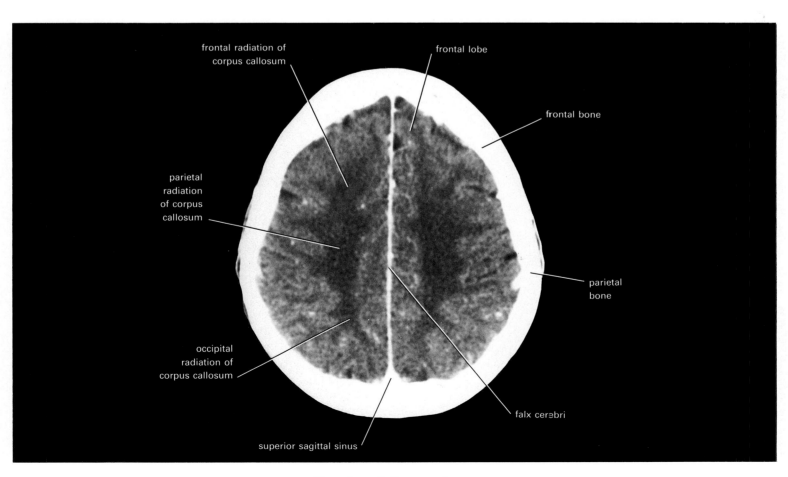

frontal radiation of corpus callosum
frontal lobe
frontal bone
parietal radiation of corpus callosum
occipital radiation of corpus callosum
parietal bone
falx cerebri
superior sagittal sinus

Section 6 from above.

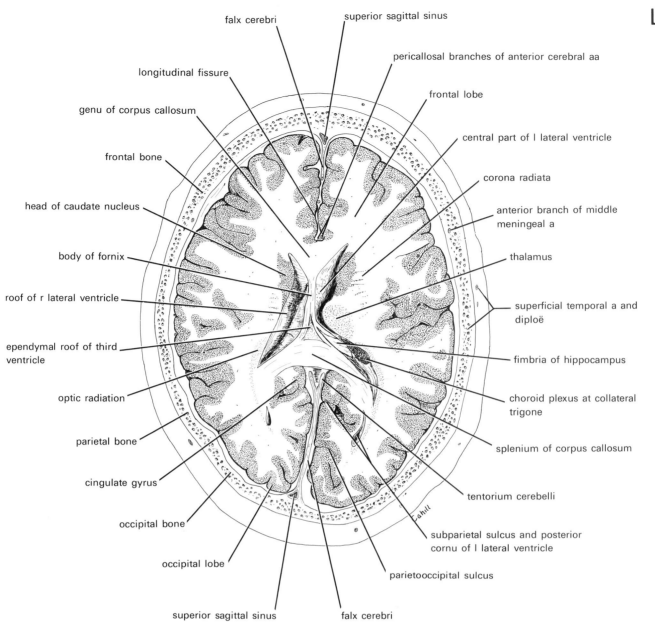

falx cerebri

superior sagittal sinus

pericallosal branches of anterior cerebral aa

longitudinal fissure

frontal lobe

genu of corpus callosum

central part of l lateral ventricle

frontal bone

corona radiata

head of caudate nucleus

anterior branch of middle meningeal a

body of fornix

thalamus

roof of r lateral ventricle

superficial temporal a and diploë

ependymal roof of third ventricle

fimbria of hippocampus

optic radiation

choroid plexus at collateral trigone

parietal bone

cingulate gyrus

splenium of corpus callosum

occipital bone

tentorium cerebelli

occipital lobe

subparietal sulcus and posterior cornu of l lateral ventricle

superior sagittal sinus

parietooccipital sulcus

falx cerebri

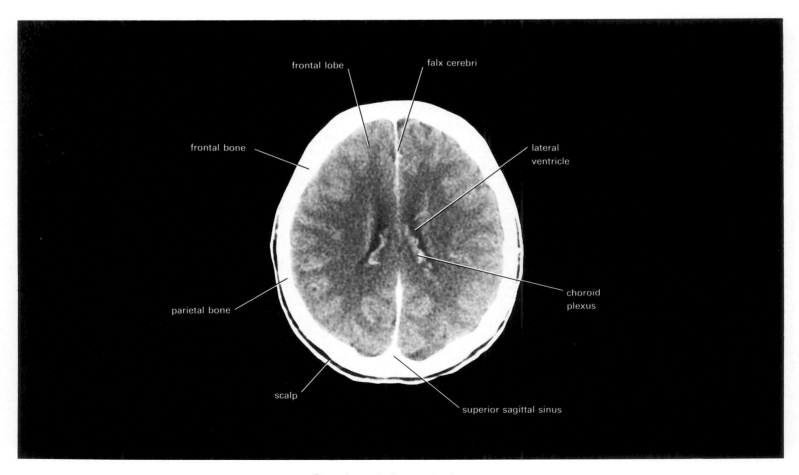

frontal lobe

falx cerebri

frontal bone

lateral ventricle

parietal bone

choroid plexus

scalp

superior sagittal sinus

Section 6 from below.

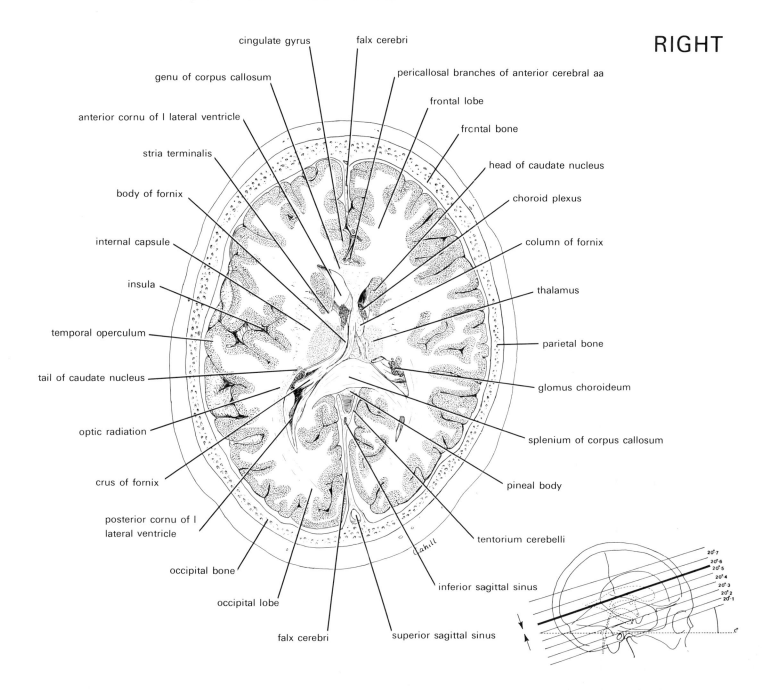

LEFT RIGHT

cingulate gyrus

falx cerebri

genu of corpus callosum

pericallosal branches of anterior cerebral aa

anterior cornu of l lateral ventricle

frontal lobe

frontal bone

stria terminalis

head of caudate nucleus

body of fornix

choroid plexus

internal capsule

column of fornix

insula

thalamus

temporal operculum

parietal bone

tail of caudate nucleus

glomus choroideum

optic radiation

splenium of corpus callosum

crus of fornix

pineal body

posterior cornu of l lateral ventricle

tentorium cerebelli

occipital bone

inferior sagittal sinus

occipital lobe

falx cerebri

superior sagittal sinus

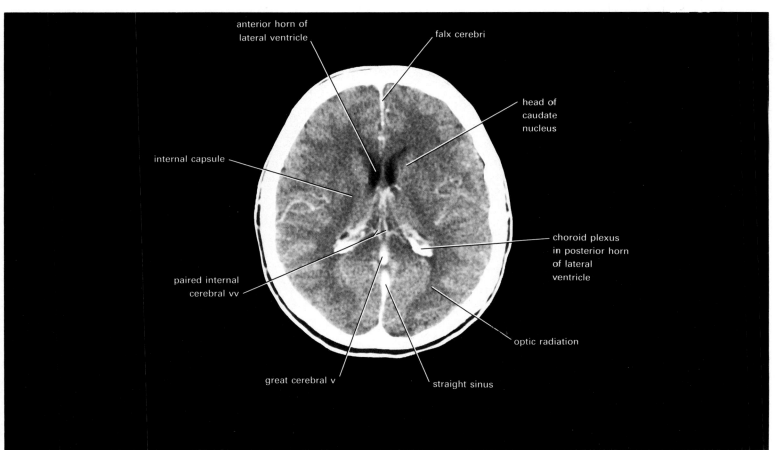

anterior horn of lateral ventricle

falx cerebri

head of caudate nucleus

internal capsule

choroid plexus in posterior horn of lateral ventricle

paired internal cerebral vv

optic radiation

great cerebral v

straight sinus

Section 5 from above.

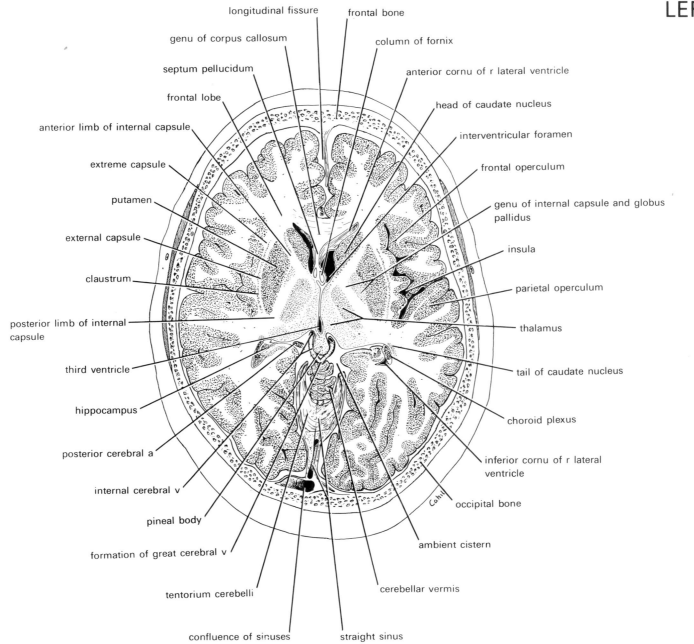

longitudinal fissure
frontal bone
genu of corpus callosum
column of fornix
septum pellucidum
anterior cornu of r lateral ventricle
frontal lobe
head of caudate nucleus
anterior limb of internal capsule
interventricular foramen
extreme capsule
frontal operculum
putamen
genu of internal capsule and globus pallidus
external capsule
insula
claustrum
parietal operculum
posterior limb of internal capsule
thalamus
third ventricle
tail of caudate nucleus
hippocampus
choroid plexus
posterior cerebral a
inferior cornu of r lateral ventricle
internal cerebral v
occipital bone
pineal body
formation of great cerebral v
ambient cistern
tentorium cerebelli
cerebellar vermis
confluence of sinuses
straight sinus

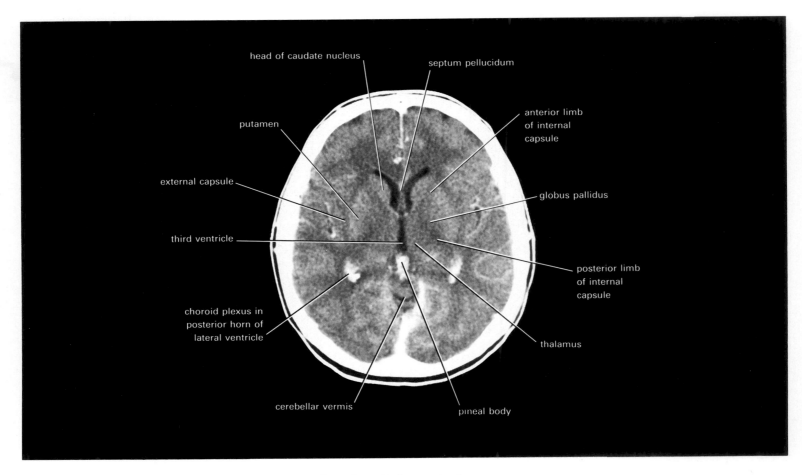

head of caudate nucleus
septum pellucidum
putamen
anterior limb of internal capsule
external capsule
globus pallidus
third ventricle
posterior limb of internal capsule
choroid plexus in posterior horn of lateral ventricle
thalamus
cerebellar vermis
pineal body

Section 5 from below.

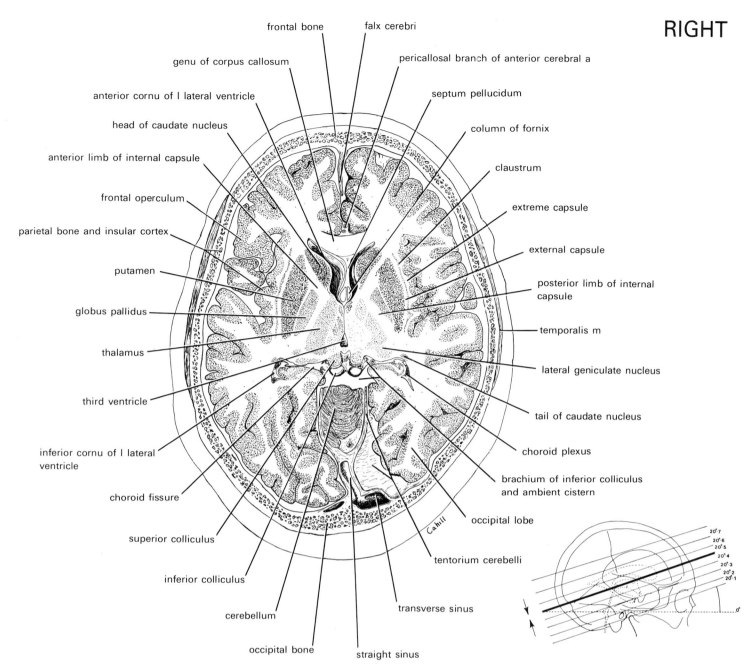

frontal bone
falx cerebri
genu of corpus callosum
pericallosal branch of anterior cerebral a
anterior cornu of I lateral ventricle
septum pellucidum
head of caudate nucleus
column of fornix
anterior limb of internal capsule
claustrum
frontal operculum
extreme capsule
parietal bone and insular cortex
external capsule
putamen
posterior limb of internal capsule
globus pallidus
temporalis m
thalamus
lateral geniculate nucleus
third ventricle
tail of caudate nucleus
inferior cornu of I lateral ventricle
choroid plexus
choroid fissure
brachium of inferior colliculus and ambient cistern
superior colliculus
occipital lobe
inferior colliculus
tentorium cerebelli
cerebellum
transverse sinus
occipital bone
straight sinus

Cahill

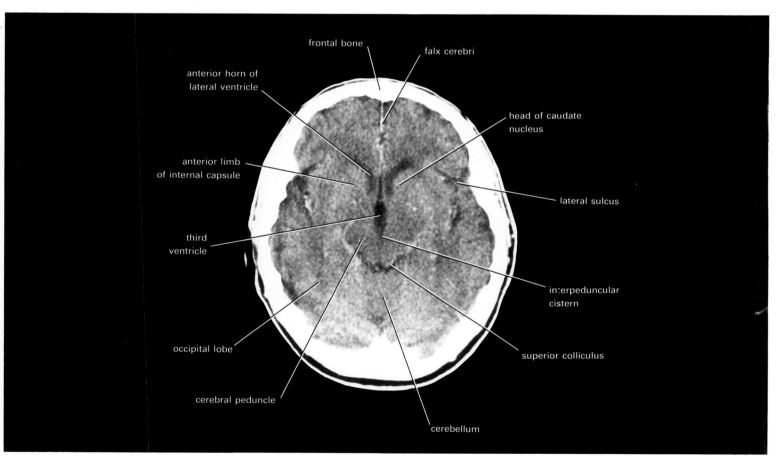

frontal bone
falx cerebri
anterior horn of lateral ventricle
head of caudate nucleus
anterior limb of internal capsule
lateral sulcus
third ventricle
interpeduncular cistern
occipital lobe
superior colliculus
cerebral peduncle
cerebellum

Section 4 from above.

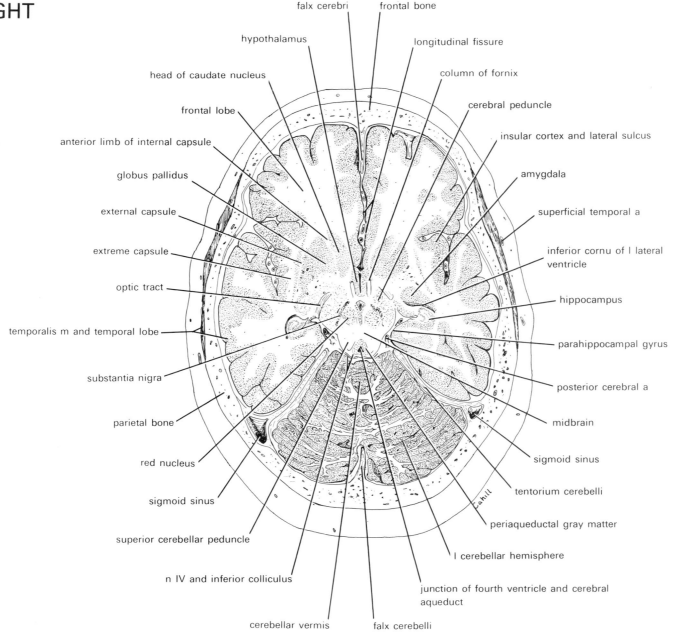

falx cerebri | frontal bone
hypothalamus | longitudinal fissure
head of caudate nucleus | column of fornix
frontal lobe | cerebral peduncle
anterior limb of internal capsule | insular cortex and lateral sulcus
globus pallidus | amygdala
external capsule | superficial temporal a
extreme capsule | inferior cornu of l lateral ventricle
optic tract | hippocampus
temporalis m and temporal lobe | parahippocampal gyrus
substantia nigra | posterior cerebral a
parietal bone | midbrain
red nucleus | sigmoid sinus
sigmoid sinus | tentorium cerebelli
superior cerebellar peduncle | periaqueductal gray matter
n IV and inferior colliculus | l cerebellar hemisphere
cerebellar vermis | junction of fourth ventricle and cerebral aqueduct
falx cerebelli

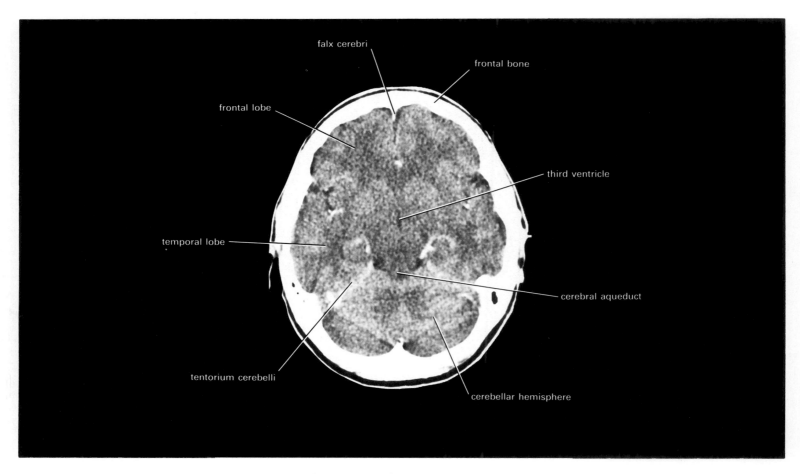

falx cerebri
frontal bone
frontal lobe
third ventricle
temporal lobe
cerebral aqueduct
tentorium cerebelli
cerebellar hemisphere

Section 4 from below.

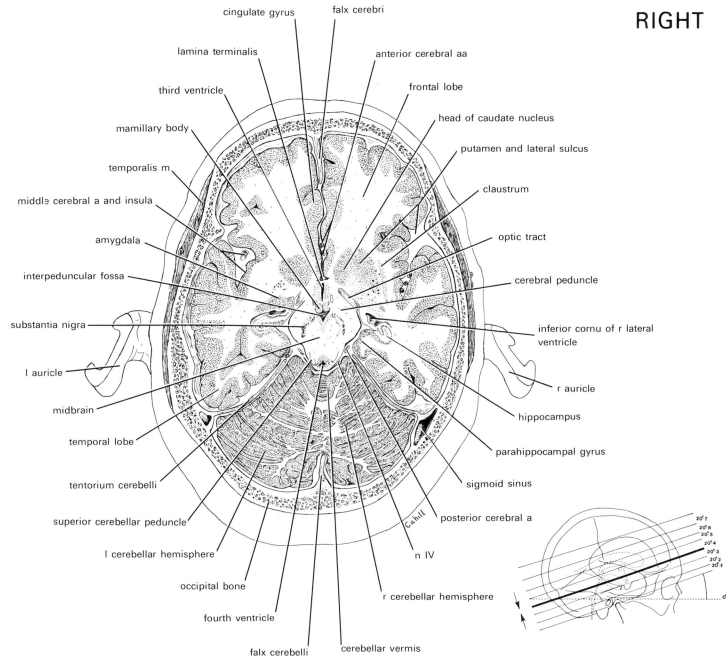

cingulate gyrus

falx cerebri

lamina terminalis

anterior cerebral aa

third ventricle

frontal lobe

mamillary body

head of caudate nucleus

temporalis m

putamen and lateral sulcus

middle cerebral a and insula

claustrum

amygdala

optic tract

interpeduncular fossa

cerebral peduncle

substantia nigra

inferior cornu of r lateral ventricle

l auricle

r auricle

midbrain

hippocampus

temporal lobe

parahippocampal gyrus

tentorium cerebelli

sigmoid sinus

superior cerebellar peduncle

posterior cerebral a

l cerebellar hemisphere

n IV

occipital bone

r cerebellar hemisphere

fourth ventricle

falx cerebelli

cerebellar vermis

Cahill

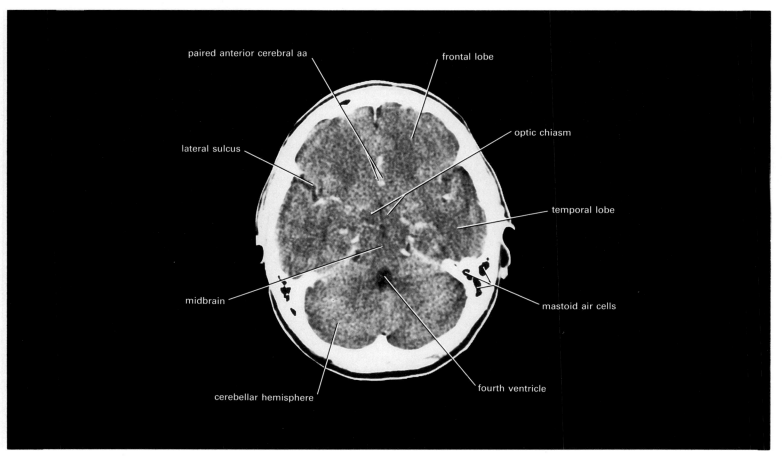

paired anterior cerebral aa

frontal lobe

lateral sulcus

optic chiasm

temporal lobe

midbrain

mastoid air cells

cerebellar hemisphere

fourth ventricle

Section 3 from above.

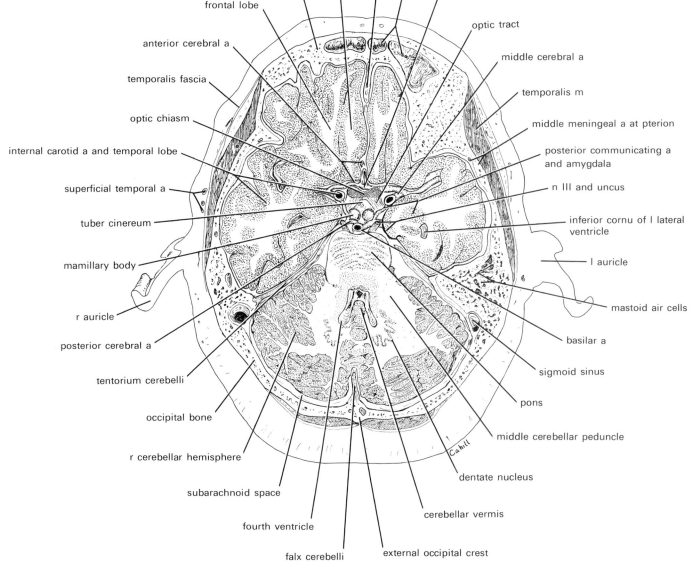

gyrus rectus
falx cerebri
frontal bone
frontal sinus
anterior communicating a
frontal lobe
optic tract
anterior cerebral a
middle cerebral a
temporalis fascia
temporalis m
optic chiasm
middle meningeal a at pterion
internal carotid a and temporal lobe
posterior communicating a and amygdala
superficial temporal a
n III and uncus
tuber cinereum
inferior cornu of l lateral ventricle
mamillary body
l auricle
r auricle
mastoid air cells
posterior cerebral a
basilar a
tentorium cerebelli
sigmoid sinus
occipital bone
pons
r cerebellar hemisphere
middle cerebellar peduncle
subarachnoid space
dentate nucleus
fourth ventricle
cerebellar vermis
falx cerebelli
external occipital crest

Cahill

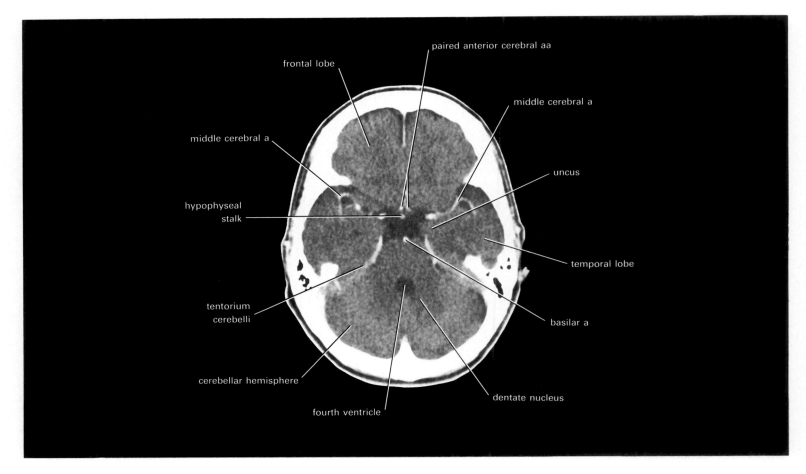

frontal lobe
paired anterior cerebral aa
middle cerebral a
middle cerebral a
uncus
hypophyseal stalk
temporal lobe
tentorium cerebelli
basilar a
cerebellar hemisphere
dentate nucleus
fourth ventricle

Section 3 from below.

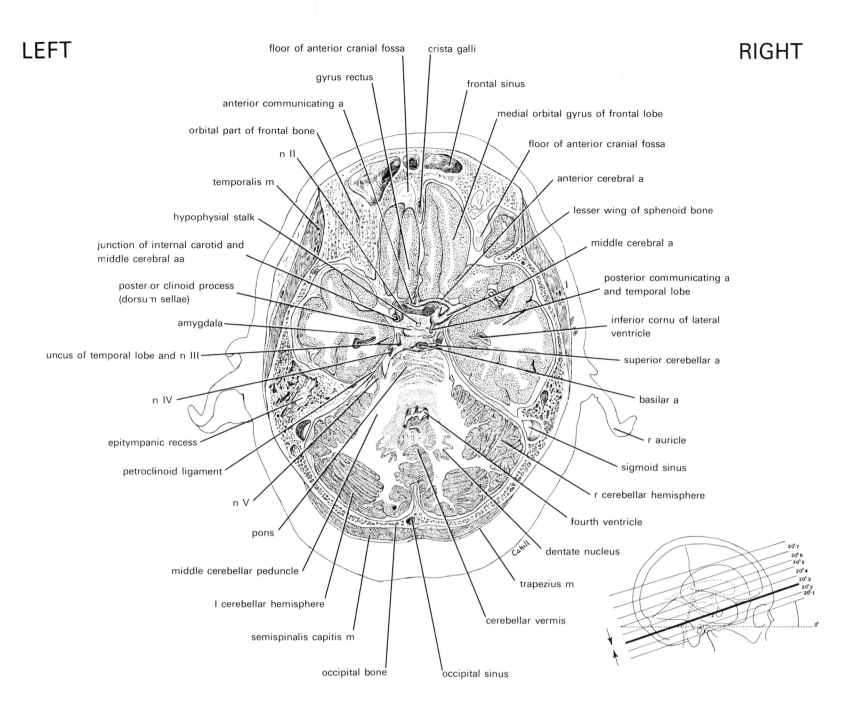

floor of anterior cranial fossa
crista galli
gyrus rectus
frontal sinus
anterior communicating a
medial orbital gyrus of frontal lobe
orbital part of frontal bone
floor of anterior cranial fossa
n II
temporalis m
anterior cerebral a
hypophysial stalk
lesser wing of sphenoid bone
junction of internal carotid and middle cerebral aa
middle cerebral a
posterior clinoid process (dorsum sellae)
posterior communicating a and temporal lobe
amygdala
inferior cornu of lateral ventricle
uncus of temporal lobe and n III
superior cerebellar a
n IV
basilar a
epitympanic recess
r auricle
petroclinoid ligament
sigmoid sinus
n V
r cerebellar hemisphere
pons
fourth ventricle
middle cerebellar peduncle
Cahill
dentate nucleus
l cerebellar hemisphere
trapezius m
semispinalis capitis m
cerebellar vermis
occipital bone
occipital sinus

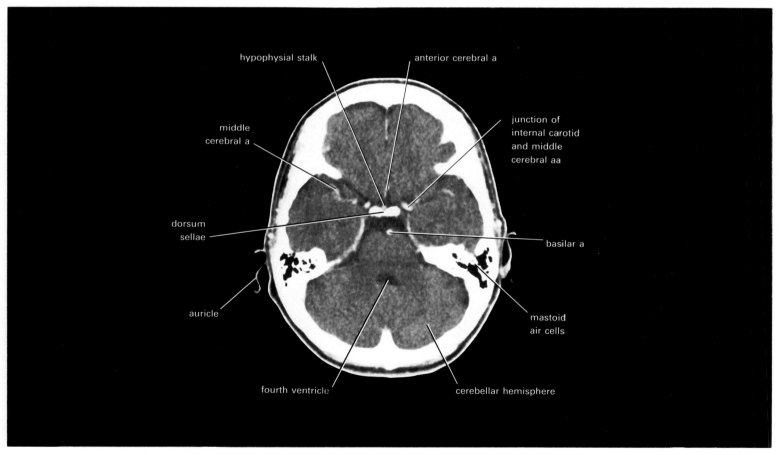

hypophysial stalk
anterior cerebral a
middle cerebral a
junction of internal carotid and middle cerebral aa
dorsum sellae
basilar a
auricle
mastoid air cells
fourth ventricle
cerebellar hemisphere

Section 2 from above.

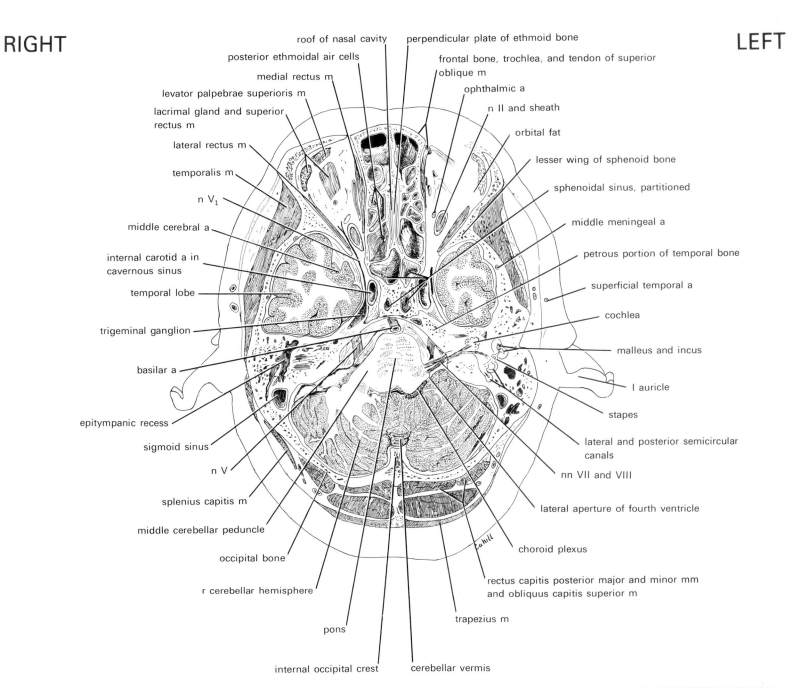

roof of nasal cavity
perpendicular plate of ethmoid bone
posterior ethmoidal air cells
frontal bone, trochlea, and tendon of superior oblique m
medial rectus m
ophthalmic a
levator palpebrae superioris m
n II and sheath
lacrimal gland and superior rectus m
orbital fat
lateral rectus m
lesser wing of sphenoid bone
temporalis m
sphenoidal sinus, partitioned
n V₁
middle meningeal a
middle cerebral a
petrous portion of temporal bone
internal carotid a in cavernous sinus
superficial temporal a
temporal lobe
cochlea
trigeminal ganglion
malleus and incus
basilar a
l auricle
epitympanic recess
stapes
sigmoid sinus
lateral and posterior semicircular canals
n V
nn VII and VIII
splenius capitis m
lateral aperture of fourth ventricle
middle cerebellar peduncle
choroid plexus
occipital bone
rectus capitis posterior major and minor mm and obliquus capitis superior m
r cerebellar hemisphere
trapezius m
pons
internal occipital crest   cerebellar vermis

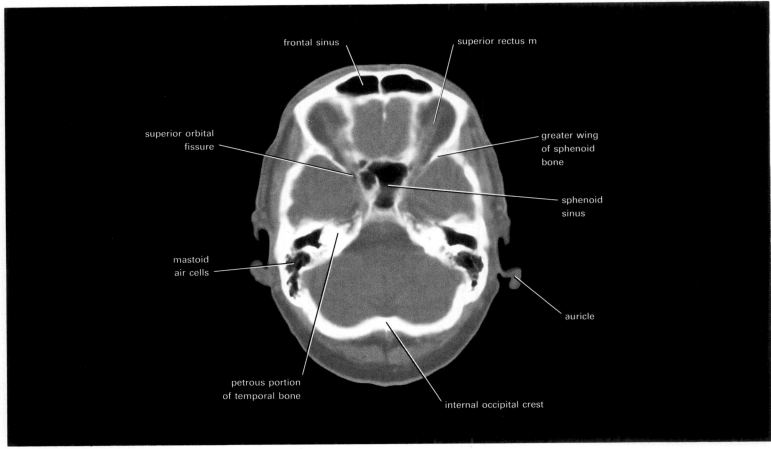

frontal sinus
superior rectus m
superior orbital fissure
greater wing of sphenoid bone
sphenoid sinus
mastoid air cells
petrous portion of temporal bone
auricle
internal occipital crest

Section 2 from below.

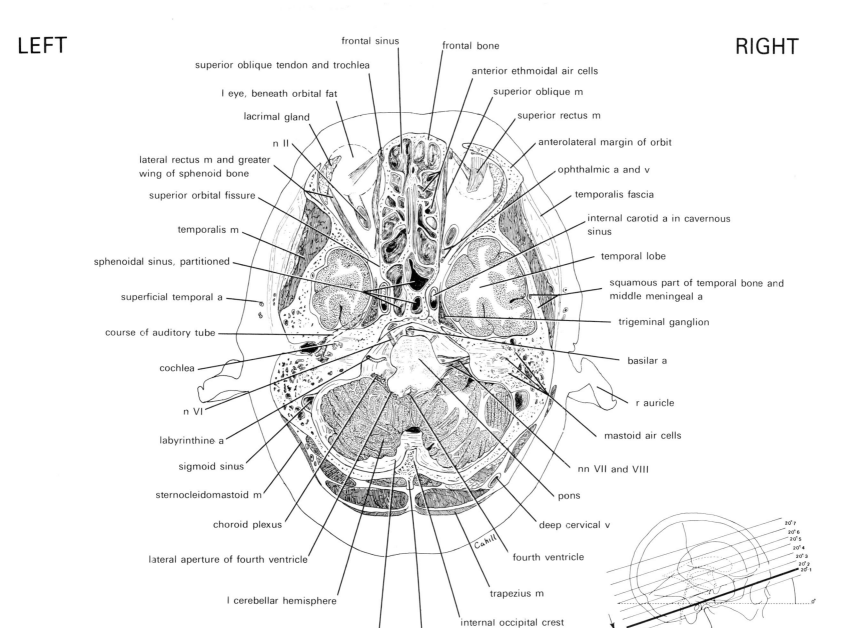

frontal sinus
frontal bone
superior oblique tendon and trochlea
anterior ethmoidal air cells
l eye, beneath orbital fat
superior oblique m
lacrimal gland
superior rectus m
n II
anterolateral margin of orbit
lateral rectus m and greater wing of sphenoid bone
ophthalmic a and v
superior orbital fissure
temporalis fascia
temporalis m
internal carotid a in cavernous sinus
sphenoidal sinus, partitioned
temporal lobe
superficial temporal a
squamous part of temporal bone and middle meningeal a
course of auditory tube
trigeminal ganglion
cochlea
basilar a
n VI
r auricle
labyrinthine a
mastoid air cells
sigmoid sinus
nn VII and VIII
sternocleidomastoid m
pons
choroid plexus
deep cervical v
lateral aperture of fourth ventricle
fourth ventricle
l cerebellar hemisphere
trapezius m
internal occipital crest
floor of posterior cranial fossa
external occipital crest
Cahill

20ʹ7
20ʹ6
20ʹ5
20ʹ4
20ʹ3
20ʹ2
20ʹ1
0ʹ

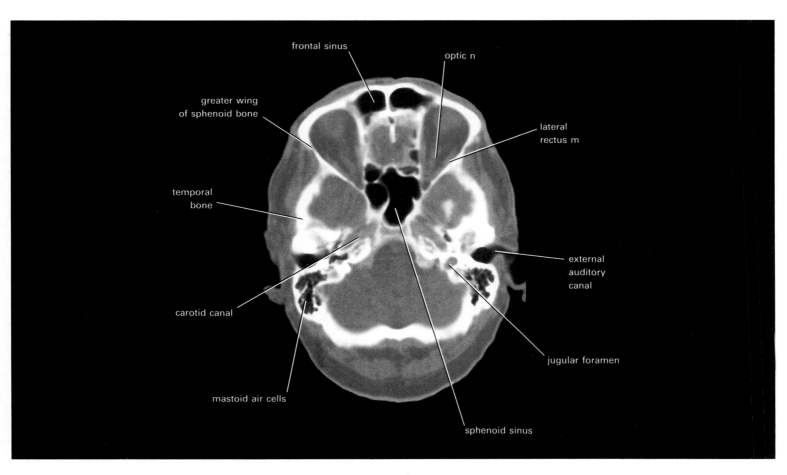

frontal sinus
optic n
greater wing of sphenoid bone
lateral rectus m
temporal bone
external auditory canal
carotid canal
jugular foramen
mastoid air cells
sphenoid sinus

Section 1 from above.

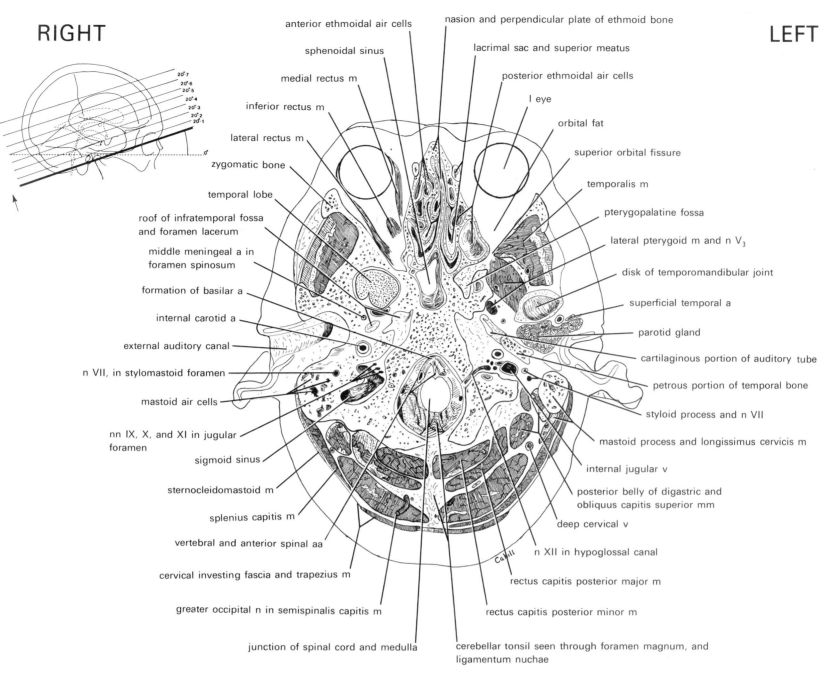

anterior ethmoidal air cells
nasion and perpendicular plate of ethmoid bone
sphenoidal sinus
lacrimal sac and superior meatus
medial rectus m
posterior ethmoidal air cells
inferior rectus m
l eye
lateral rectus m
orbital fat
zygomatic bone
superior orbital fissure
temporal lobe
temporalis m
roof of infratemporal fossa
and foramen lacerum
pterygopalatine fossa
middle meningeal a in
foramen spinosum
lateral pterygoid m and n V$_3$
formation of basilar a
disk of temporomandibular joint
internal carotid a
superficial temporal a
external auditory canal
parotid gland
n VII, in stylomastoid foramen
cartilaginous portion of auditory tube
mastoid air cells
petrous portion of temporal bone
nn IX, X, and XI in jugular
foramen
styloid process and n VII
sigmoid sinus
mastoid process and longissimus cervicis m
sternocleidomastoid m
internal jugular v
splenius capitis m
posterior belly of digastric and
obliquus capitis superior mm
vertebral and anterior spinal aa
deep cervical v
cervical investing fascia and trapezius m
n XII in hypoglossal canal
greater occipital n in semispinalis capitis m
rectus capitis posterior major m
rectus capitis posterior minor m
junction of spinal cord and medulla
cerebellar tonsil seen through foramen magnum, and
ligamentum nuchae

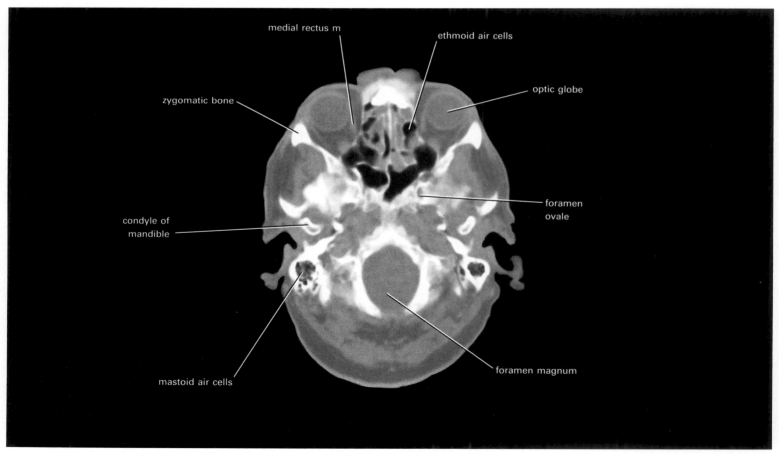

medial rectus m
ethmoid air cells
zygomatic bone
optic globe
condyle of
mandible
foramen
ovale
mastoid air cells
foramen magnum

Section 1 from below.

The Head and Neck 0° From Orbitomeatal Plane

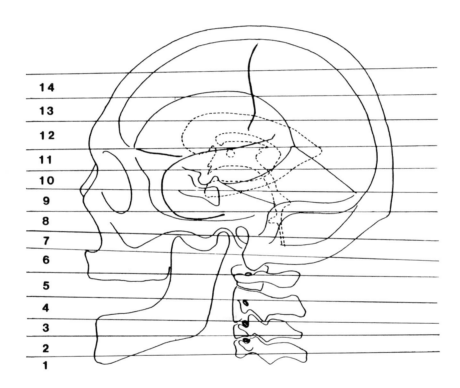

LEFT

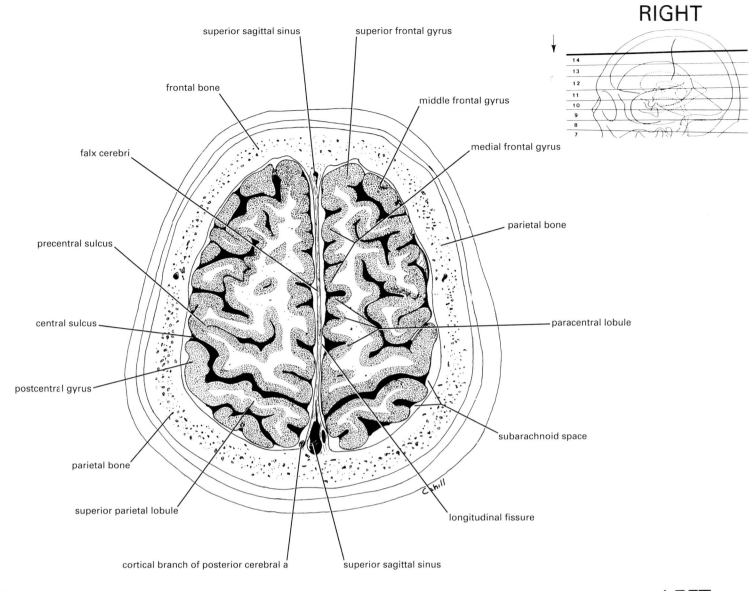

superior sagittal sinus

superior frontal gyrus

frontal bone

middle frontal gyrus

falx cerebri

medial frontal gyrus

parietal bone

precentral sulcus

central sulcus

paracentral lobule

postcentral gyrus

subarachnoid space

parietal bone

superior parietal lobule

longitudinal fissure

cortical branch of posterior cerebral a

superior sagittal sinus

RIGHT   LEFT

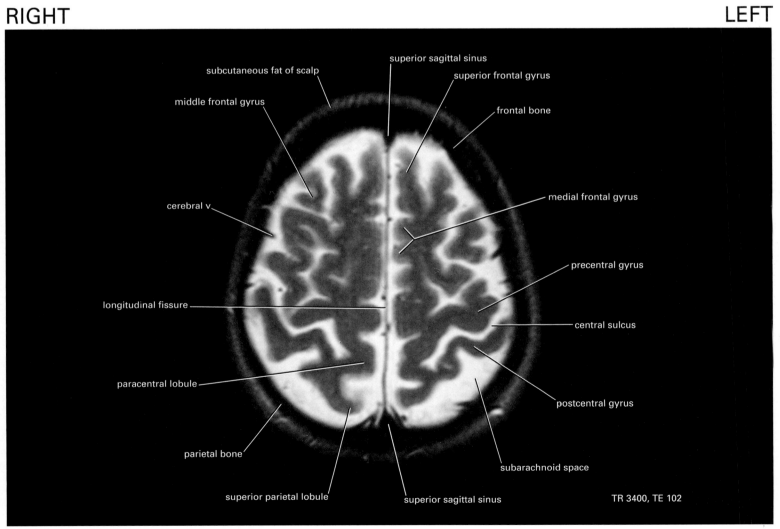

subcutaneous fat of scalp

superior sagittal sinus

superior frontal gyrus

middle frontal gyrus

frontal bone

cerebral v

medial frontal gyrus

precentral gyrus

longitudinal fissure

central sulcus

paracentral lobule

postcentral gyrus

parietal bone

subarachnoid space

superior parietal lobule

superior sagittal sinus

TR 3400, TE 102

Section 14, anatomy from above, MR image from below.

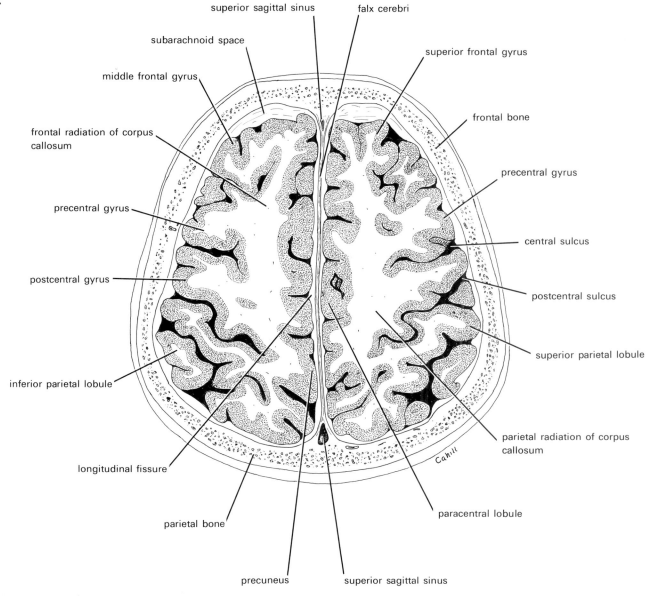

superior sagittal sinus

falx cerebri

subarachnoid space

superior frontal gyrus

middle frontal gyrus

frontal bone

frontal radiation of corpus callosum

precentral gyrus

precentral gyrus

central sulcus

postcentral gyrus

postcentral sulcus

superior parietal lobule

inferior parietal lobule

parietal radiation of corpus callosum

longitudinal fissure

paracentral lobule

parietal bone

precuneus

superior sagittal sinus

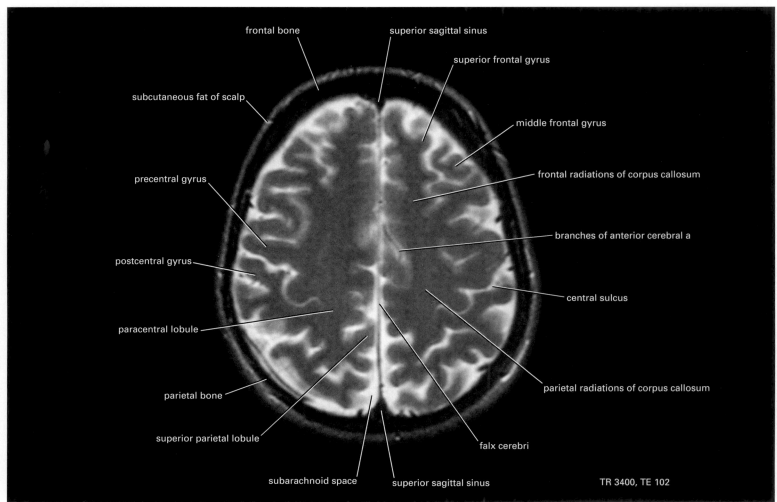

frontal bone

superior sagittal sinus

subcutaneous fat of scalp

superior frontal gyrus

middle frontal gyrus

precentral gyrus

frontal radiations of corpus callosum

branches of anterior cerebral a

postcentral gyrus

central sulcus

paracentral lobule

parietal radiations of corpus callosum

parietal bone

superior parietal lobule

falx cerebri

subarachnoid space

superior sagittal sinus

TR 3400, TE 102

Section 14 from below.

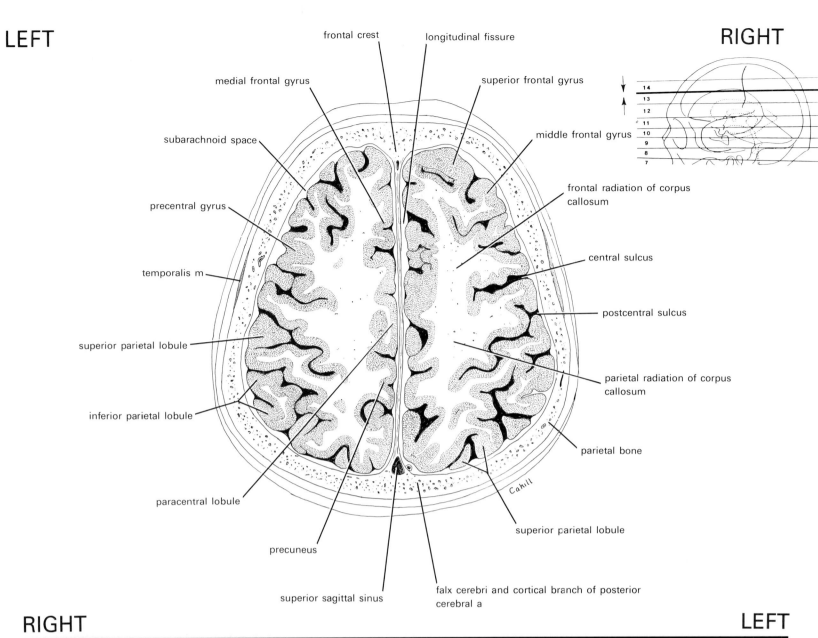

frontal crest

longitudinal fissure

medial frontal gyrus

superior frontal gyrus

subarachnoid space

middle frontal gyrus

frontal radiation of corpus callosum

precentral gyrus

central sulcus

temporalis m

postcentral sulcus

superior parietal lobule

inferior parietal lobule

parietal radiation of corpus callosum

parietal bone

Cahill

paracentral lobule

superior parietal lobule

precuneus

superior sagittal sinus

falx cerebri and cortical branch of posterior cerebral a

RIGHT

LEFT

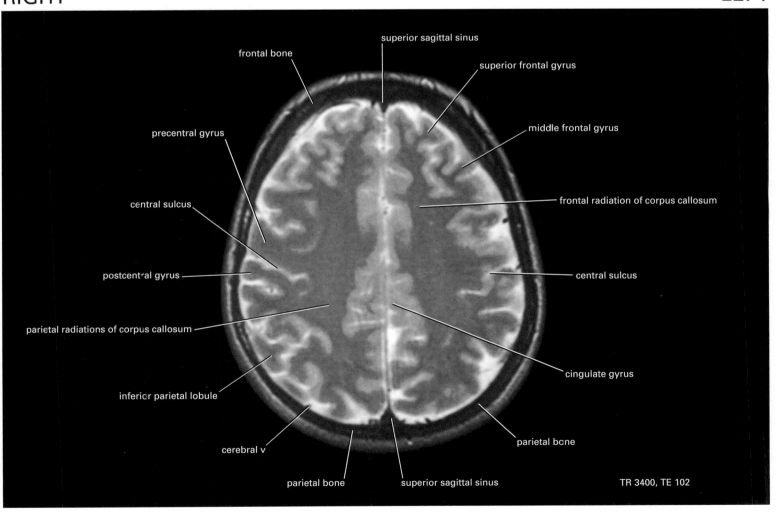

frontal bone

superior sagittal sinus

superior frontal gyrus

precentral gyrus

middle frontal gyrus

central sulcus

frontal radiation of corpus callosum

postcentral gyrus

central sulcus

parietal radiations of corpus callosum

cingulate gyrus

inferior parietal lobule

parietal bone

cerebral v

parietal bone

superior sagittal sinus

TR 3400, TE 102

Section 13, anatomy from above, MR image from below.

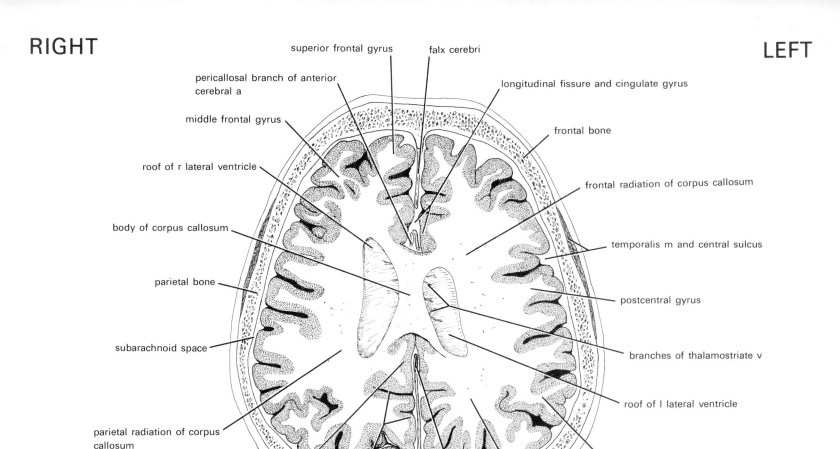

superior frontal gyrus

falx cerebri

pericallosal branch of anterior cerebral a

longitudinal fissure and cingulate gyrus

middle frontal gyrus

frontal bone

roof of r lateral ventricle

frontal radiation of corpus callosum

body of corpus callosum

temporalis m and central sulcus

parietal bone

postcentral gyrus

subarachnoid space

branches of thalamostriate v

roof of l lateral ventricle

parietal radiation of corpus callosum

inferior parietal lobule

cingulate gyrus

occipital radiation of corpus callosum

subparietal sulcus and precuneus

inferior sagittal sinus

superior sagittal sinus

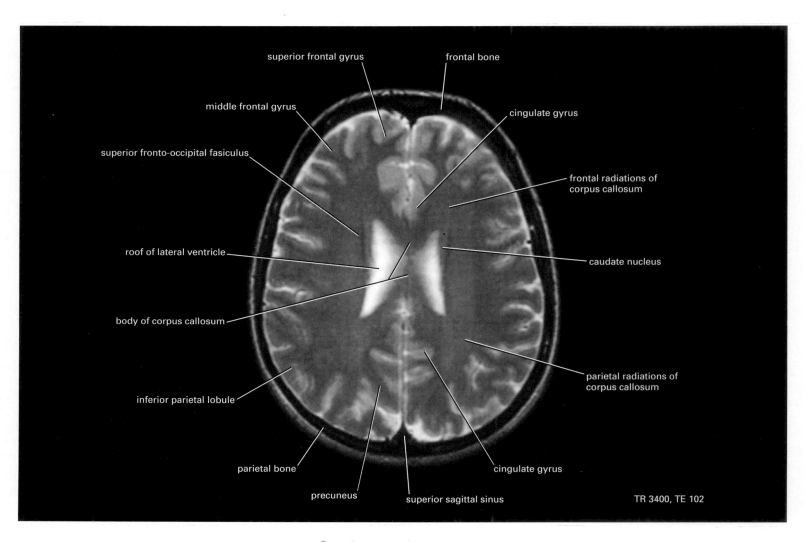

superior frontal gyrus

frontal bone

middle frontal gyrus

cingulate gyrus

superior fronto-occipital fasiculus

frontal radiations of corpus callosum

roof of lateral ventricle

caudate nucleus

body of corpus callosum

parietal radiations of corpus callosum

inferior parietal lobule

parietal bone

cingulate gyrus

precuneus

superior sagittal sinus

TR 3400, TE 102

Section 13 from below.

frontal crest

falx cerebri

frontal bone and superior frontal gyrus

pericallosal branches of
anterior cerebral aa

middle frontal gyrus

r lateral ventricle

body of corpus callosum

head of caudate nucleus, seen through
ventricle

precentral gyrus

temporalis m

postcentral gyrus

anterior branch of middle
meningeal a

subarachnoid space

caudate nucleus

thalamostriate v

fornix

thalamus, seen through l lateral
ventricle

posterior branch of middle
meningeal a

body of fornix

choroid plexus

falx cerebri

diploë

superior sagittal sinus

inferior sagittal sinus and cuneus

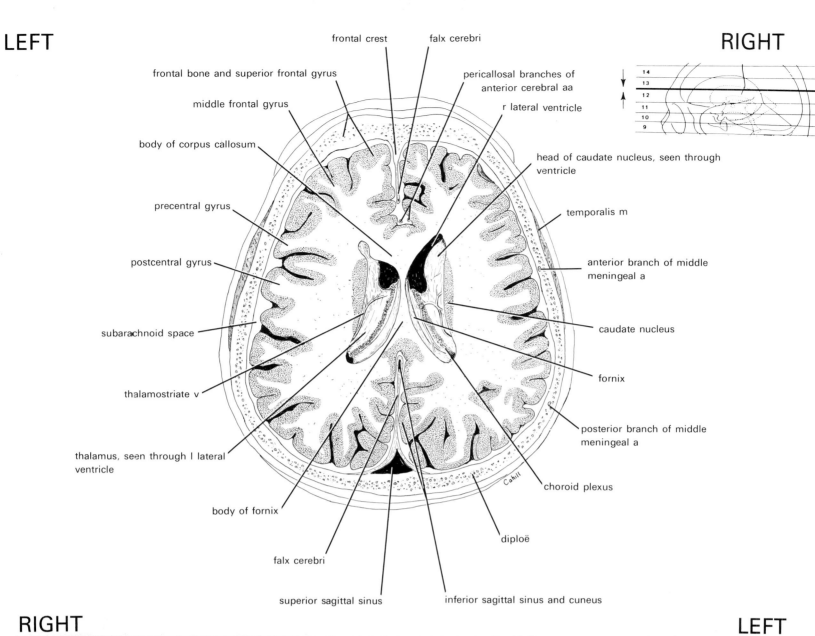

superior frontal gyrus

frontal crest

cingulate gyrus

middle frontal gyrus

frontal bone

genu of corpus callosum

lateral ventricle

caudate nucleus

insular cortex

splenium of corpus callosum

cingulate gyrus

parietal bone

falx cerebri

cuneus

superior sagittal sinus

TR 3400, TE 102

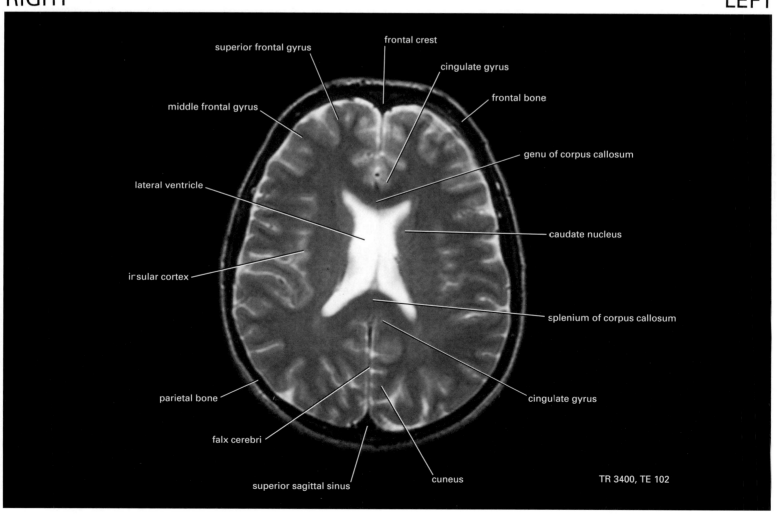

Section 12, anatomy from above, MR image from below.

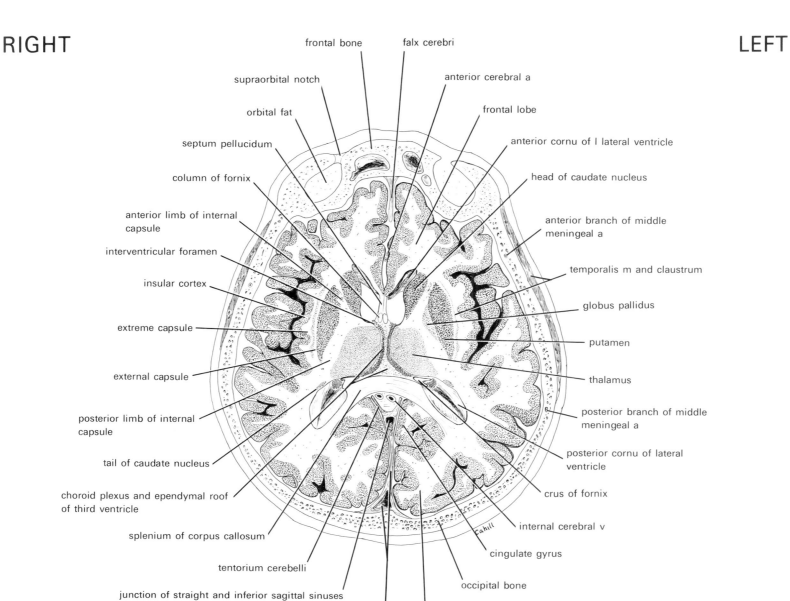

frontal bone
falx cerebri
supraorbital notch
anterior cerebral a
orbital fat
frontal lobe
septum pellucidum
anterior cornu of l lateral ventricle
column of fornix
head of caudate nucleus
anterior limb of internal capsule
anterior branch of middle meningeal a
interventricular foramen
temporalis m and claustrum
insular cortex
globus pallidus
extreme capsule
putamen
external capsule
thalamus
posterior limb of internal capsule
posterior branch of middle meningeal a
tail of caudate nucleus
posterior cornu of lateral ventricle
choroid plexus and ependymal roof of third ventricle
crus of fornix
splenium of corpus callosum
internal cerebral v
tentorium cerebelli
cingulate gyrus
junction of straight and inferior sagittal sinuses
occipital bone
falx cerebri and superior sagittal sinus
occipital lobe

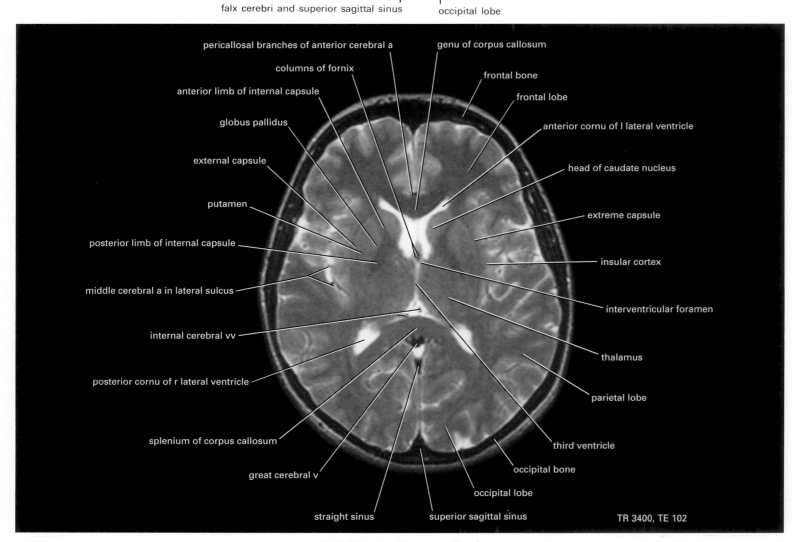

pericallosal branches of anterior cerebral a
genu of corpus callosum
columns of fornix
frontal bone
anterior limb of internal capsule
frontal lobe
globus pallidus
anterior cornu of l lateral ventricle
external capsule
head of caudate nucleus
putamen
extreme capsule
posterior limb of internal capsule
insular cortex
middle cerebral a in lateral sulcus
interventricular foramen
internal cerebral vv
thalamus
posterior cornu of r lateral ventricle
parietal lobe
splenium of corpus callosum
third ventricle
great cerebral v
occipital bone
straight sinus
occipital lobe
superior sagittal sinus
TR 3400, TE 102

Section 12 from below.

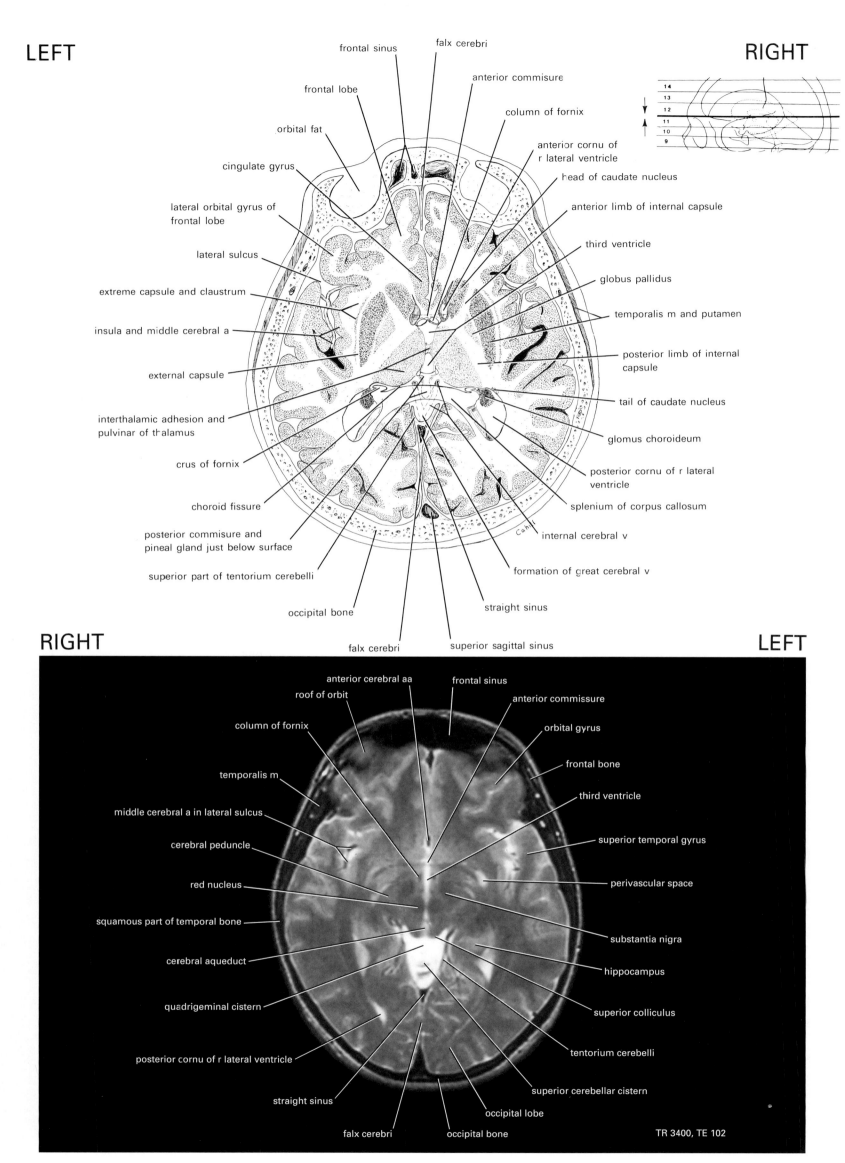

LEFT

RIGHT

frontal sinus
falx cerebri
anterior commisure
frontal lobe
column of fornix
orbital fat
anterior cornu of
r lateral ventricle
cingulate gyrus
Head of caudate nucleus
lateral orbital gyrus of
frontal lobe
anterior limb of internal capsule
lateral sulcus
third ventricle
extreme capsule and claustrum
globus pallidus
temporalis m and putamen
insula and middle cerebral a
posterior limb of internal
capsule
external capsule
tail of caudate nucleus
interthalamic adhesion and
pulvinar of thalamus
glomus choroideum
crus of fornix
posterior cornu of r lateral
ventricle
choroid fissure
splenium of corpus callosum
posterior commisure and
pineal gland just below surface
internal cerebral v
superior part of tentorium cerebelli
formation of great cerebral v
occipital bone
straight sinus
falx cerebri
superior sagittal sinus

RIGHT

LEFT

anterior cerebral aa
frontal sinus
roof of orbit
anterior commissure
column of fornix
orbital gyrus
frontal bone
temporalis m
third ventricle
middle cerebral a in lateral sulcus
cerebral peduncle
superior temporal gyrus
red nucleus
perivascular space
squamous part of temporal bone
substantia nigra
cerebral aqueduct
hippocampus
quadrigeminal cistern
superior colliculus
posterior cornu of r lateral ventricle
tentorium cerebelli
straight sinus
superior cerebellar cistern
falx cerebri
occipital lobe
occipital bone
TR 3400, TE 102

Section 11, anatomy from above, MR image from below.

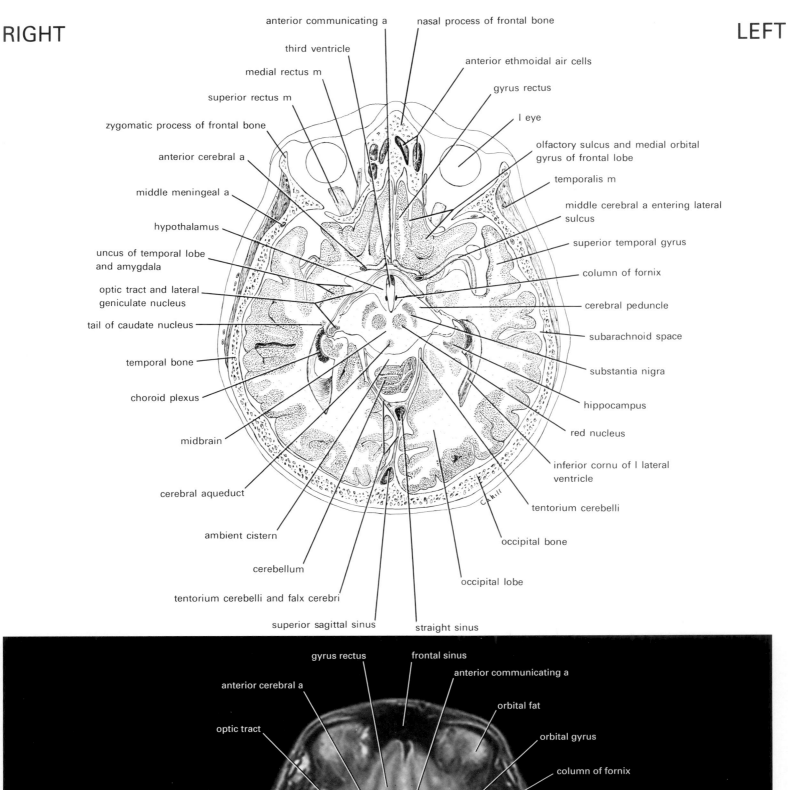

anterior communicating a
nasal process of frontal bone
third ventricle
anterior ethmoidal air cells
medial rectus m
gyrus rectus
superior rectus m
l eye
zygomatic process of frontal bone
olfactory sulcus and medial orbital gyrus of frontal lobe
anterior cerebral a
temporalis m
middle meningeal a
middle cerebral a entering lateral sulcus
hypothalamus
superior temporal gyrus
uncus of temporal lobe and amygdala
column of fornix
optic tract and lateral geniculate nucleus
cerebral peduncle
tail of caudate nucleus
subarachnoid space
temporal bone
substantia nigra
choroid plexus
hippocampus
midbrain
red nucleus
cerebral aqueduct
inferior cornu of l lateral ventricle
ambient cistern
tentorium cerebelli
cerebellum
occipital bone
tentorium cerebelli and falx cerebri
occipital lobe
superior sagittal sinus
straight sinus

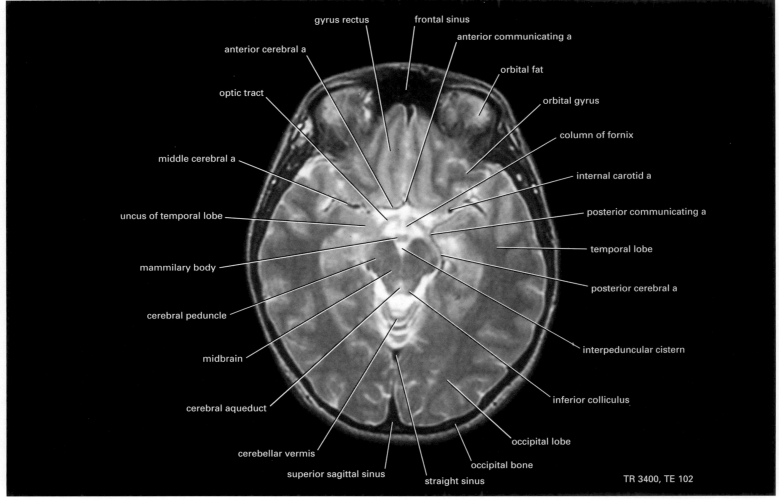

gyrus rectus
frontal sinus
anterior cerebral a
anterior communicating a
orbital fat
optic tract
orbital gyrus
column of fornix
middle cerebral a
internal carotid a
uncus of temporal lobe
posterior communicating a
mammilary body
temporal lobe
cerebral peduncle
posterior cerebral a
midbrain
interpeduncular cistern
cerebral aqueduct
inferior colliculus
cerebellar vermis
occipital lobe
superior sagittal sinus
occipital bone
straight sinus
TR 3400, TE 102

Section 11 from below.

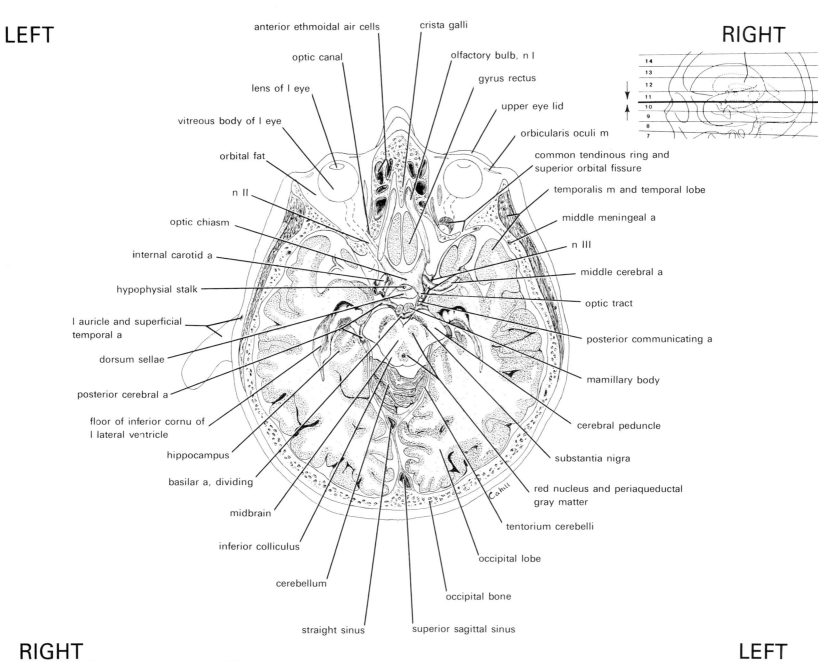

anterior ethmoidal air cells
crista galli
optic canal
olfactory bulb, n I
lens of l eye
gyrus rectus
vitreous body of l eye
upper eye lid
orbital fat
orbicularis oculi m
n II
common tendinous ring and superior orbital fissure
optic chiasm
temporalis m and temporal lobe
internal carotid a
middle meningeal a
hypophysial stalk
n III
l auricle and superficial temporal a
middle cerebral a
dorsum sellae
optic tract
posterior cerebral a
posterior communicating a
floor of inferior cornu of l lateral ventricle
mamillary body
hippocampus
cerebral peduncle
basilar a, dividing
substantia nigra
midbrain
red nucleus and periaqueductal gray matter
inferior colliculus
tentorium cerebelli
cerebellum
occipital lobe
straight sinus
occipital bone
superior sagittal sinus

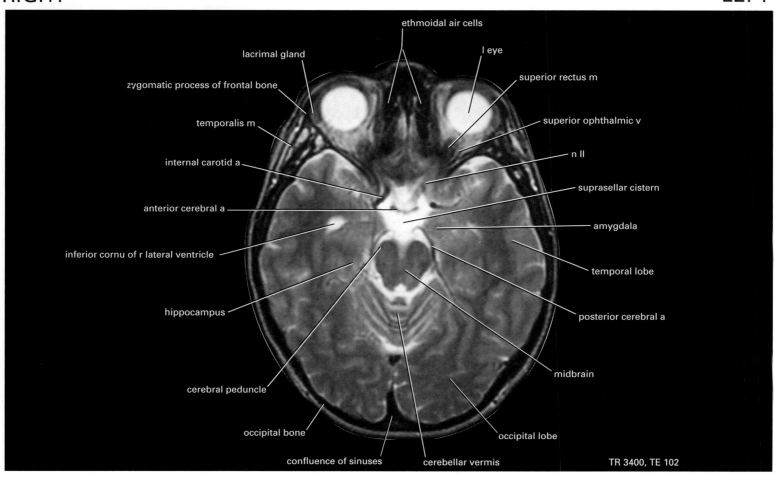

ethmoidal air cells
lacrimal gland
l eye
zygomatic process of frontal bone
superior rectus m
temporalis m
superior ophthalmic v
internal carotid a
n II
anterior cerebral a
suprasellar cistern
inferior cornu of r lateral ventricle
amygdala
hippocampus
temporal lobe
cerebral peduncle
posterior cerebral a
occipital bone
midbrain
confluence of sinuses
cerebellar vermis
occipital lobe
TR 3400, TE 102

Section 10, anatomy from above, MR image from below.

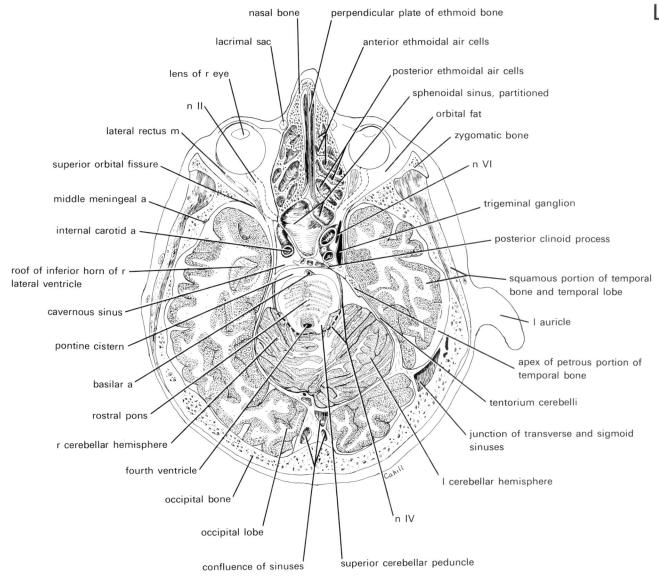

nasal bone

perpendicular plate of ethmoid bone

lacrimal sac

anterior ethmoidal air cells

lens of r eye

posterior ethmoidal air cells

n II

sphenoidal sinus, partitioned

lateral rectus m

orbital fat

superior orbital fissure

zygomatic bone

middle meningeal a

n VI

internal carotid a

trigeminal ganglion

roof of inferior horn of r lateral ventricle

posterior clinoid process

cavernous sinus

squamous portion of temporal bone and temporal lobe

pontine cistern

l auricle

basilar a

apex of petrous portion of temporal bone

rostral pons

tentorium cerebelli

r cerebellar hemisphere

junction of transverse and sigmoid sinuses

fourth ventricle

l cerebellar hemisphere

occipital bone

n IV

occipital lobe

confluence of sinuses

superior cerebellar peduncle

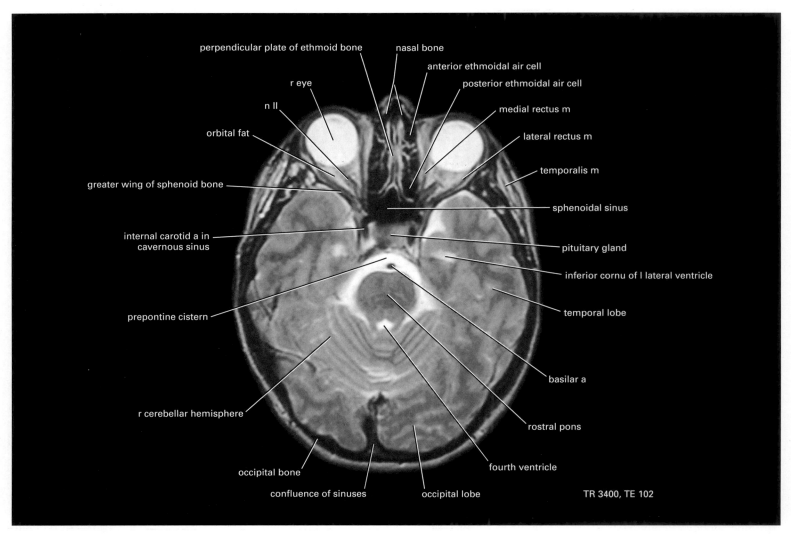

perpendicular plate of ethmoid bone

nasal bone

r eye

anterior ethmoidal air cell

n II

posterior ethmoidal air cell

orbital fat

medial rectus m

lateral rectus m

greater wing of sphenoid bone

temporalis m

sphenoidal sinus

internal carotid a in cavernous sinus

pituitary gland

inferior cornu of l lateral ventricle

temporal lobe

prepontine cistern

basilar a

r cerebellar hemisphere

rostral pons

occipital bone

fourth ventricle

confluence of sinuses

occipital lobe

TR 3400, TE 102

Section 10 from below.

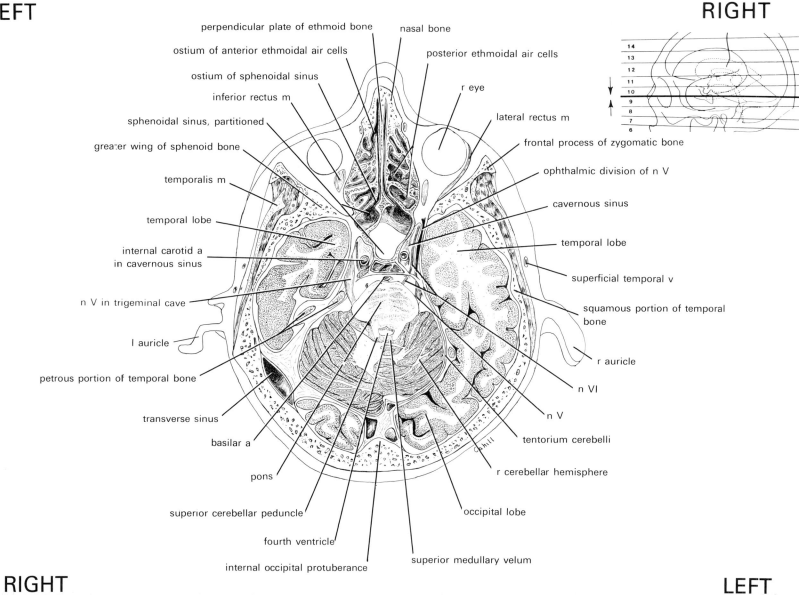

perpendicular plate of ethmoid bone
nasal bone
ostium of anterior ethmoidal air cells
posterior ethmoidal air cells
ostium of sphenoidal sinus
r eye
inferior rectus m
lateral rectus m
sphenoidal sinus, partitioned
frontal process of zygomatic bone
greater wing of sphenoid bone
ophthalmic division of n V
temporalis m
cavernous sinus
temporal lobe
temporal lobe
internal carotid a
in cavernous sinus
superficial temporal v
n V in trigeminal cave
squamous portion of temporal
bone
l auricle
r auricle
petrous portion of temporal bone
n VI
transverse sinus
n V
basilar a
tentorium cerebelli
pons
r cerebellar hemisphere
superior cerebellar peduncle
occipital lobe
fourth ventricle
superior medullary velum
internal occipital protuberance

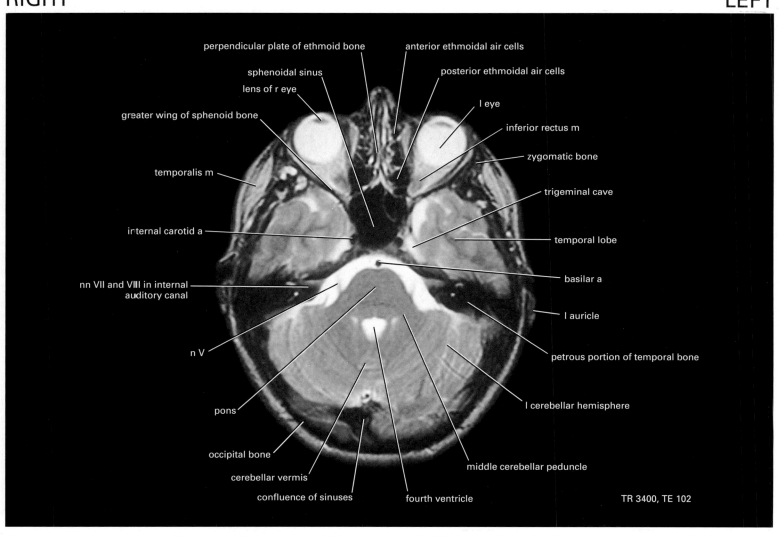

perpendicular plate of ethmoid bone
anterior ethmoidal air cells
sphenoidal sinus
posterior ethmoidal air cells
lens of r eye
l eye
greater wing of sphenoid bone
inferior rectus m
zygomatic bone
temporalis m
trigeminal cave
internal carotid a
temporal lobe
basilar a
nn VII and VIII in internal
auditory canal
l auricle
n V
petrous portion of temporal bone
pons
l cerebellar hemisphere
occipital bone
middle cerebellar peduncle
cerebellar vermis
confluence of sinuses
fourth ventricle
TR 3400, TE 102

Section 9, anatomy from above, MR image from below.

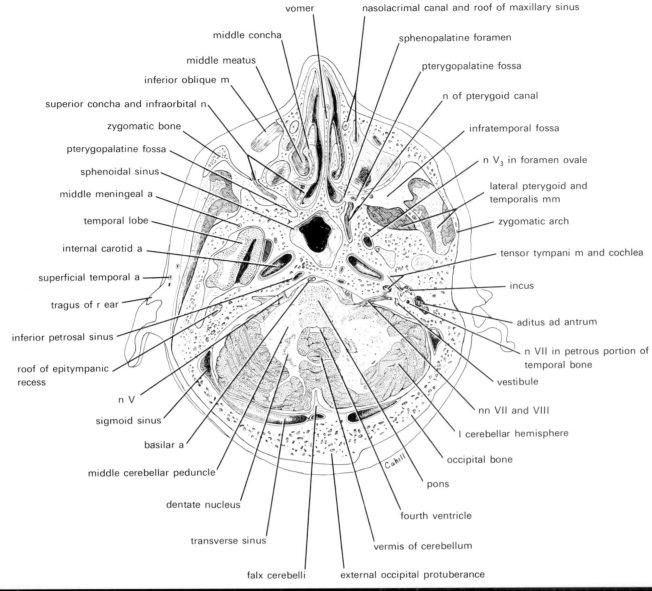

vomer
nasolacrimal canal and roof of maxillary sinus
middle concha
sphenopalatine foramen
middle meatus
pterygopalatine fossa
inferior oblique m
superior concha and infraorbital n
n of pterygoid canal
zygomatic bone
infratemporal fossa
pterygopalatine fossa
n V₃ in foramen ovale
sphenoidal sinus
lateral pterygoid and temporalis mm
middle meningeal a
zygomatic arch
temporal lobe
tensor tympani m and cochlea
internal carotid a
incus
superficial temporal a
tragus of r ear
aditus ad antrum
inferior petrosal sinus
n VII in petrous portion of temporal bone
roof of epitympanic recess
vestibule
n V
nn VII and VIII
sigmoid sinus
l cerebellar hemisphere
basilar a
occipital bone
middle cerebellar peduncle
pons
dentate nucleus
fourth ventricle
transverse sinus
vermis of cerebellum
falx cerebelli
external occipital protuberance

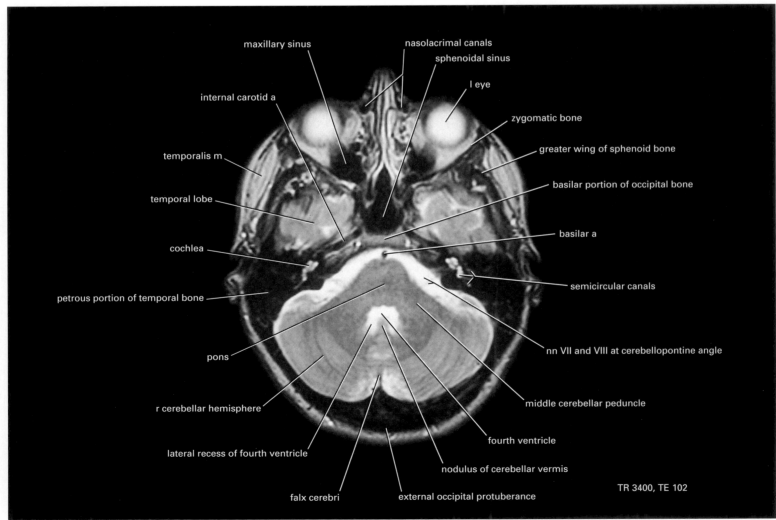

maxillary sinus
nasolacrimal canals
sphenoidal sinus
internal carotid a
l eye
zygomatic bone
greater wing of sphenoid bone
temporalis m
basilar portion of occipital bone
temporal lobe
basilar a
cochlea
semicircular canals
petrous portion of temporal bone
pons
nn VII and VIII at cerebellopontine angle
r cerebellar hemisphere
middle cerebellar peduncle
lateral recess of fourth ventricle
fourth ventricle
falx cerebri
nodulus of cerebellar vermis
external occipital protuberance
TR 3400, TE 102

Section 9 from below.

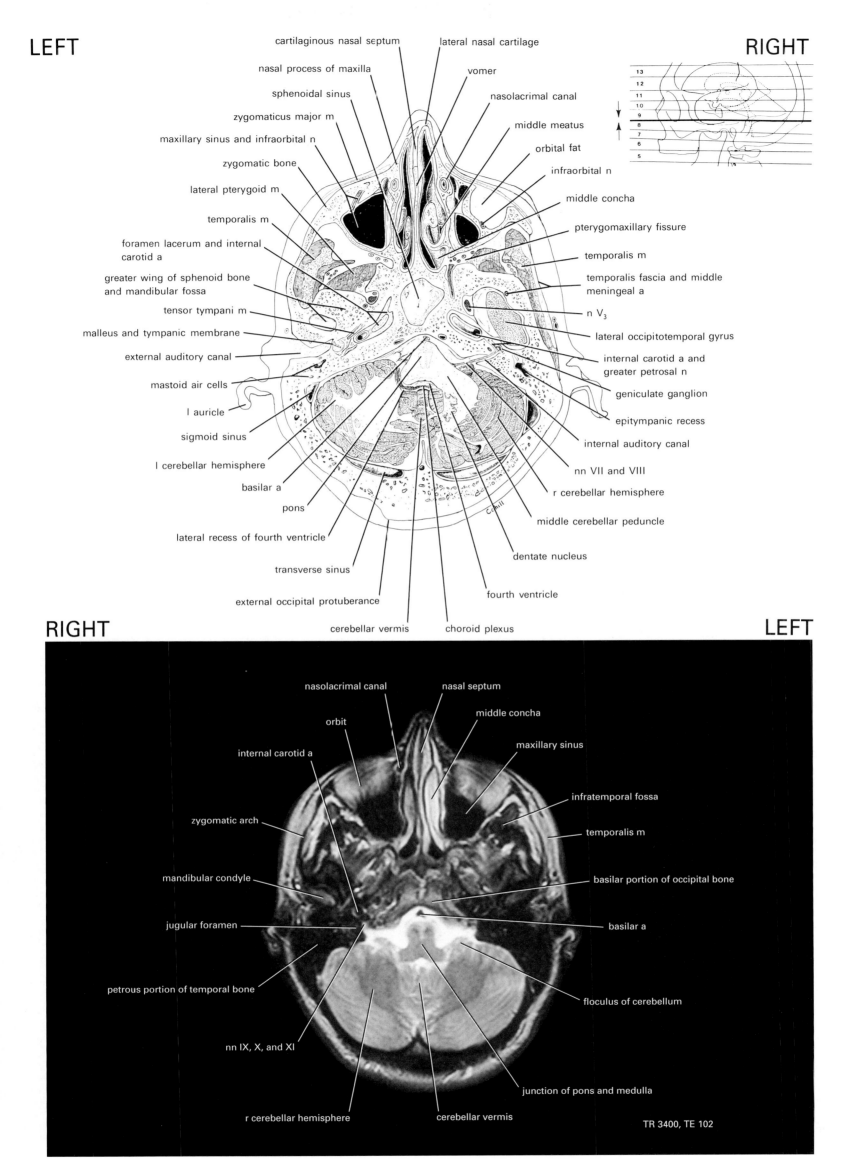

cartilaginous nasal septum
lateral nasal cartilage
nasal process of maxilla
vomer
sphenoidal sinus
nasolacrimal canal
zygomaticus major m
middle meatus
maxillary sinus and infraorbital n
orbital fat
zygomatic bone
infraorbital n
lateral pterygoid m
middle concha
temporalis m
pterygomaxillary fissure
foramen lacerum and internal carotid a
temporalis m
greater wing of sphenoid bone and mandibular fossa
temporalis fascia and middle meningeal a
tensor tympani m
n V₃
malleus and tympanic membrane
lateral occipitotemporal gyrus
external auditory canal
internal carotid a and greater petrosal n
mastoid air cells
geniculate ganglion
l auricle
epitympanic recess
sigmoid sinus
internal auditory canal
l cerebellar hemisphere
nn VII and VIII
basilar a
r cerebellar hemisphere
pons
middle cerebellar peduncle
lateral recess of fourth ventricle
dentate nucleus
transverse sinus
fourth ventricle
external occipital protuberance
cerebellar vermis
choroid plexus

nasolacrimal canal
nasal septum
orbit
middle concha
internal carotid a
maxillary sinus
zygomatic arch
infratemporal fossa
temporalis m
mandibular condyle
basilar portion of occipital bone
jugular foramen
basilar a
petrous portion of temporal bone
floculus of cerebellum
nn IX, X, and XI
junction of pons and medulla
r cerebellar hemisphere
cerebellar vermis

TR 3400, TE 102

Section 8, anatomy from above, MR image from below.

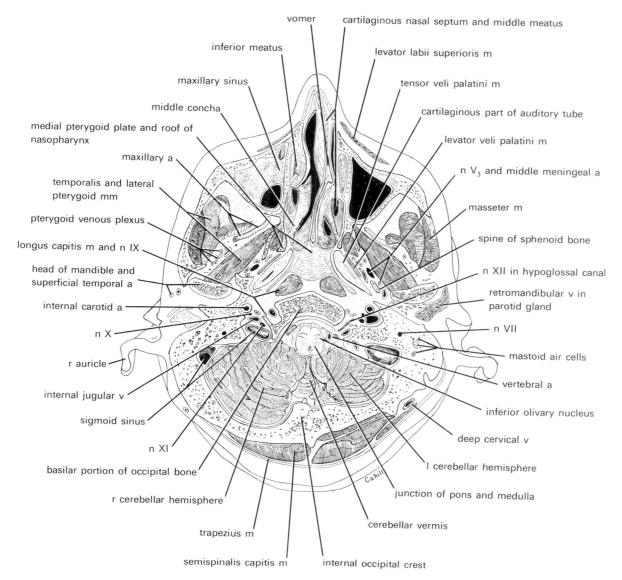

vomer

cartilaginous nasal septum and middle meatus

inferior meatus

levator labii superioris m

maxillary sinus

tensor veli palatini m

middle concha

cartilaginous part of auditory tube

medial pterygoid plate and roof of nasopharynx

levator veli palatini m

maxillary a

n V₃ and middle meningeal a

temporalis and lateral pterygoid mm

masseter m

pterygoid venous plexus

spine of sphenoid bone

longus capitis m and n IX

n XII in hypoglossal canal

head of mandible and superficial temporal a

retromandibular v in parotid gland

internal carotid a

n VII

n X

mastoid air cells

r auricle

internal jugular v

vertebral a

sigmoid sinus

inferior olivary nucleus

n XI

deep cervical v

basilar portion of occipital bone

l cerebellar hemisphere

r cerebellar hemisphere

junction of pons and medulla

trapezius m

cerebellar vermis

semispinalis capitis m

internal occipital crest

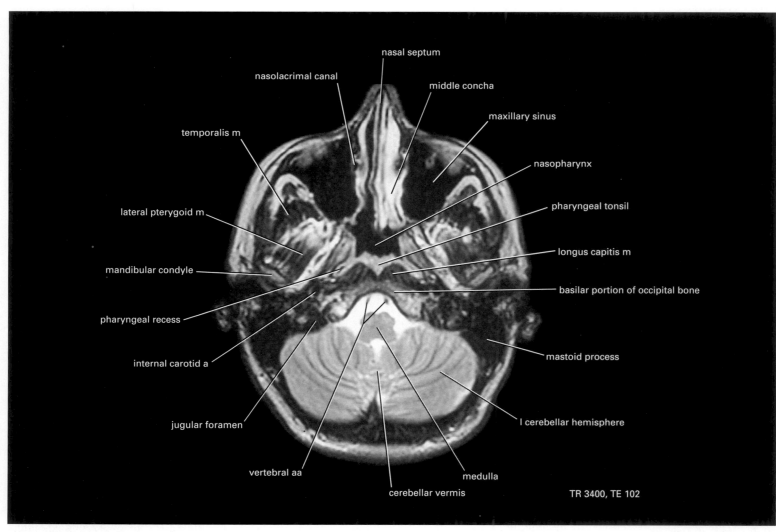

nasal septum

nasolacrimal canal

middle concha

temporalis m

maxillary sinus

nasopharynx

lateral pterygoid m

pharyngeal tonsil

mandibular condyle

longus capitis m

pharyngeal recess

basilar portion of occipital bone

internal carotid a

mastoid process

jugular foramen

l cerebellar hemisphere

vertebral aa

medulla

cerebellar vermis

TR 3400, TE 102

Section 8 from below.

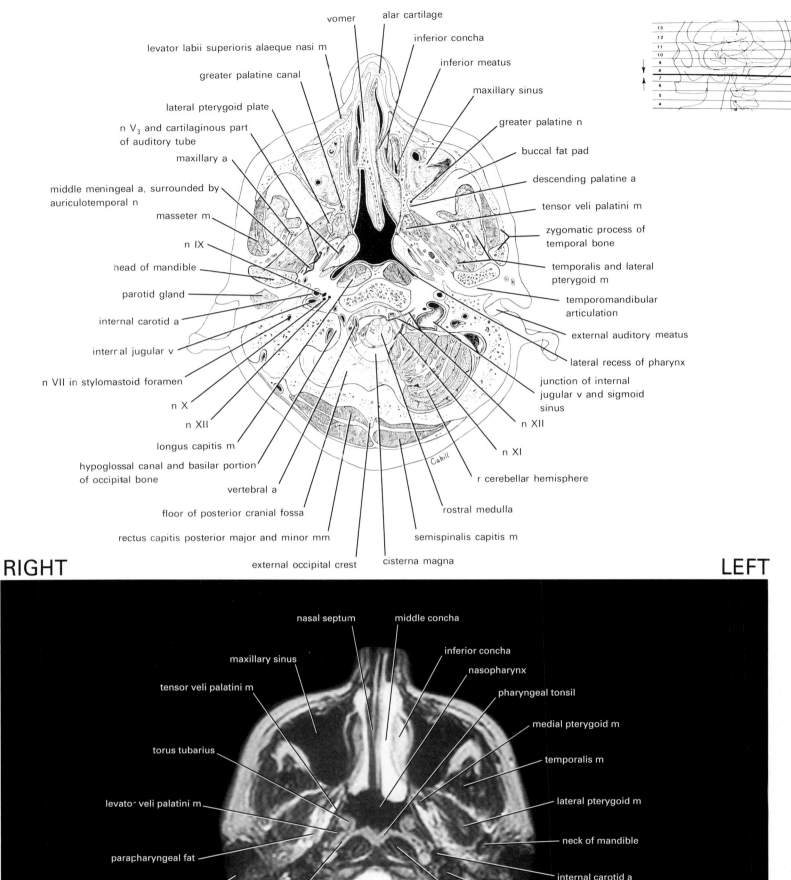

vomer
alar cartilage
levator labii superioris alaeque nasi m
inferior concha
greater palatine canal
inferior meatus
lateral pterygoid plate
maxillary sinus
n V₃ and cartilaginous part
of auditory tube
greater palatine n
maxillary a
buccal fat pad
middle meningeal a, surrounded by
descending palatine a
auriculotemporal n
tensor veli palatini m
masseter m
zygomatic process of
temporal bone
n IX
head of mandible
temporalis and lateral
pterygoid m
parotid gland
temporomandibular
articulation
internal carotid a
external auditory meatus
internal jugular v
lateral recess of pharynx
n VII in stylomastoid foramen
junction of internal
jugular v and sigmoid
sinus
n X
n XII
n XII
longus capitis m
n XI
hypoglossal canal and basilar portion
of occipital bone
r cerebellar hemisphere
vertebral a
floor of posterior cranial fossa
rostral medulla
rectus capitis posterior major and minor mm
semispinalis capitis m
external occipital crest
cisterna magna

Cahill

RIGHT

LEFT

nasal septum
middle concha
maxillary sinus
inferior concha
tensor veli palatini m
nasopharynx
pharyngeal tonsil
torus tubarius
medial pterygoid m
temporalis m
levator veli palatini m
lateral pterygoid m
parapharyngeal fat
neck of mandible
r auricle
internal carotid a
bulb of internal jugular v
longus capitis m
pharyngeal recess
n XII in hypoglossal canal
l cerebellar hemisphere
vertebral a
medulla
cerebellar tonsil
posterior inferior cerebellar a

TR 3400, TE 102

Section 7, anatomy from above, MR image from below.

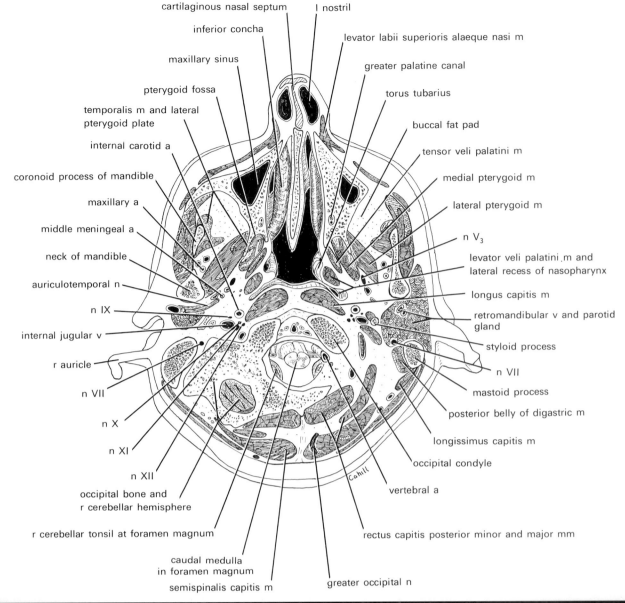

cartilaginous nasal septum
l nostril
inferior concha
levator labii superioris alaeque nasi m
maxillary sinus
greater palatine canal
pterygoid fossa
torus tubarius
temporalis m and lateral pterygoid plate
buccal fat pad
internal carotid a
tensor veli palatini m
coronoid process of mandible
medial pterygoid m
maxillary a
lateral pterygoid m
middle meningeal a
n V₃
neck of mandible
levator veli palatini m and lateral recess of nasopharynx
auriculotemporal n
longus capitis m
n IX
retromandibular v and parotid gland
internal jugular v
styloid process
r auricle
n VII
n VII
mastoid process
n X
posterior belly of digastric m
n XI
longissimus capitis m
n XII
occipital condyle
occipital bone and r cerebellar hemisphere
vertebral a
r cerebellar tonsil at foramen magnum
rectus capitis posterior minor and major mm
caudal medulla in foramen magnum
semispinalis capitis m
greater occipital n

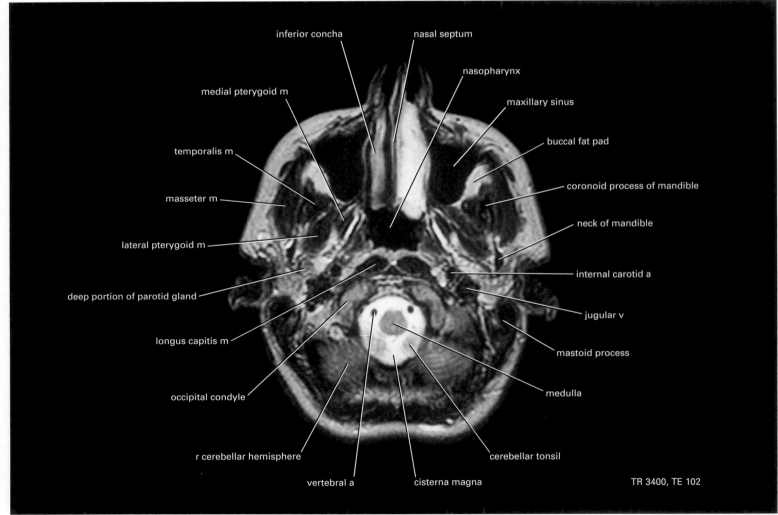

inferior concha
nasal septum
nasopharynx
medial pterygoid m
maxillary sinus
temporalis m
buccal fat pad
masseter m
coronoid process of mandible
lateral pterygoid m
neck of mandible
deep portion of parotid gland
internal carotid a
jugular v
longus capitis m
mastoid process
occipital condyle
medulla
r cerebellar hemisphere
cerebellar tonsil
vertebral a
cisterna magna
TR 3400, TE 102

Section 7 from below.

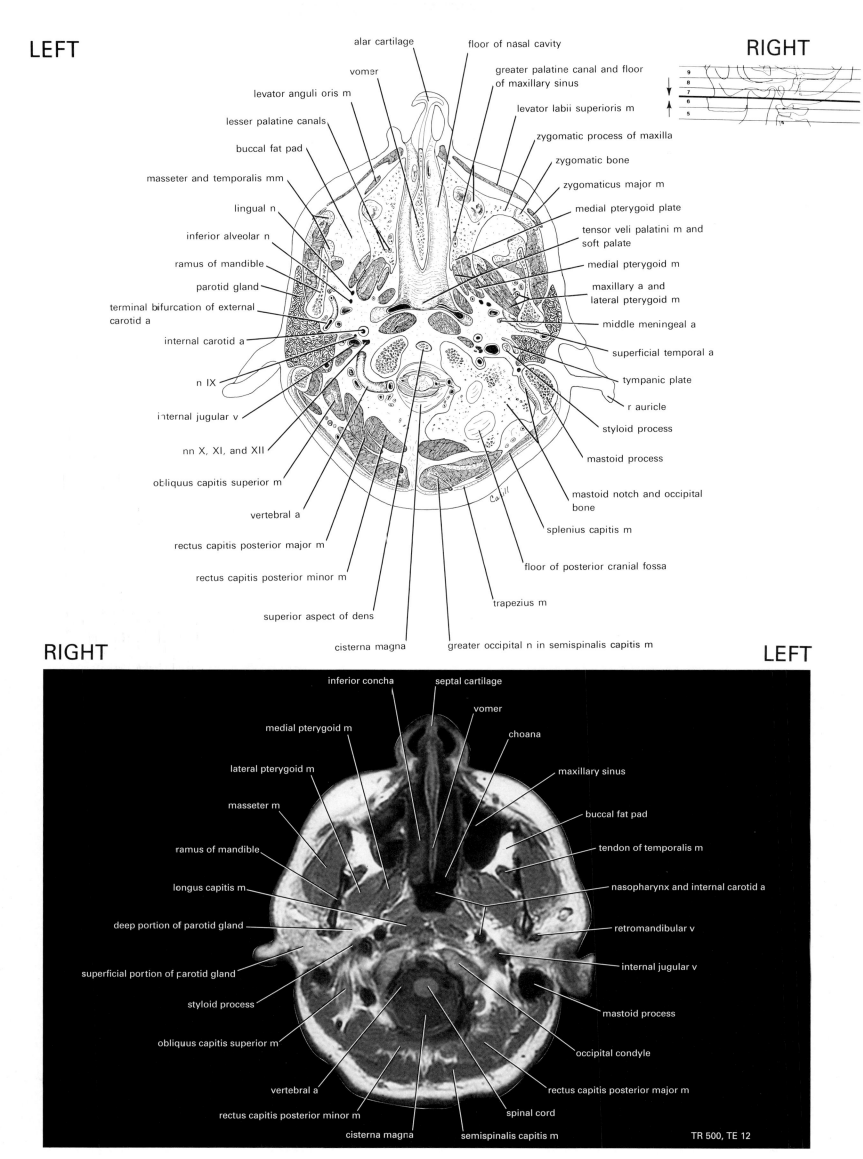

alar cartilage
vomer
levator anguli oris m
lesser palatine canals
buccal fat pad
masseter and temporalis mm
lingual n
inferior alveolar n
ramus of mandible
parotid gland
terminal bifurcation of external carotid a
internal carotid a
n IX
internal jugular v
nn X, XI, and XII
obliquus capitis superior m
vertebral a
rectus capitis posterior major m
rectus capitis posterior minor m
superior aspect of dens
cisterna magna

floor of nasal cavity
greater palatine canal and floor of maxillary sinus
levator labii superioris m
zygomatic process of maxilla
zygomatic bone
zygomaticus major m
medial pterygoid plate
tensor veli palatini m and soft palate
medial pterygoid m
maxillary a and lateral pterygoid m
middle meningeal a
superficial temporal a
tympanic plate
r auricle
styloid process
mastoid process
mastoid notch and occipital bone
splenius capitis m
floor of posterior cranial fossa
trapezius m
greater occipital n in semispinalis capitis m

RIGHT

LEFT

inferior concha
septal cartilage
vomer
medial pterygoid m
choana
lateral pterygoid m
maxillary sinus
masseter m
buccal fat pad
ramus of mandible
tendon of temporalis m
longus capitis m
nasopharynx and internal carotid a
deep portion of parotid gland
retromandibular v
superficial portion of parotid gland
internal jugular v
styloid process
mastoid process
obliquus capitis superior m
occipital condyle
vertebral a
rectus capitis posterior major m
rectus capitis posterior minor m
spinal cord
cisterna magna
semispinalis capitis m

TR 500, TE 12

Section 6, anatomy from above, MR image from below.

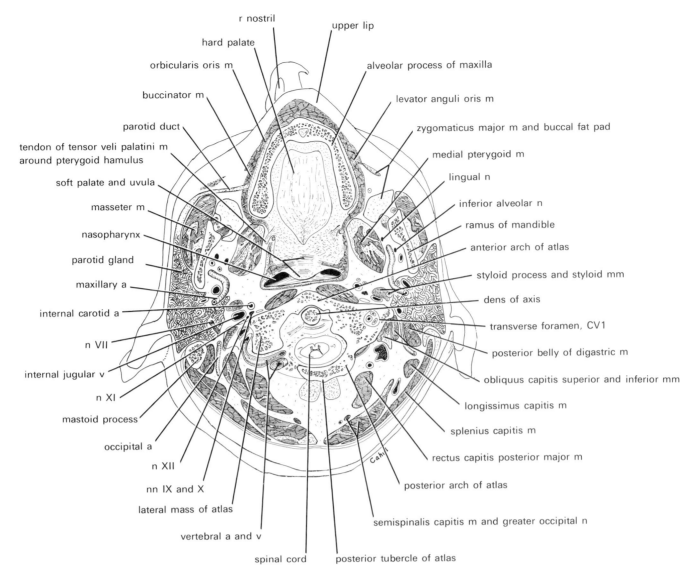

r nostril
upper lip
hard palate
orbicularis oris m
alveolar process of maxilla
buccinator m
levator anguli oris m
parotid duct
zygomaticus major m and buccal fat pad
tendon of tensor veli palatini m
around pterygoid hamulus
medial pterygoid m
soft palate and uvula
lingual n
masseter m
inferior alveolar n
nasopharynx
ramus of mandible
parotid gland
anterior arch of atlas
maxillary a
styloid process and styloid mm
internal carotid a
dens of axis
n VII
transverse foramen, CV1
internal jugular v
posterior belly of digastric m
n XI
obliquus capitis superior and inferior mm
mastoid process
longissimus capitis m
occipital a
splenius capitis m
n XII
rectus capitis posterior major m
nn IX and X
posterior arch of atlas
lateral mass of atlas
semispinalis capitis m and greater occipital n
vertebral a and v
spinal cord
posterior tubercle of atlas

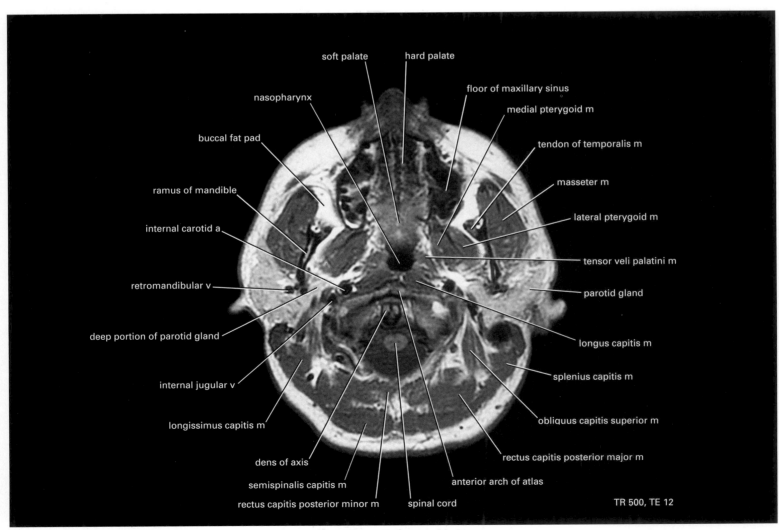

soft palate
hard palate
nasopharynx
floor of maxillary sinus
medial pterygoid m
buccal fat pad
tendon of temporalis m
ramus of mandible
masseter m
internal carotid a
lateral pterygoid m
retromandibular v
tensor veli palatini m
parotid gland
deep portion of parotid gland
longus capitis m
internal jugular v
splenius capitis m
longissimus capitis m
obliquus capitis superior m
dens of axis
rectus capitis posterior major m
semispinalis capitis m
anterior arch of atlas
rectus capitis posterior minor m
spinal cord
TR 500, TE 12

Section 6 from below.

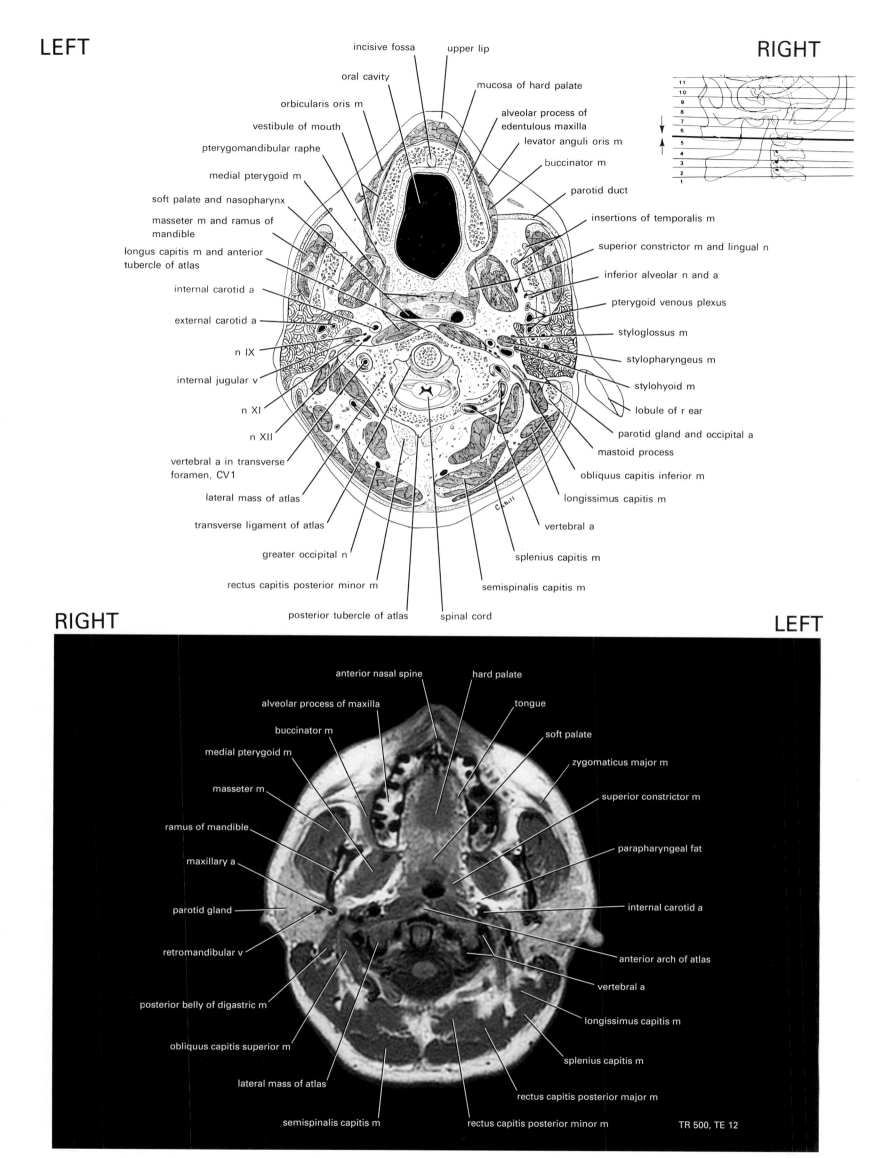

incisive fossa
upper lip
oral cavity
mucosa of hard palate
orbicularis oris m
alveolar process of
edentulous maxilla
vestibule of mouth
levator anguli oris m
pterygomandibular raphe
buccinator m
medial pterygoid m
parotid duct
soft palate and nasopharynx
insertions of temporalis m
masseter m and ramus of
mandible
superior constrictor m and lingual n
longus capitis m and anterior
tubercle of atlas
inferior alveolar n and a
pterygoid venous plexus
internal carotid a
styloglossus m
external carotid a
stylopharyngeus m
n IX
stylohyoid m
internal jugular v
lobule of r ear
n XI
parotid gland and occipital a
n XII
mastoid process
vertebral a in transverse
foramen, CV1
obliquus capitis inferior m
lateral mass of atlas
longissimus capitis m
transverse ligament of atlas
vertebral a
greater occipital n
splenius capitis m
rectus capitis posterior minor m
semispinalis capitis m
posterior tubercle of atlas
spinal cord

RIGHT

LEFT

anterior nasal spine
hard palate
alveolar process of maxilla
tongue
buccinator m
soft palate
medial pterygoid m
zygomaticus major m
masseter m
superior constrictor m
ramus of mandible
parapharyngeal fat
maxillary a
parotid gland
internal carotid a
retromandibular v
anterior arch of atlas
vertebral a
posterior belly of digastric m
longissimus capitis m
obliquus capitis superior m
splenius capitis m
lateral mass of atlas
rectus capitis posterior major m
semispinalis capitis m
rectus capitis posterior minor m
TR 500, TE 12

Section 5, anatomy from above, MR image from below.

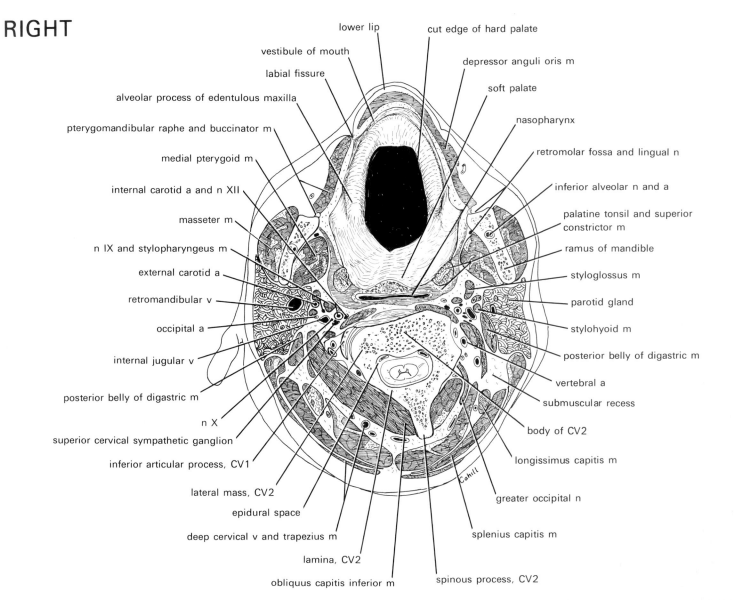

lower lip
vestibule of mouth
labial fissure
alveolar process of edentulous maxilla
pterygomandibular raphe and buccinator m
medial pterygoid m
internal carotid a and n XII
masseter m
n IX and stylopharyngeus m
external carotid a
retromandibular v
occipital a
internal jugular v
posterior belly of digastric m
n X
superior cervical sympathetic ganglion
inferior articular process, CV1
lateral mass, CV2
epidural space
deep cervical v and trapezius m
lamina, CV2
obliquus capitis inferior m

cut edge of hard palate
depressor anguli oris m
soft palate
nasopharynx
retromolar fossa and lingual n
inferior alveolar n and a
palatine tonsil and superior constrictor m
ramus of mandible
styloglossus m
parotid gland
stylohyoid m
posterior belly of digastric m
vertebral a
submuscular recess
body of CV2
longissimus capitis m
greater occipital n
splenius capitis m

spinous process, CV2

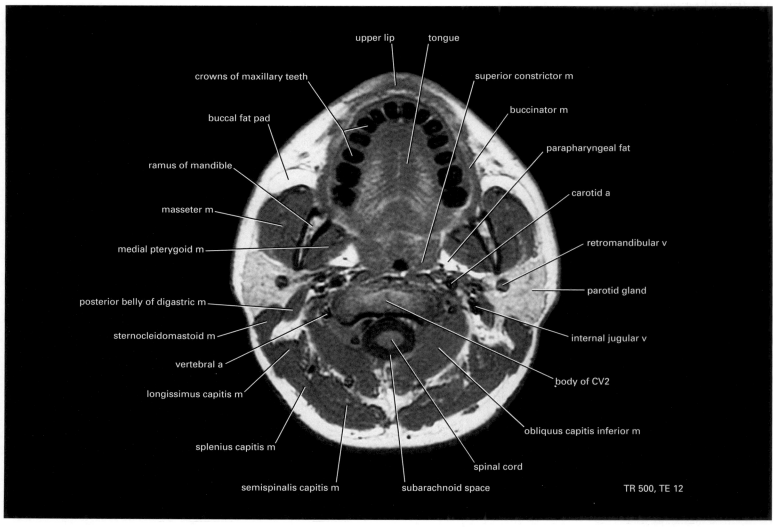

upper lip
tongue
crowns of maxillary teeth
superior constrictor m
buccal fat pad
buccinator m
parapharyngeal fat
ramus of mandible
masseter m
carotid a
medial pterygoid m
retromandibular v
posterior belly of digastric m
parotid gland
sternocleidomastoid m
internal jugular v
vertebral a
longissimus capitis m
body of CV2
obliquus capitis inferior m
splenius capitis m
spinal cord
semispinalis capitis m
subarachnoid space

TR 500, TE 12

Section 5 from below.

LEFT

lower lip
mucosa of floor of mouth
orbicularis oris m
tongue
buccal mucosa
depressor anguli oris m
lingual n
buccinator m
ramus of mandible
oropharynx
masseter m
palatoglossus m
medial pterygoid m
inferior alveolar a and n
styloglossus m
palatine tonsil
n IX and stylopharyngeus m
palatopharyngeus m
external carotid a
superior constrictor m
parotid gland
retromandibular v
n XII
stylohyoid m
internal jugular v
parotid gland
internal carotid a
longus capitis m
nn X and XI
posterior belly of digastric m
sternocleidomastoid m
inferior articular process, CV1
vertebral a
lateral mass, CV2
sympathetic trunk
cervical investing fascia
splenius capitis m
lamina, CV2
trapezius m
semispinalis capitis m
spinal cord
obliquus capitis inferior m

RIGHT

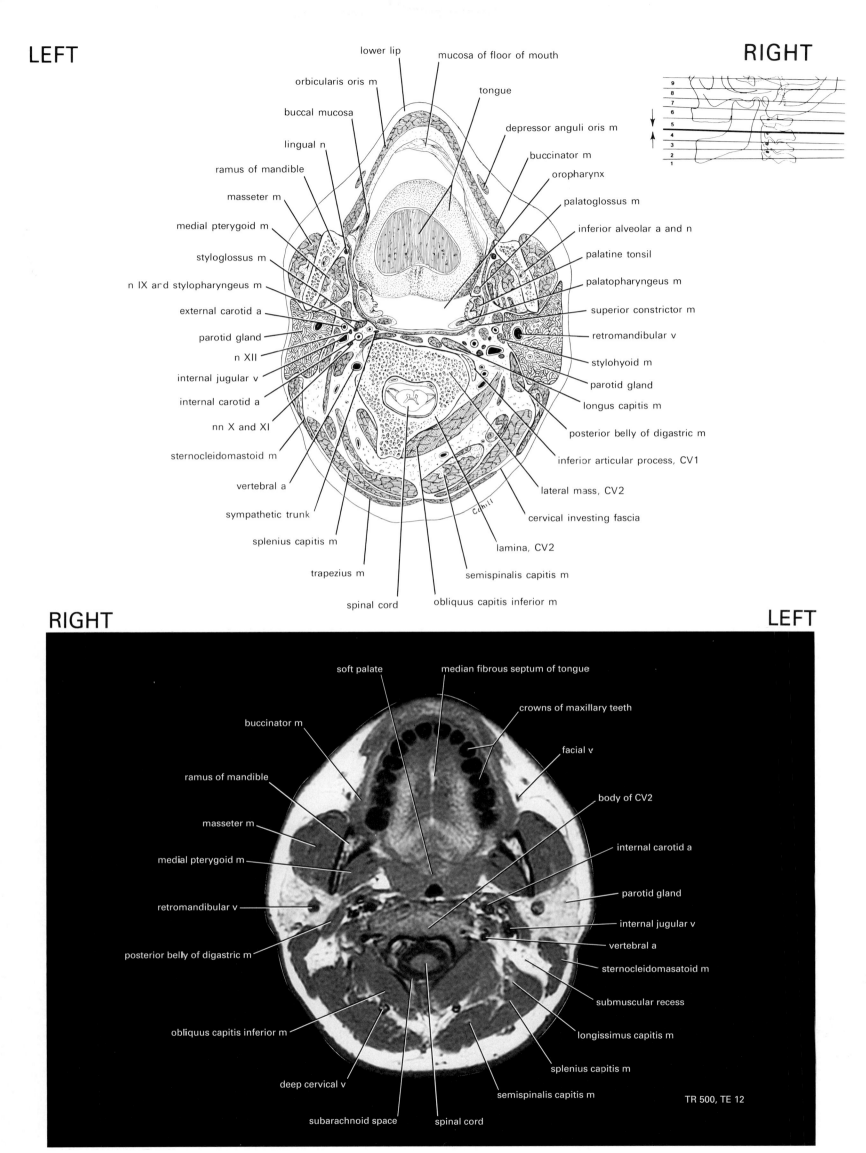

RIGHT

soft palate
median fibrous septum of tongue
buccinator m
crowns of maxillary teeth
facial v
ramus of mandible
body of CV2
masseter m
internal carotid a
medial pterygoid m
parotid gland
retromandibular v
internal jugular v
vertebral a
posterior belly of digastric m
sternocleidomasatoid m
submuscular recess
obliquus capitis inferior m
longissimus capitis m
splenius capitis m
deep cervical v
semispinalis capitis m
subarachnoid space
spinal cord

LEFT

TR 500, TE 12

Section 4, anatomy from above, MR image from below.

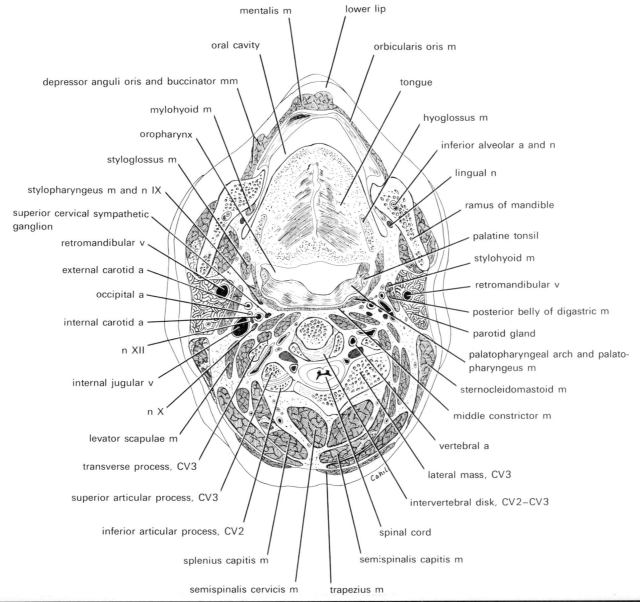

mentalis m
lower lip
oral cavity
orbicularis oris m
depressor anguli oris and buccinator mm
tongue
mylohyoid m
hyoglossus m
oropharynx
inferior alveolar a and n
styloglossus m
lingual n
stylopharyngeus m and n IX
ramus of mandible
superior cervical sympathetic ganglion
palatine tonsil
retromandibular v
stylohyoid m
external carotid a
retromandibular v
occipital a
posterior belly of digastric m
internal carotid a
parotid gland
n XII
palatopharyngeal arch and palato-pharyngeus m
internal jugular v
sternocleidomastoid m
n X
middle constrictor m
levator scapulae m
vertebral a
transverse process, CV3
lateral mass, CV3
superior articular process, CV3
intervertebral disk, CV2–CV3
inferior articular process, CV2
spinal cord
splenius capitis m
semispinalis capitis m
semispinalis cervicis m
trapezius m

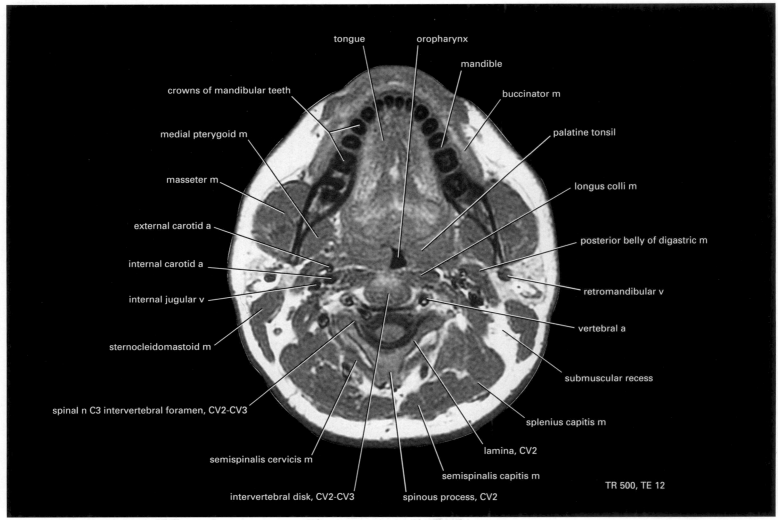

tongue
oropharynx
mandible
crowns of mandibular teeth
buccinator m
medial pterygoid m
palatine tonsil
masseter m
longus colli m
external carotid a
posterior belly of digastric m
internal carotid a
retromandibular v
internal jugular v
vertebral a
sternocleidomastoid m
submuscular recess
spinal n C3 intervertebral foramen, CV2-CV3
splenius capitis m
semispinalis cervicis m
lamina, CV2
intervertebral disk, CV2-CV3
semispinalis capitis m
spinous process, CV2
TR 500, TE 12

Section 4 from below.

median fibrous septum of tongue

sublingual fold and genioglossus m

alveolar process of edentulous mandible

oropharynx

transverse m of tongue

hyoglossus m

depressor anguli oris m

lingual n

mylohyoid m

stylopharyngeus m

ramus of mandible

n IX

inferior alveolar canal

external carotid a

masseter m

internal carotid a

facial a

n XII

medial pterygoid m

n X

palatine tonsil

internal jugular v

retromandibular v

n XI

parotid gland

sympathetic trunk

posterior belly of digastric m

longus capitis m

middle constrictor m

levator scapulae m

sternocleidomastoid m

vertebral a

body of CV2 and longus colli m

lateral mass, CV3

spinal n, C3

semispinalis cervicis m

superior articular process, CV3

semispinalis capitis m

inferior articular process, CV2

lamina, CV3

spinal cord and dura mater

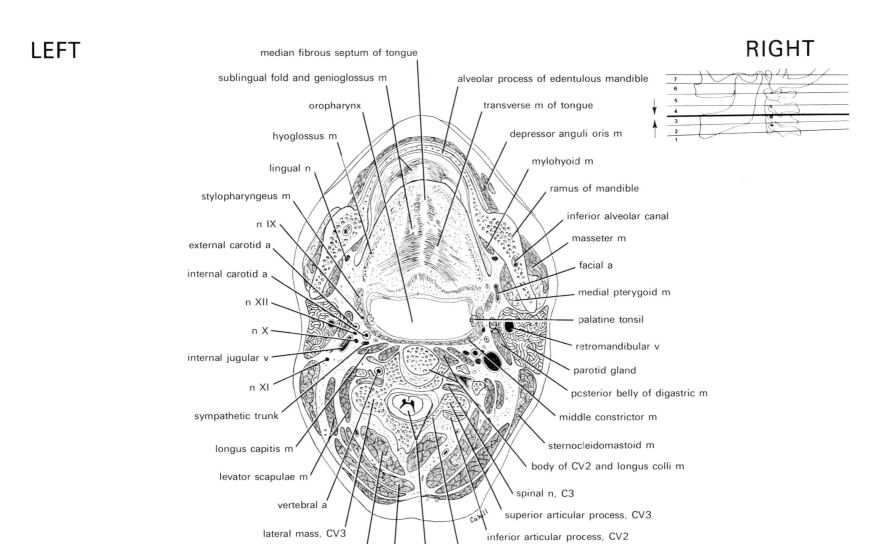

alveolar process of mandible

tongue

oropharynx

medial pterygoid m

buccinator m

palatine tonsil

masseter m

internal carotid a

retromandibular v

posterior belly of digastric m

sternocleidomastoid m

internal jugular v

levator scapulae m

splenius capitis m

vertebral a

inferior articular process, CV3

semispinalis capitis m

spinal cord

TR 500, TE 12

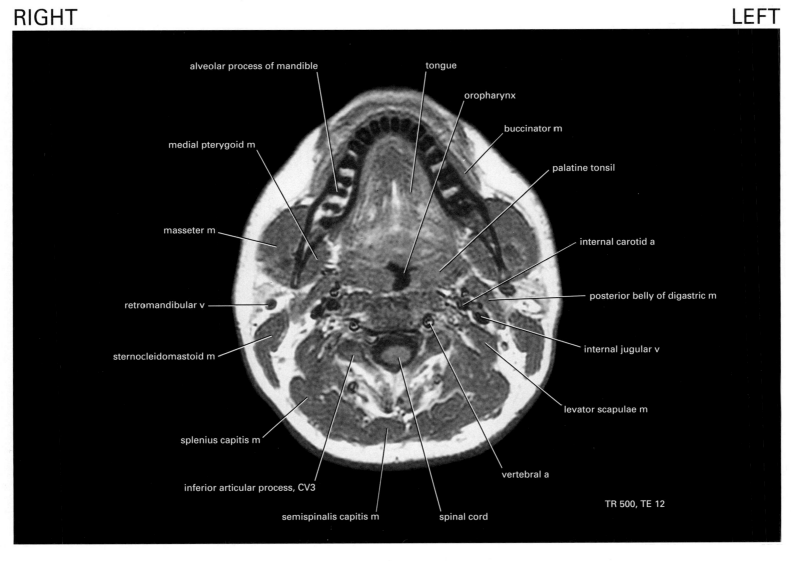

Section 3, anatomy from above, MR image from below.

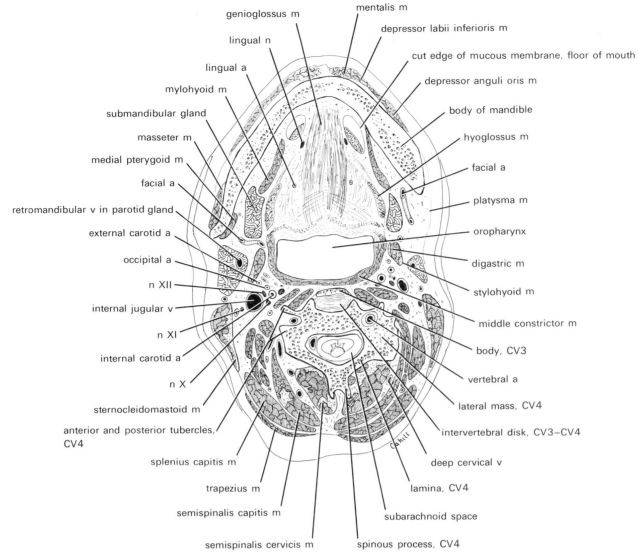

genioglossus m
mentalis m
lingual n
depressor labii inferioris m
lingual a
cut edge of mucous membrane, floor of mouth
mylohyoid m
depressor anguli oris m
submandibular gland
body of mandible
masseter m
hyoglossus m
medial pterygoid m
facial a
facial a
platysma m
retromandibular v in parotid gland
oropharynx
external carotid a
digastric m
occipital a
stylohyoid m
n XII
middle constrictor m
internal jugular v
body, CV3
n XI
vertebral a
internal carotid a
lateral mass, CV4
n X
intervertebral disk, CV3–CV4
sternocleidomastoid m
deep cervical v
anterior and posterior tubercles, CV4
lamina, CV4
splenius capitis m
subarachnoid space
trapezius m
spinous process, CV4
semispinalis capitis m
semispinalis cervicis m

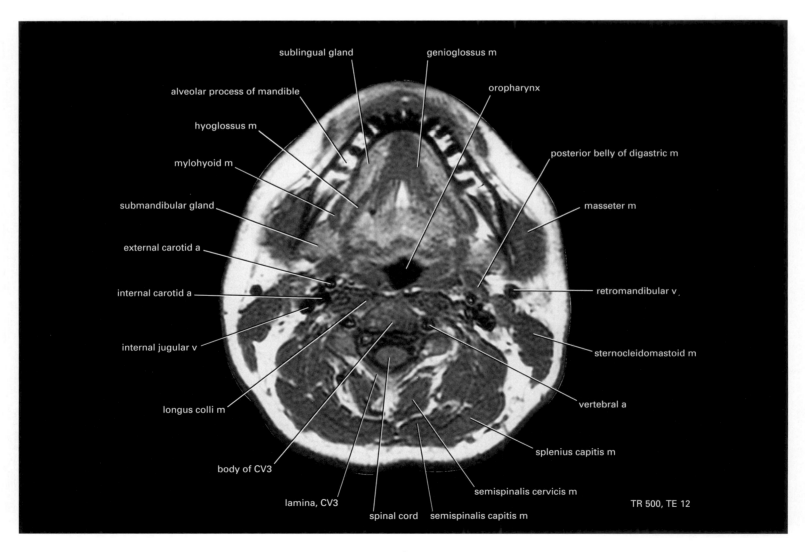

sublingual gland
genioglossus m
alveolar process of mandible
oropharynx
hyoglossus m
posterior belly of digastric m
mylohyoid m
masseter m
submandibular gland
external carotid a
internal carotid a
retromandibular v
internal jugular v
sternocleidomastoid m
longus colli m
vertebral a
body of CV3
splenius capitis m
lamina, CV3
semispinalis cervicis m
spinal cord
semispinalis capitis m

TR 500, TE 12

Section 3 from below.

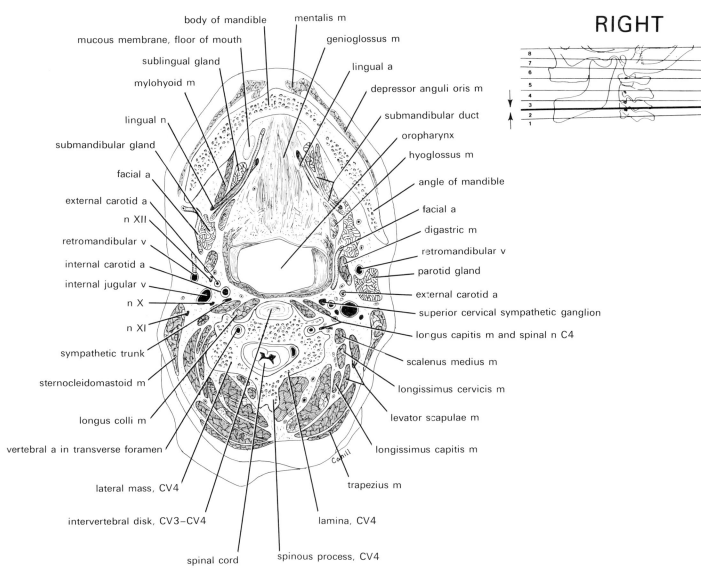

body of mandible

mentalis m

mucous membrane, floor of mouth

genioglossus m

sublingual gland

lingual a

mylohyoid m

depressor anguli oris m

lingual n

submandibular duct

submandibular gland

oropharynx

facial a

hyoglossus m

external carotid a

angle of mandible

n XII

facial a

retromandibular v

digastric m

internal carotid a

retromandibular v

internal jugular v

parotid gland

n X

external carotid a

n XI

superior cervical sympathetic ganglion

sympathetic trunk

longus capitis m and spinal n C4

sternocleidomastoid m

scalenus medius m

longissimus cervicis m

longus colli m

levator scapulae m

vertebral a in transverse foramen

longissimus capitis m

lateral mass, CV4

trapezius m

intervertebral disk, CV3–CV4

lamina, CV4

spinal cord

spinous process, CV4

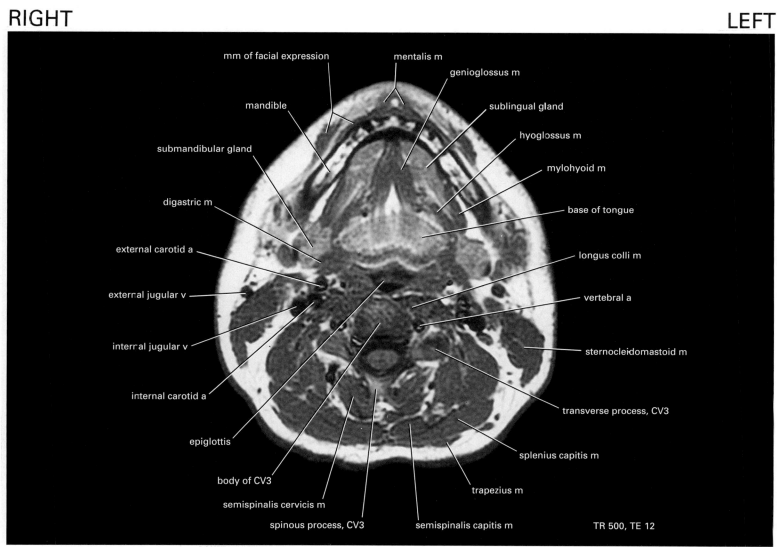

mm of facial expression

mentalis m

genioglossus m

mandible

sublingual gland

submandibular gland

hyoglossus m

mylohyoid m

digastric m

base of tongue

external carotid a

longus colli m

external jugular v

vertebral a

internal jugular v

sternocleidomastoid m

internal carotid a

transverse process, CV3

epiglottis

splenius capitis m

body of CV3

trapezius m

semispinalis cervicis m

semispinalis capitis m

spinous process, CV3

TR 500, TE 12

Section 2, anatomy from above, MR image from below.

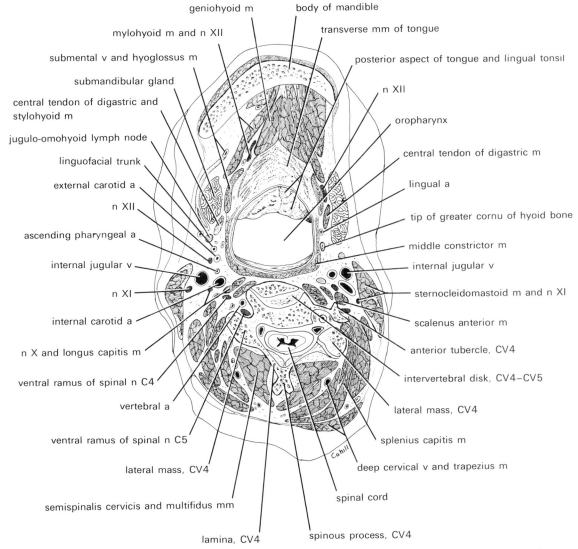

geniohyoid m
body of mandible
mylohyoid m and n XII
transverse mm of tongue
submental v and hyoglossus m
posterior aspect of tongue and lingual tonsil
submandibular gland
n XII
central tendon of digastric and stylohyoid m
oropharynx
jugulo-omohyoid lymph node
central tendon of digastric m
linguofacial trunk
lingual a
external carotid a
tip of greater cornu of hyoid bone
n XII
middle constrictor m
ascending pharyngeal a
internal jugular v
internal jugular v
sternocleidomastoid m and n XI
n XI
scalenus anterior m
internal carotid a
anterior tubercle, CV4
n X and longus capitis m
intervertebral disk, CV4–CV5
ventral ramus of spinal n C4
lateral mass, CV4
vertebral a
splenius capitis m
ventral ramus of spinal n C5
deep cervical v and trapezius m
lateral mass, CV4
spinal cord
semispinalis cervicis and multifidus mm
lamina, CV4
spinous process, CV4

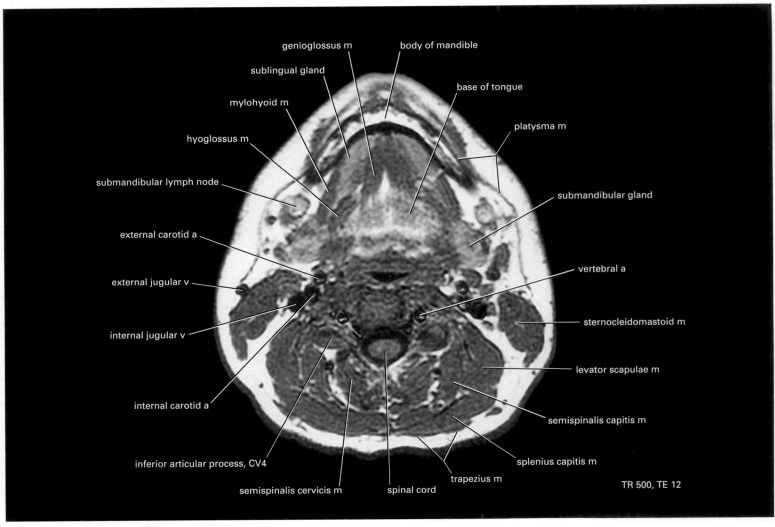

genioglossus m
body of mandible
sublingual gland
base of tongue
mylohyoid m
platysma m
hyoglossus m
submandibular lymph node
submandibular gland
external carotid a
vertebral a
external jugular v
sternocleidomastoid m
internal jugular v
levator scapulae m
internal carotid a
semispinalis capitis m
splenius capitis m
inferior articular process, CV4
trapezius m
semispinalis cervicis m
spinal cord
TR 500, TE 12

Section 2 from below.

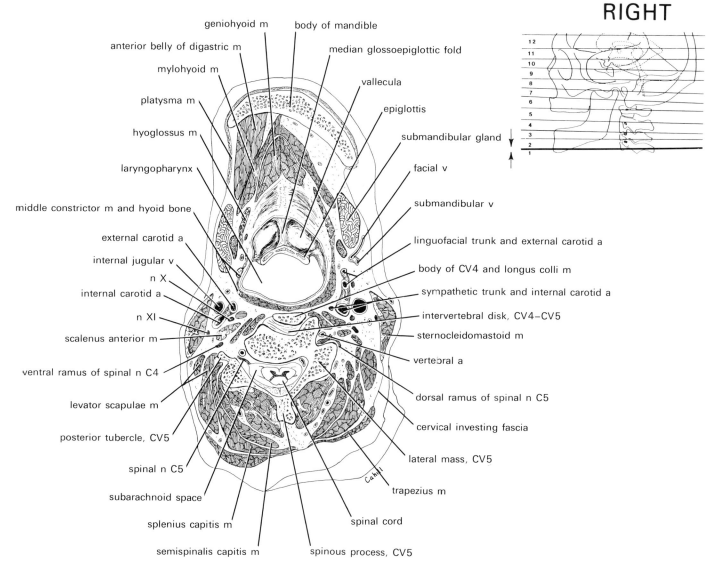

geniohyoid m
body of mandible
anterior belly of digastric m
median glossoepiglottic fold
mylohyoid m
vallecula
platysma m
epiglottis
hyoglossus m
submandibular gland
laryngopharynx
facial v
middle constrictor m and hyoid bone
submandibular v
external carotid a
linguofacial trunk and external carotid a
internal jugular v
body of CV4 and longus colli m
n X
sympathetic trunk and internal carotid a
internal carotid a
intervertebral disk, CV4–CV5
n XI
sternocleidomastoid m
scalenus anterior m
vertebral a
ventral ramus of spinal n C4
dorsal ramus of spinal n C5
levator scapulae m
cervical investing fascia
posterior tubercle, CV5
lateral mass, CV5
spinal n C5
trapezius m
subarachnoid space
spinal cord
splenius capitis m
semispinalis capitis m
spinous process, CV5

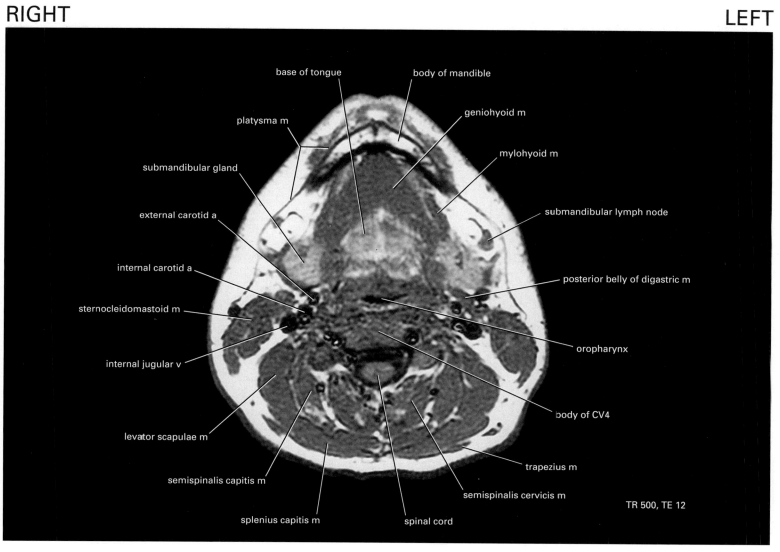

base of tongue
body of mandible
platysma m
geniohyoid m
submandibular gland
mylohyoid m
external carotid a
submandibular lymph node
internal carotid a
posterior belly of digastric m
sternocleidomastoid m
internal jugular v
oropharynx
levator scapulae m
body of CV4
semispinalis capitis m
trapezius m
splenius capitis m
semispinalis cervicis m
spinal cord
TR 500, TE 12

Section 1, anatomy from above, MR image from below.

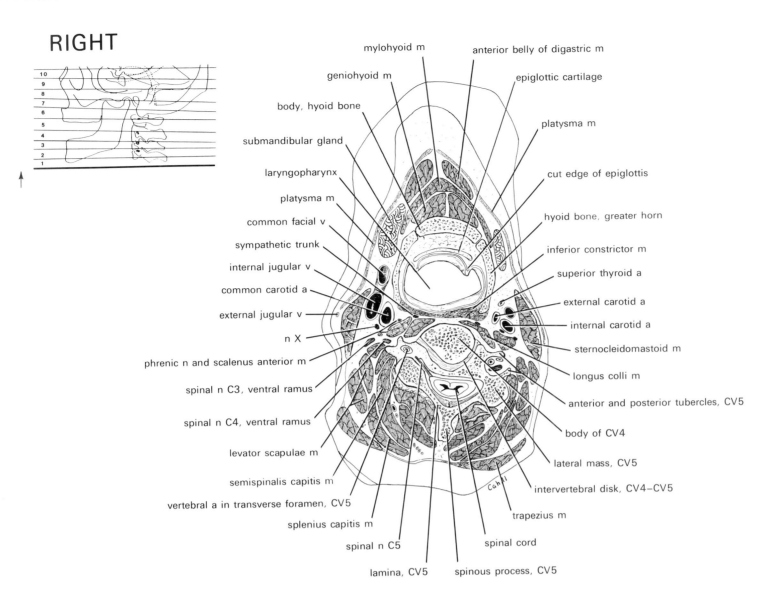

mylohyoid m
anterior belly of digastric m
geniohyoid m
epiglottic cartilage
body, hyoid bone
platysma m
submandibular gland
cut edge of epiglottis
laryngopharynx
platysma m
hyoid bone, greater horn
common facial v
inferior constrictor m
sympathetic trunk
superior thyroid a
internal jugular v
external carotid a
common carotid a
internal carotid a
external jugular v
sternocleidomastoid m
n X
longus colli m
phrenic n and scalenus anterior m
anterior and posterior tubercles, CV5
spinal n C3, ventral ramus
body of CV4
spinal n C4, ventral ramus
lateral mass, CV5
levator scapulae m
intervertebral disk, CV4–CV5
semispinalis capitis m
trapezius m
vertebral a in transverse foramen, CV5
splenius capitis m
spinal cord
spinal n C5
lamina, CV5
spinous process, CV5

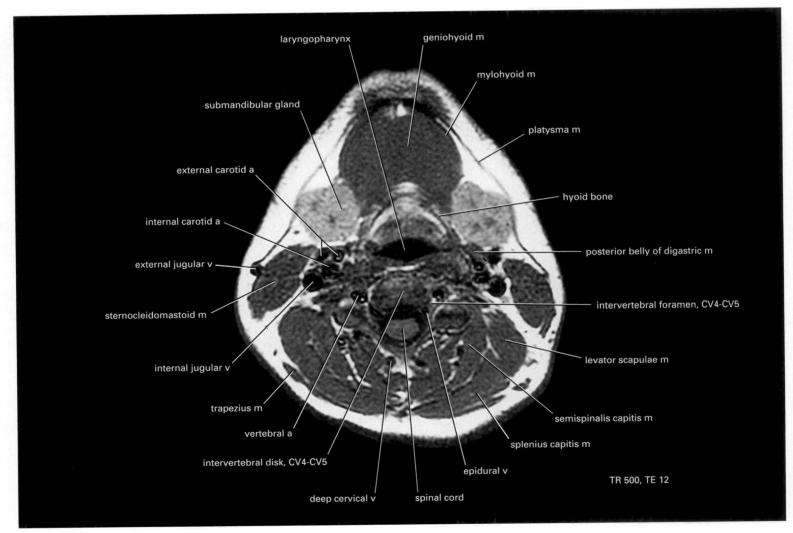

laryngopharynx
geniohyoid m
mylohyoid m
submandibular gland
platysma m
external carotid a
hyoid bone
internal carotid a
external jugular v
posterior belly of digastric m
sternocleidomastoid m
intervertebral foramen, CV4-CV5
internal jugular v
levator scapulae m
trapezius m
semispinalis capitis m
vertebral a
splenius capitis m
intervertebral disk, CV4-CV5
epidural v
TR 500, TE 12
deep cervical v
spinal cord

Section 1 from below.

The Head and Neck in Sagittal Planes

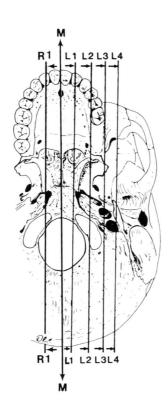

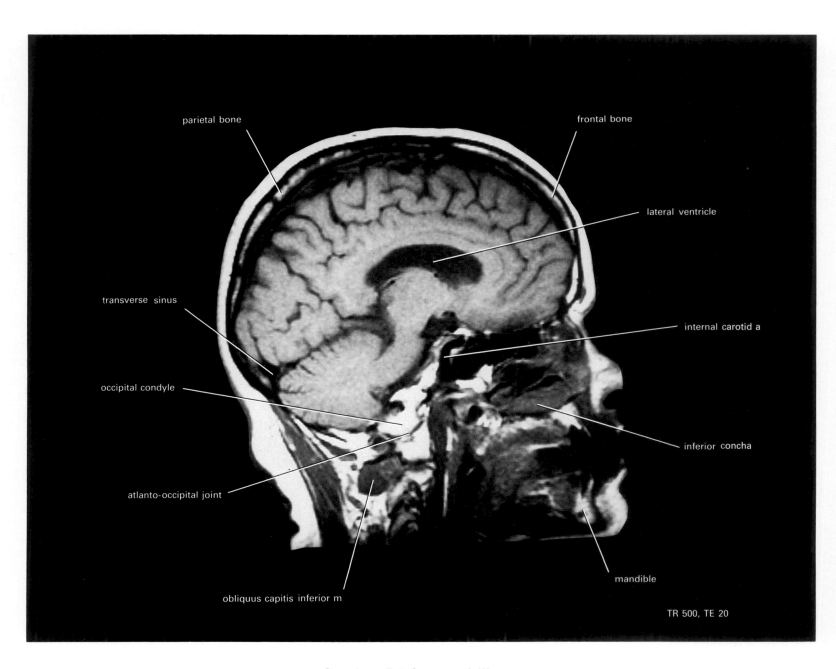

Section R1 from midline.

BONES, MUSCLES, VESSELS, AND VISCERA

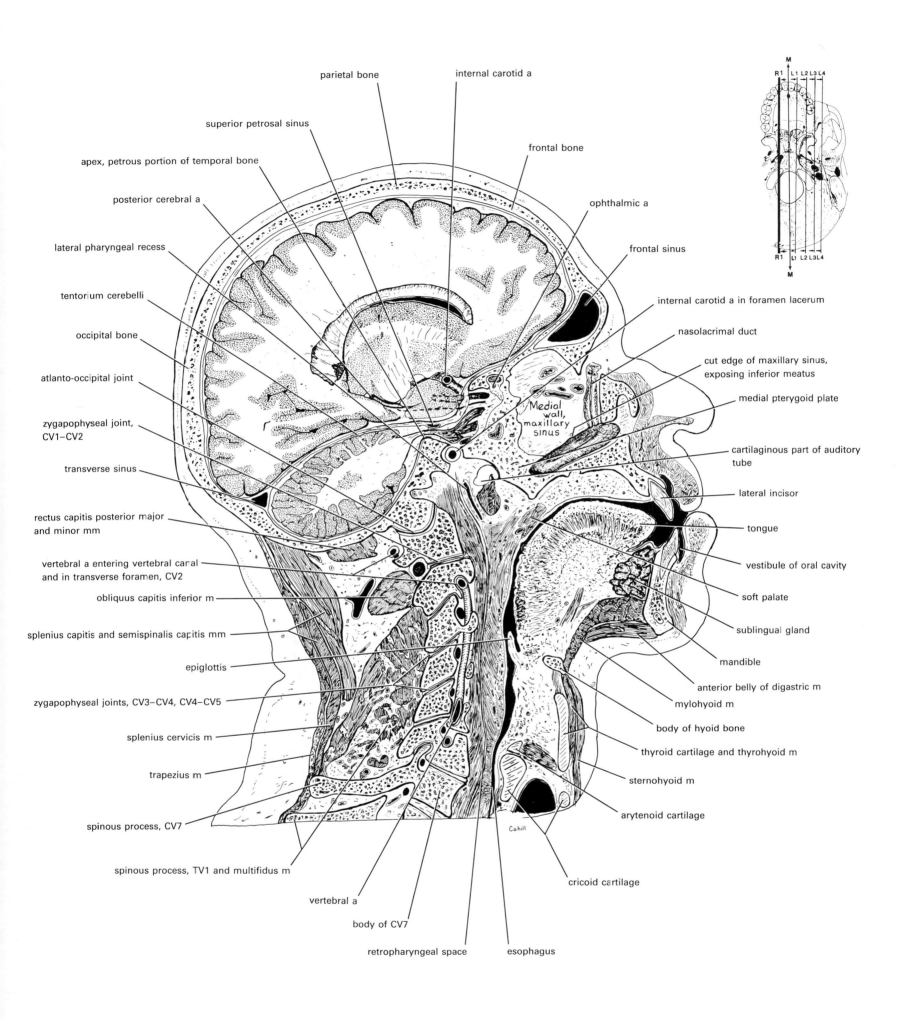

parietal bone

internal carotid a

superior petrosal sinus

frontal bone

apex, petrous portion of temporal bone

ophthalmic a

posterior cerebral a

frontal sinus

lateral pharyngeal recess

internal carotid a in foramen lacerum

tentorium cerebelli

nasolacrimal duct

occipital bone

cut edge of maxillary sinus, exposing inferior meatus

atlanto-occipital joint

Medial wall, maxillary sinus

medial pterygoid plate

zygapophyseal joint, CV1–CV2

cartilaginous part of auditory tube

transverse sinus

lateral incisor

rectus capitis posterior major and minor mm

tongue

vertebral a entering vertebral caral and in transverse foramen, CV2

vestibule of oral cavity

obliquus capitis inferior m

soft palate

splenius capitis and semispinalis capitis mm

sublingual gland

epiglottis

mandible

zygapophyseal joints, CV3–CV4, CV4–CV5

anterior belly of digastric m

splenius cervicis m

mylohyoid m

trapezius m

body of hyoid bone

thyroid cartilage and thyrohyoid m

spinous process, CV7

sternohyoid m

arytenoid cartilage

spinous process, TV1 and multifidus m

cricoid cartilage

vertebral a

body of CV7

retropharyngeal space

esophagus

Cahill

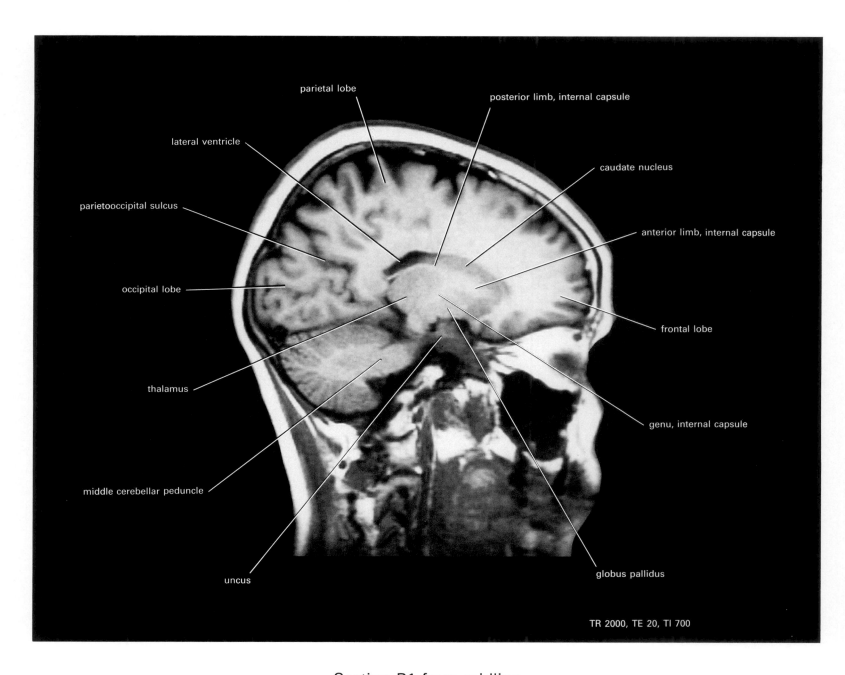

Section R1 from midline.

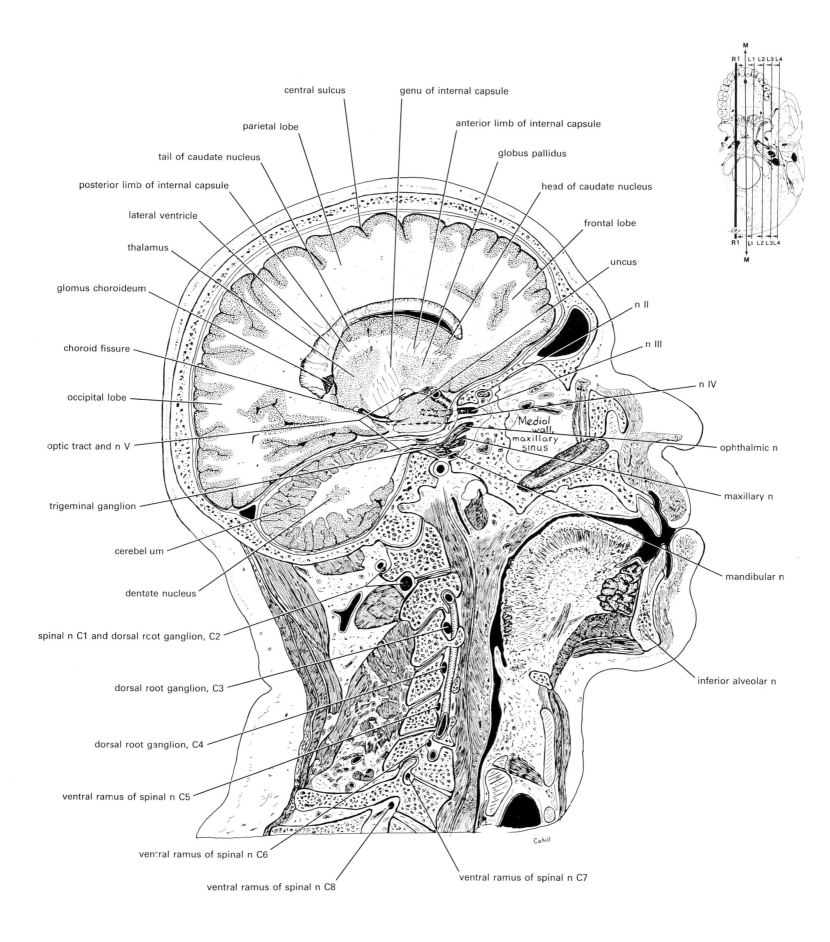

central sulcus

genu of internal capsule

parietal lobe

anterior limb of internal capsule

tail of caudate nucleus

globus pallidus

posterior limb of internal capsule

head of caudate nucleus

lateral ventricle

frontal lobe

thalamus

uncus

glomus choroideum

n II

choroid fissure

n III

occipital lobe

n IV

optic tract and n V

Medial wall, maxillary sinus

ophthalmic n

trigeminal ganglion

maxillary n

cerebellum

mandibular n

dentate nucleus

spinal n C1 and dorsal root ganglion, C2

dorsal root ganglion, C3

inferior alveolar n

dorsal root ganglion, C4

ventral ramus of spinal n C5

ventral ramus of spinal n C6

ventral ramus of spinal n C8

ventral ramus of spinal n C7

Cahill

Section R1 from midline.

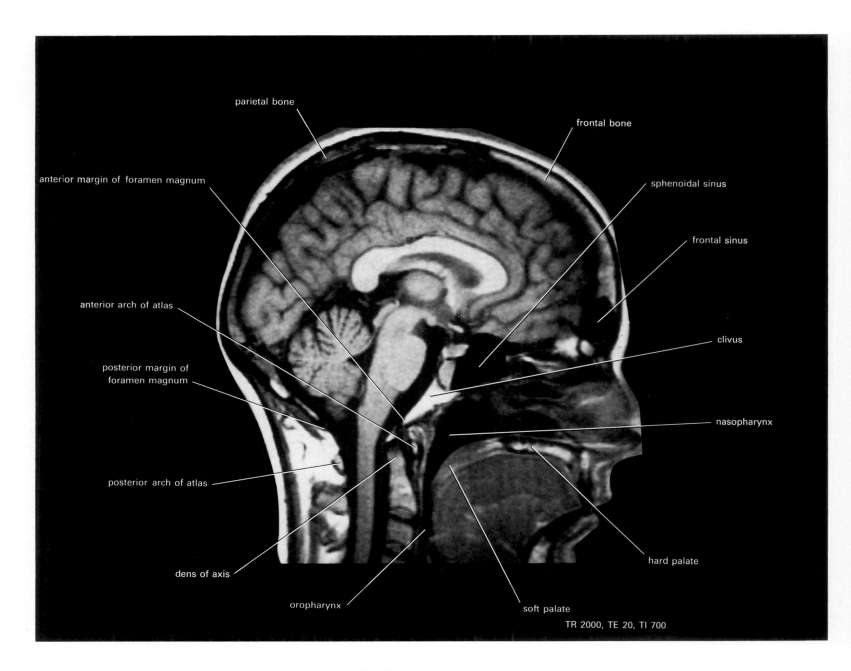

parietal bone

frontal bone

anterior margin of foramen magnum

sphenoidal sinus

frontal sinus

anterior arch of atlas

clivus

posterior margin of
foramen magnum

nasopharynx

posterior arch of atlas

hard palate

dens of axis

oropharynx

soft palate

TR 2000, TE 20, TI 700

Median Section

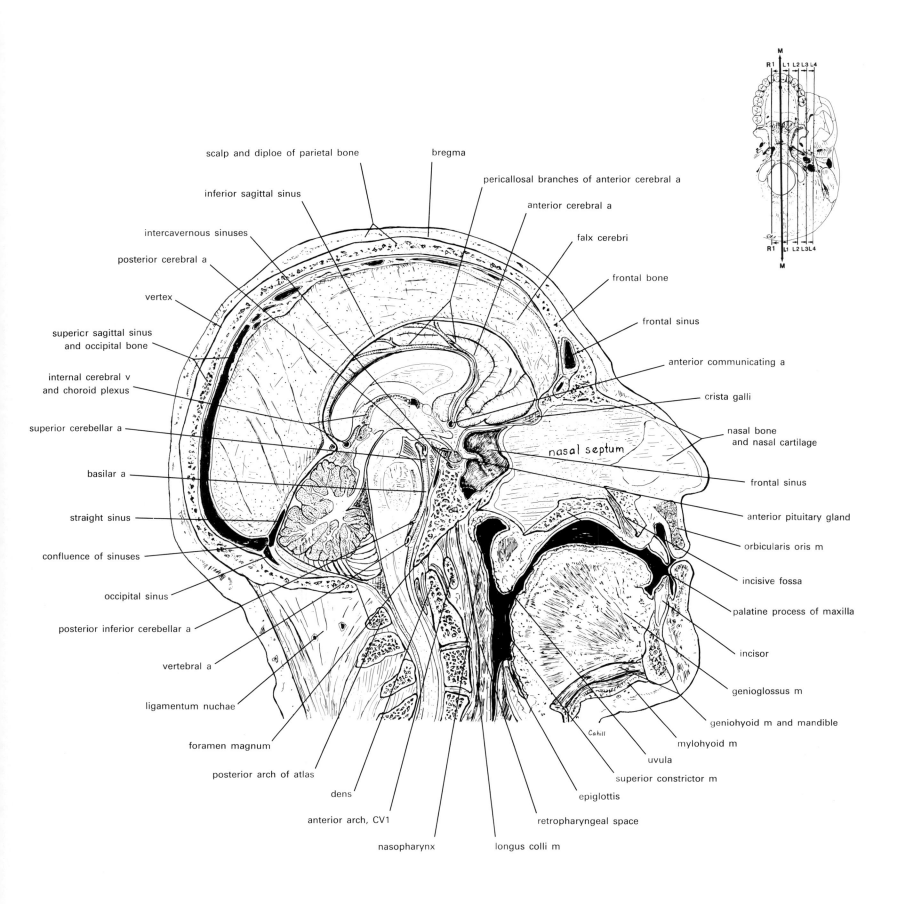

scalp and diploe of parietal bone

bregma

inferior sagittal sinus

pericallosal branches of anterior cerebral a

intercavernous sinuses

anterior cerebral a

posterior cerebral a

falx cerebri

vertex

frontal bone

superior sagittal sinus
and occipital bone

frontal sinus

internal cerebral v
and choroid plexus

anterior communicating a

superior cerebellar a

crista galli

basilar a

nasal bone
and nasal cartilage

nasal septum

straight sinus

frontal sinus

confluence of sinuses

anterior pituitary gland

occipital sinus

orbicularis oris m

posterior inferior cerebellar a

incisive fossa

vertebral a

palatine process of maxilla

ligamentum nuchae

incisor

foramen magnum

genioglossus m

posterior arch of atlas

geniohyoid m and mandible

dens

mylohyoid m

anterior arch, CV1

uvula

nasopharynx

superior constrictor m

epiglottis

retropharyngeal space

longus colli m

Cahill

Median Section

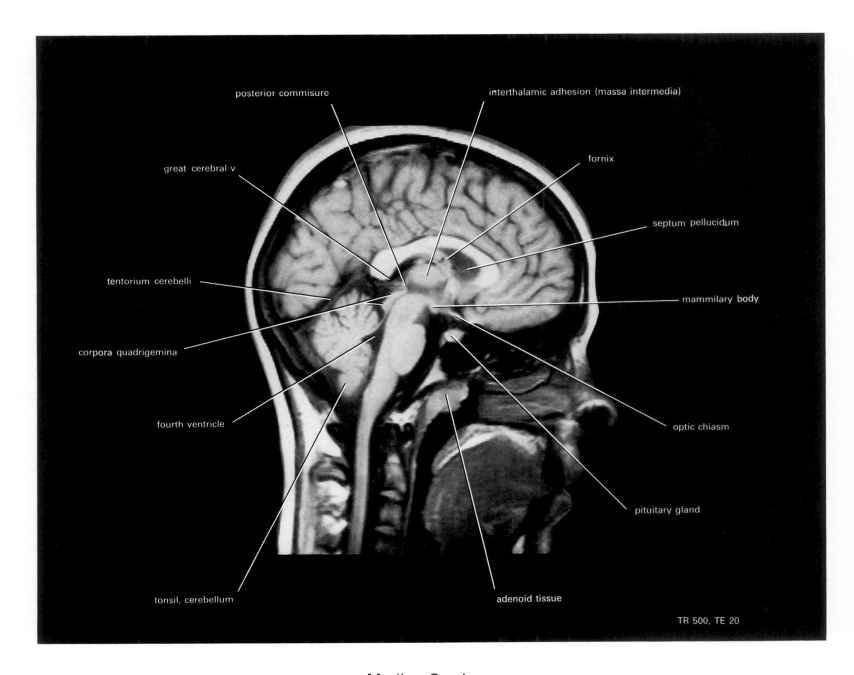

posterior commisure

interthalamic adhesion (massa intermedia)

great cerebral v

fornix

septum pellucidum

tentorium cerebelli

mammilary body

corpora quadrigemina

optic chiasm

fourth ventricle

pituitary gland

tonsil, cerebellum

adenoid tissue

TR 500, TE 20

Median Section

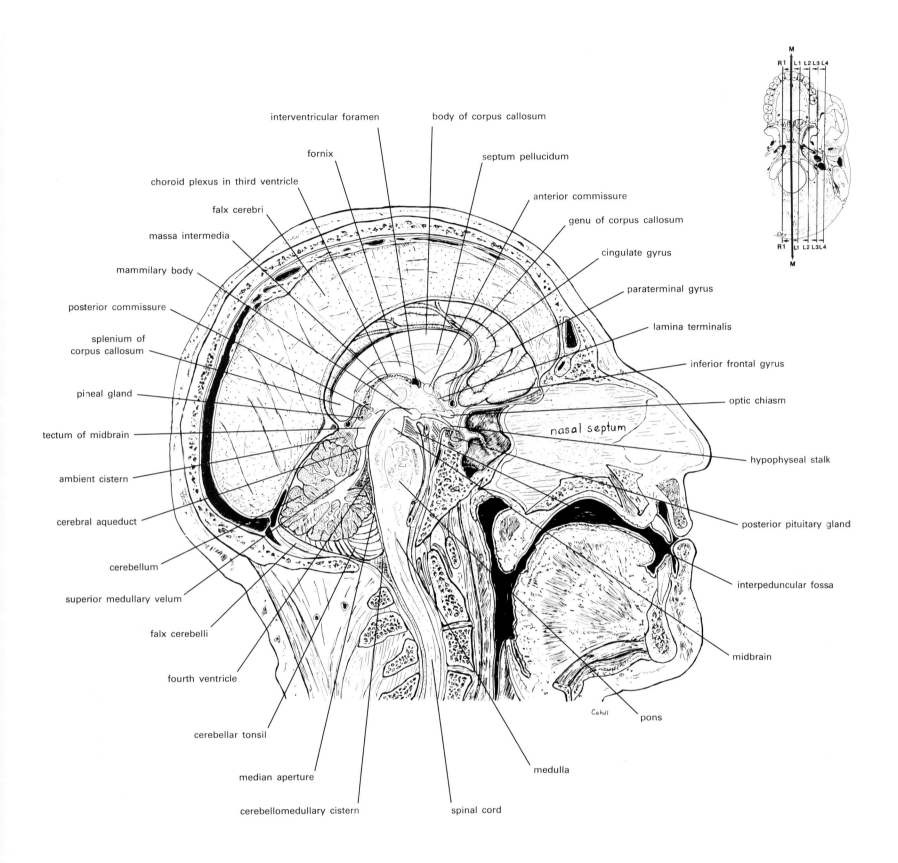

interventricular foramen

body of corpus callosum

fornix

septum pellucidum

choroid plexus in third ventricle

anterior commissure

falx cerebri

genu of corpus callosum

massa intermedia

cingulate gyrus

mammilary body

paraterminal gyrus

posterior commissure

lamina terminalis

splenium of corpus callosum

inferior frontal gyrus

pineal gland

optic chiasm

tectum of midbrain

nasal septum

ambient cistern

hypophyseal stalk

cerebral aqueduct

cerebellum

posterior pituitary gland

superior medullary velum

interpeduncular fossa

falx cerebelli

fourth ventricle

midbrain

cerebellar tonsil

Cahill

pons

median aperture

cerebellomedullary cistern

medulla

spinal cord

Median Section

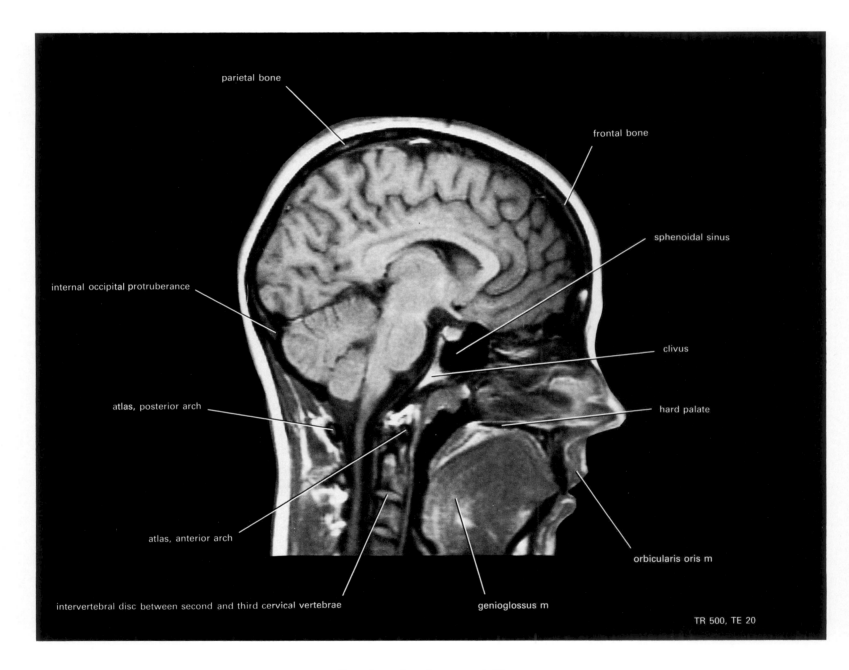

parietal bone

frontal bone

sphenoidal sinus

internal occipital protruberance

clivus

atlas, posterior arch

hard palate

atlas, anterior arch

orbicularis oris m

intervertebral disc between second and third cervical vertebrae

genioglossus m

TR 500, TE 20

Section L1 from midline.

BONES AND MUSCLES

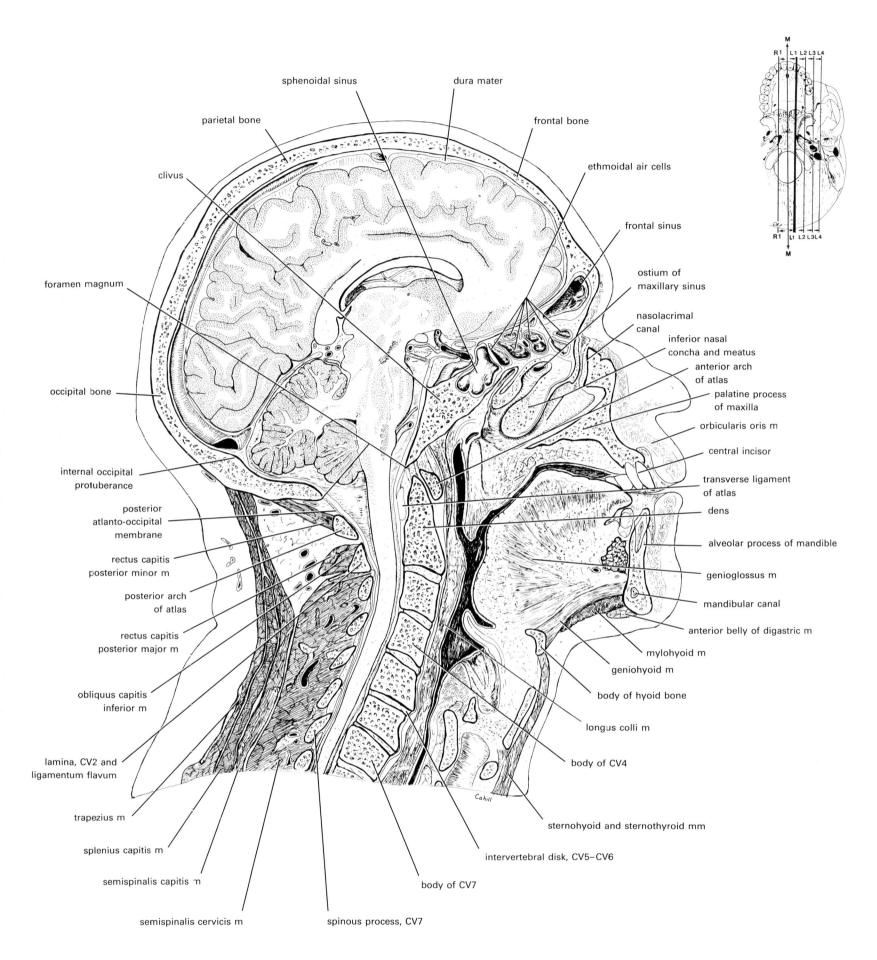

sphenoidal sinus

dura mater

parietal bone

frontal bone

clivus

ethmoidal air cells

frontal sinus

foramen magnum

ostium of
maxillary sinus

nasolacrimal
canal

inferior nasal
concha and meatus

anterior arch
of atlas

occipital bone

palatine process
of maxilla

orbicularis oris m

central incisor

internal occipital
protuberance

transverse ligament
of atlas

dens

posterior
atlanto-occipital
membrane

alveolar process of mandible

rectus capitis
posterior minor m

genioglossus m

mandibular canal

posterior arch
of atlas

anterior belly of digastric m

rectus capitis
posterior major m

mylohyoid m

geniohyoid m

obliquus capitis
inferior m

body of hyoid bone

longus colli m

lamina, CV2 and
ligamentum flavum

body of CV4

trapezius m

sternohyoid and sternothyroid mm

splenius capitis m

intervertebral disk, CV5–CV6

semispinalis capitis m

body of CV7

semispinalis cervicis m

spinous process, CV7

Section L1 from midline.

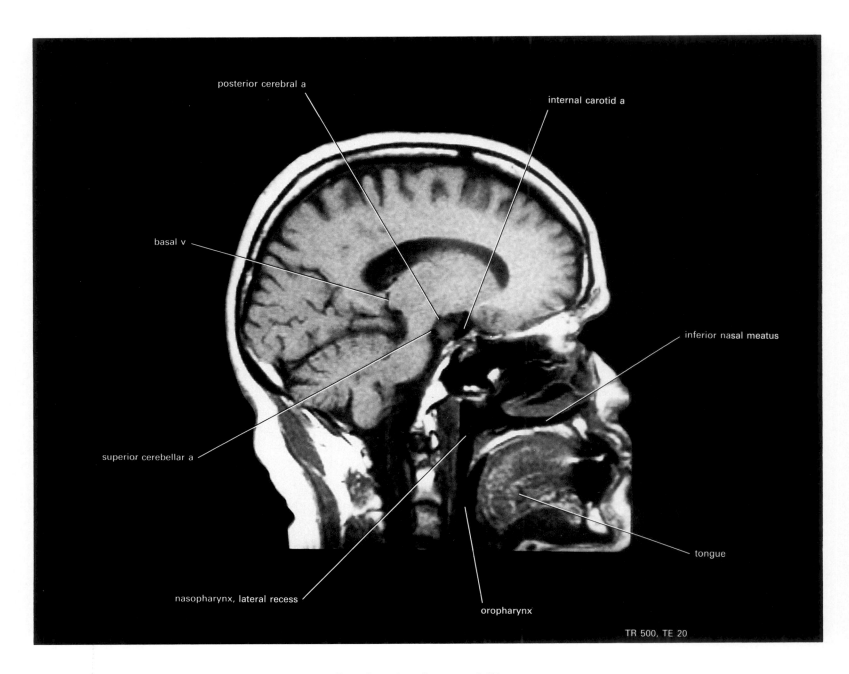

Section L1 from midline.

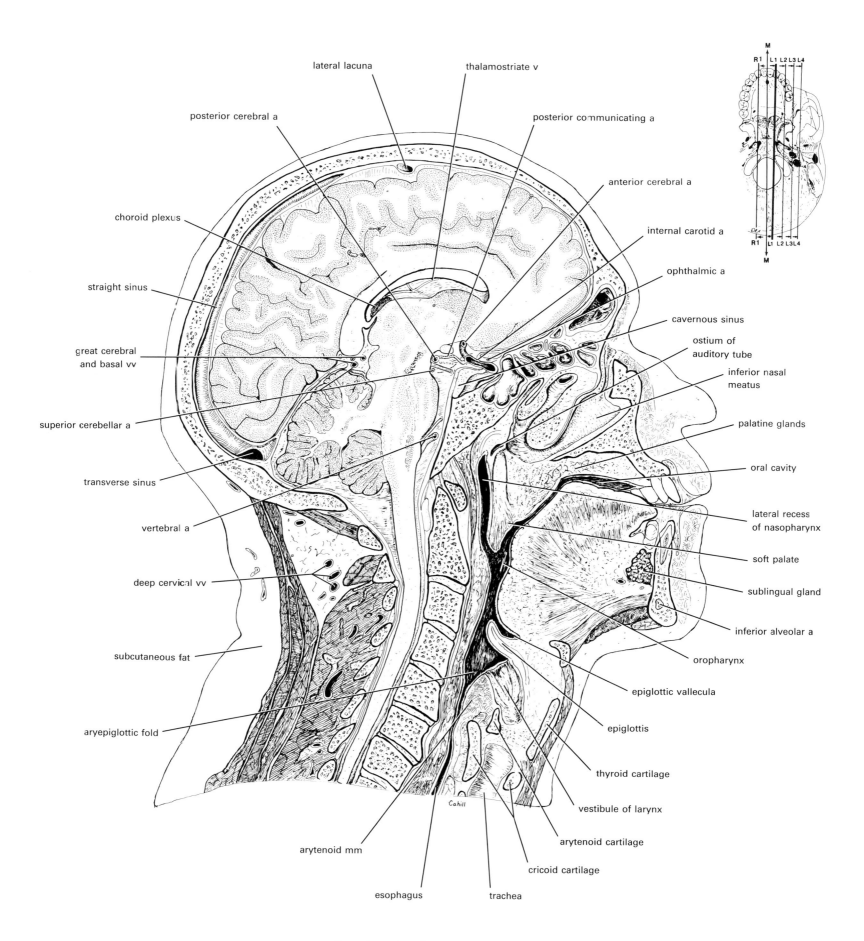

lateral lacuna

thalamostriate v

posterior cerebral a

posterior communicating a

anterior cerebral a

choroid plexus

internal carotid a

ophthalmic a

straight sinus

cavernous sinus

ostium of
auditory tube

great cerebral
and basal vv

inferior nasal
meatus

superior cerebellar a

palatine glands

oral cavity

transverse sinus

lateral recess
of nasopharynx

vertebral a

soft palate

sublingual gland

deep cervical vv

inferior alveolar a

subcutaneous fat

oropharynx

epiglottic vallecula

aryepiglottic fold

epiglottis

thyroid cartilage

vestibule of larynx

arytenoid mm

arytenoid cartilage

cricoid cartilage

esophagus

trachea

Cahill

Section L1 from midline.

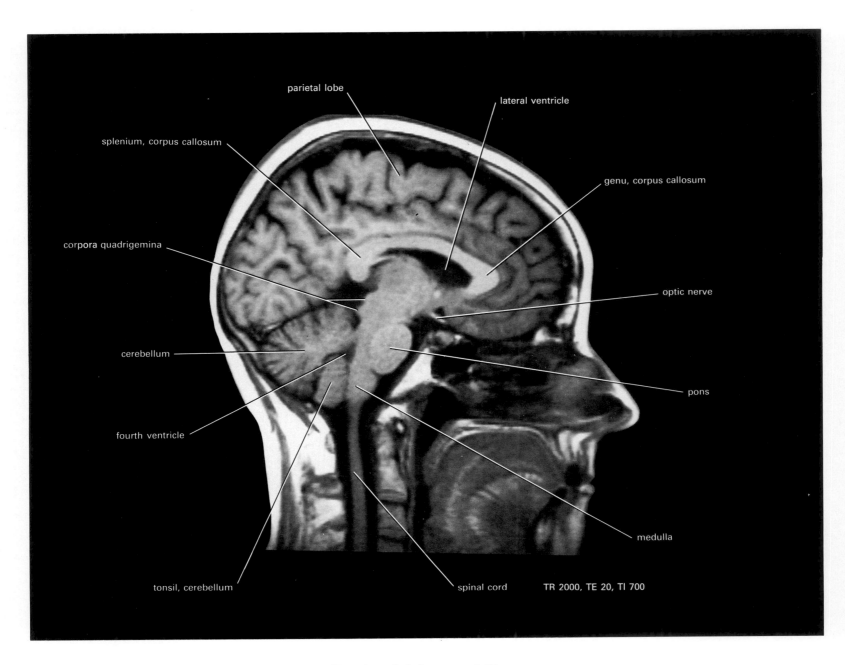

Section L1 from midline.

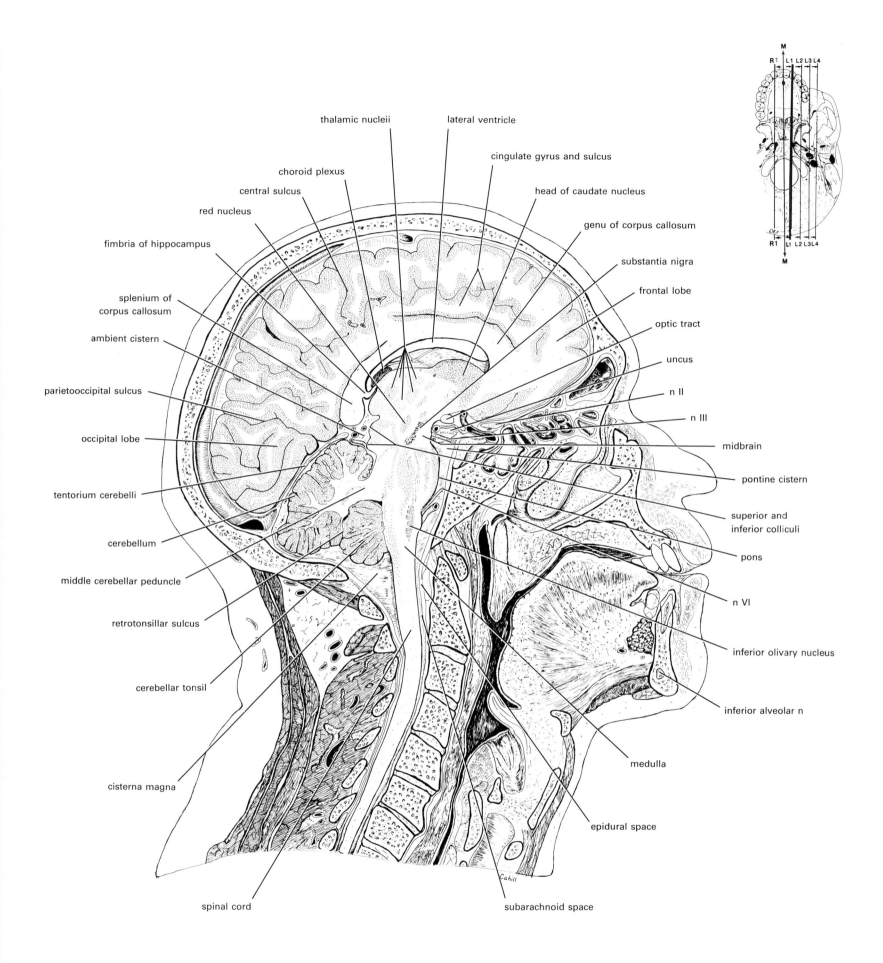

thalamic nucleii

lateral ventricle

cingulate gyrus and sulcus

choroid plexus

central sulcus

head of caudate nucleus

red nucleus

genu of corpus callosum

fimbria of hippocampus

substantia nigra

frontal lobe

splenium of
corpus callosum

optic tract

ambient cistern

uncus

n II

parietooccipital sulcus

n III

midbrain

occipital lobe

pontine cistern

tentorium cerebelli

superior and
inferior colliculi

cerebellum

pons

middle cerebellar peduncle

n VI

retrotonsillar sulcus

inferior olivary nucleus

cerebellar tonsil

inferior alveolar n

medulla

cisterna magna

epidural space

spinal cord

subarachnoid space

Section L1 from midline.

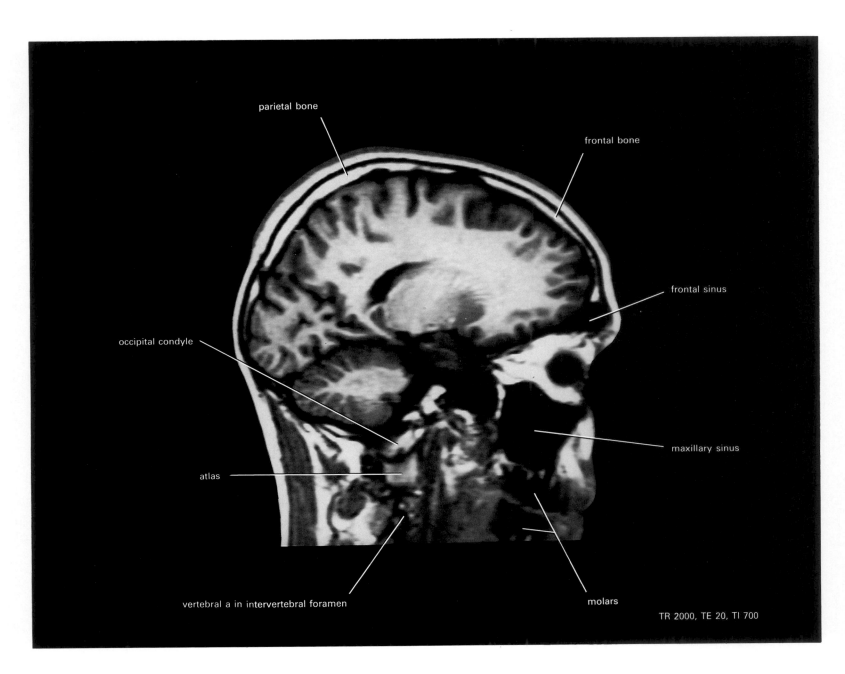

Section L2 from midline.

BONES AND JOINTS

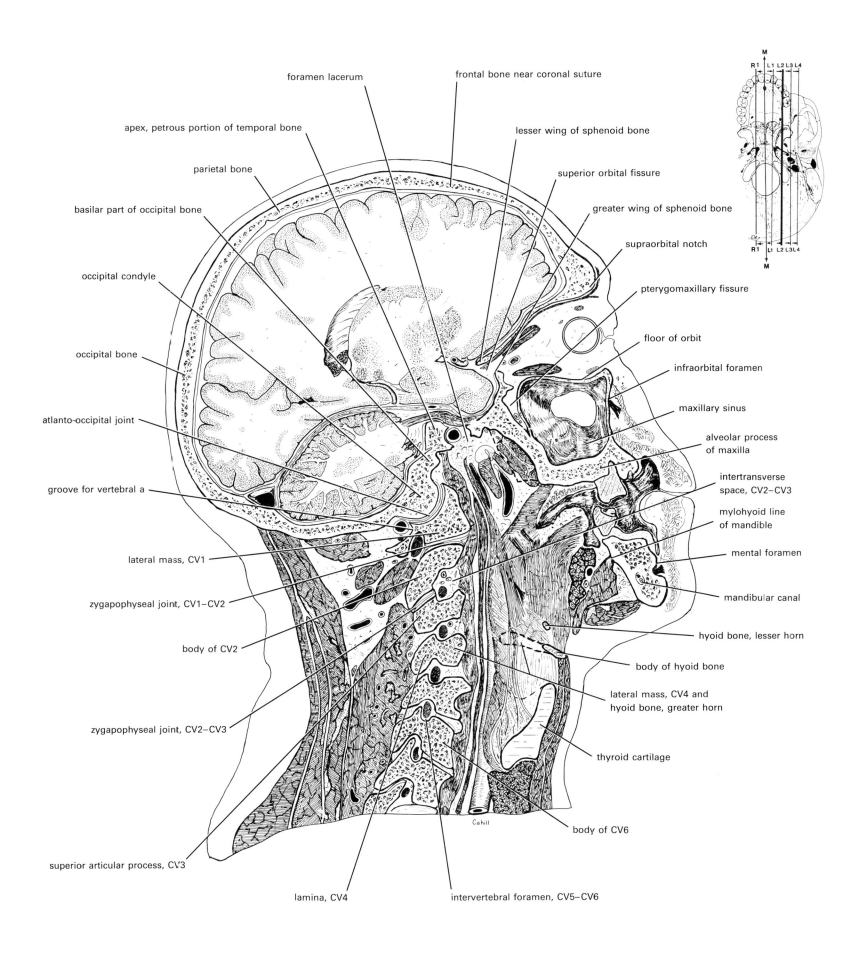

foramen lacerum

frontal bone near coronal suture

apex, petrous portion of temporal bone

lesser wing of sphenoid bone

parietal bone

superior orbital fissure

basilar part of occipital bone

greater wing of sphenoid bone

supraorbital notch

occipital condyle

pterygomaxillary fissure

occipital bone

floor of orbit

infraorbital foramen

atlanto-occipital joint

maxillary sinus

alveolar process
of maxilla

groove for vertebral a

intertransverse
space, CV2–CV3

mylohyoid line
of mandible

lateral mass, CV1

mental foramen

zygapophyseal joint, CV1–CV2

mandibular canal

body of CV2

hyoid bone, lesser horn

body of hyoid bone

lateral mass, CV4 and
hyoid bone, greater horn

zygapophyseal joint, CV2–CV3

thyroid cartilage

body of CV6

superior articular process, CV3

lamina, CV4

intervertebral foramen, CV5–CV6

Cahill

Section L2 from midline.

MUSCLES

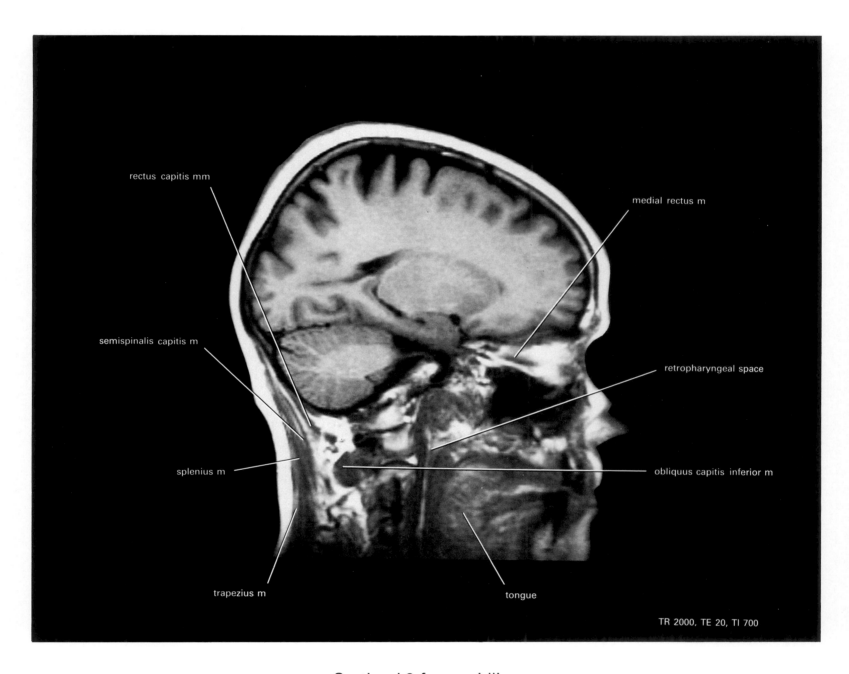

rectus capitis mm

medial rectus m

semispinalis capitis m

retropharyngeal space

splenius m

obliquus capitis inferior m

trapezius m

tongue

TR 2000, TE 20, TI 700

Section L2 from midline.

MUSCLES

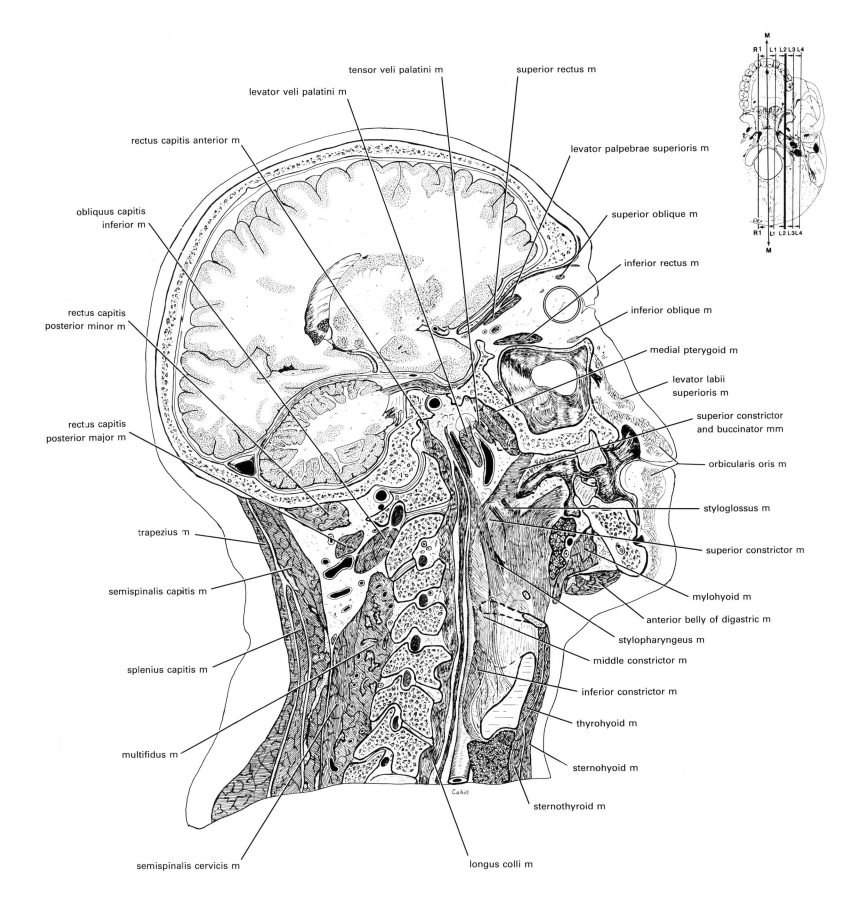

tensor veli palatini m

superior rectus m

levator veli palatini m

levator palpebrae superioris m

rectus capitis anterior m

superior oblique m

obliquus capitis inferior m

inferior rectus m

inferior oblique m

rectus capitis posterior minor m

medial pterygoid m

levator labii superioris m

superior constrictor and buccinator mm

rectus capitis posterior major m

orbicularis oris m

styloglossus m

trapezius m

superior constrictor m

semispinalis capitis m

mylohyoid m

anterior belly of digastric m

splenius capitis m

stylopharyngeus m

middle constrictor m

inferior constrictor m

thyrohyoid m

multifidus m

sternohyoid m

sternothyroid m

semispinalis cervicis m

longus colli m

Section L2 from midline.

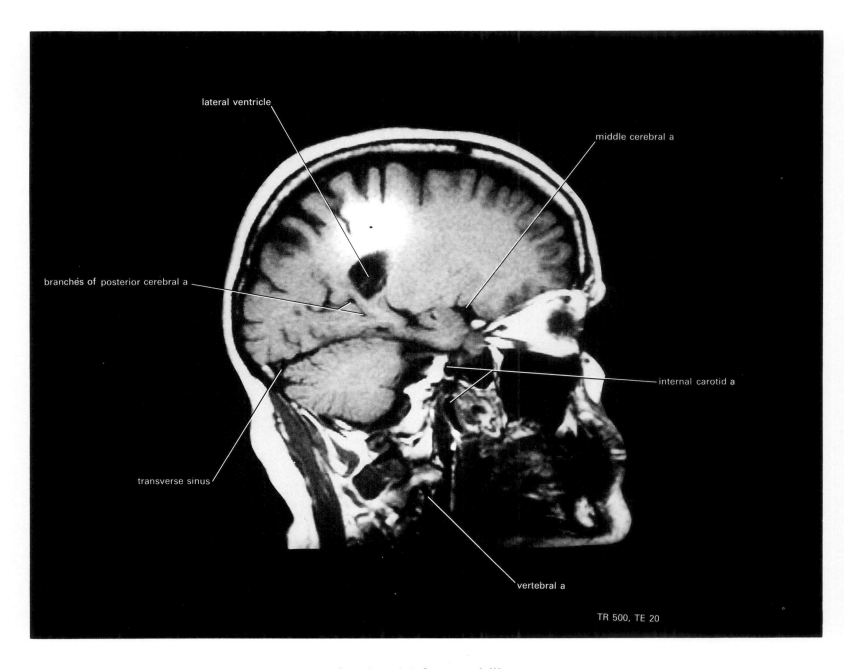

lateral ventricle

middle cerebral a

branches of posterior cerebral a

internal carotid a

transverse sinus

vertebral a

TR 500, TE 20

Section L2 from midline.

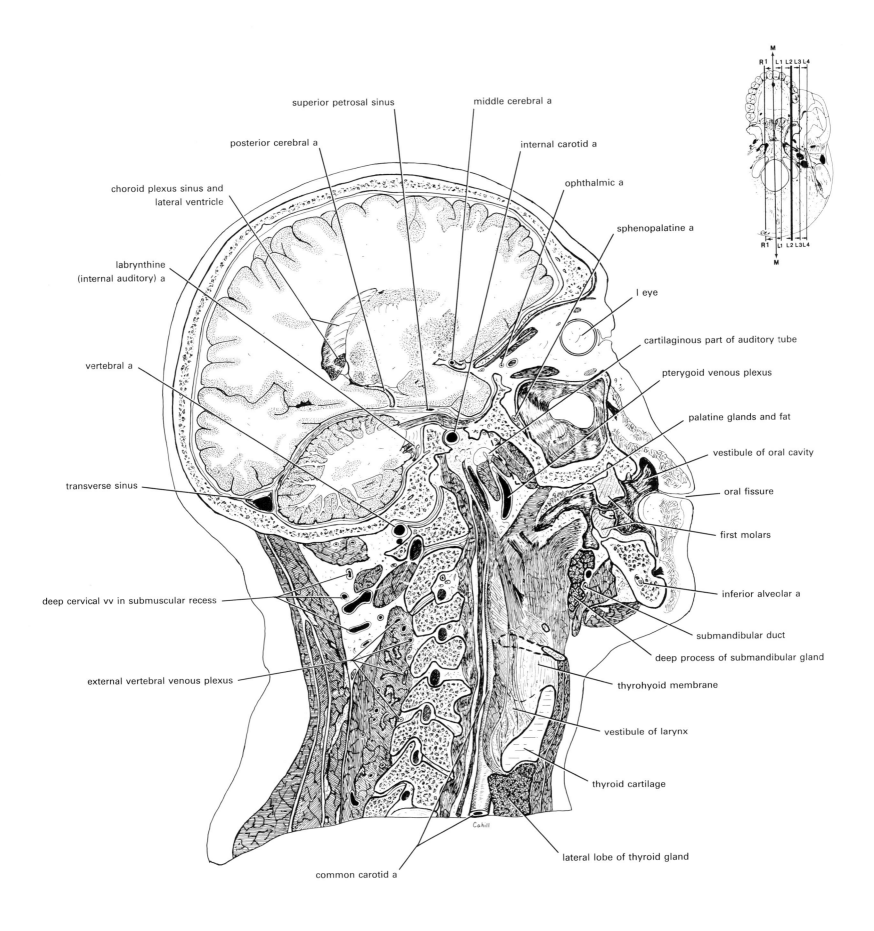

superior petrosal sinus

middle cerebral a

posterior cerebral a

internal carotid a

choroid plexus sinus and
lateral ventricle

ophthalmic a

sphenopalatine a

labrynthine
(internal auditory) a

l eye

cartilaginous part of auditory tube

vertebral a

pterygoid venous plexus

palatine glands and fat

vestibule of oral cavity

transverse sinus

oral fissure

first molars

deep cervical vv in submuscular recess

inferior alveolar a

submandibular duct

external vertebral venous plexus

deep process of submandibular gland

thyrohyoid membrane

vestibule of larynx

thyroid cartilage

common carotid a

lateral lobe of thyroid gland

Section L2 from midline.

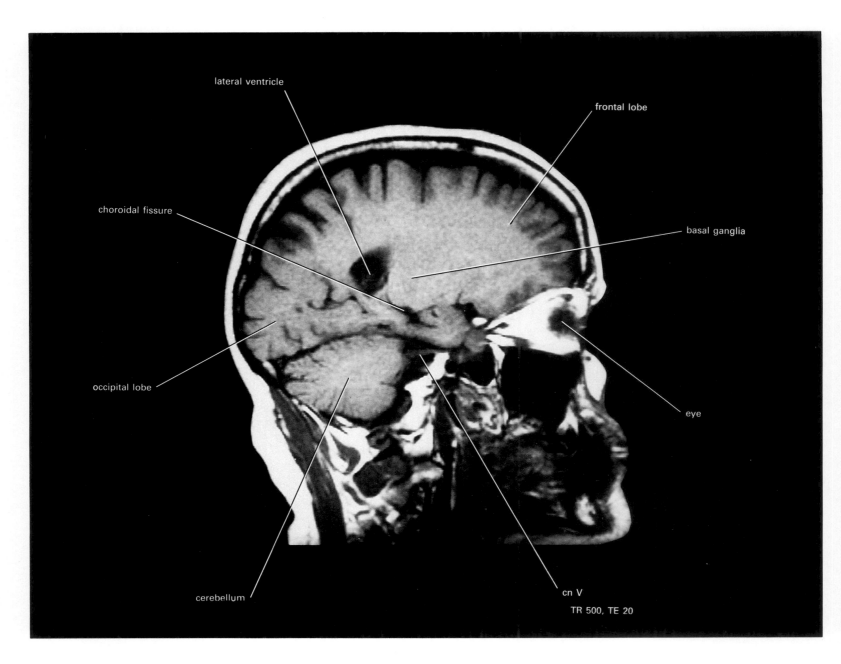

Section L2 from midline.

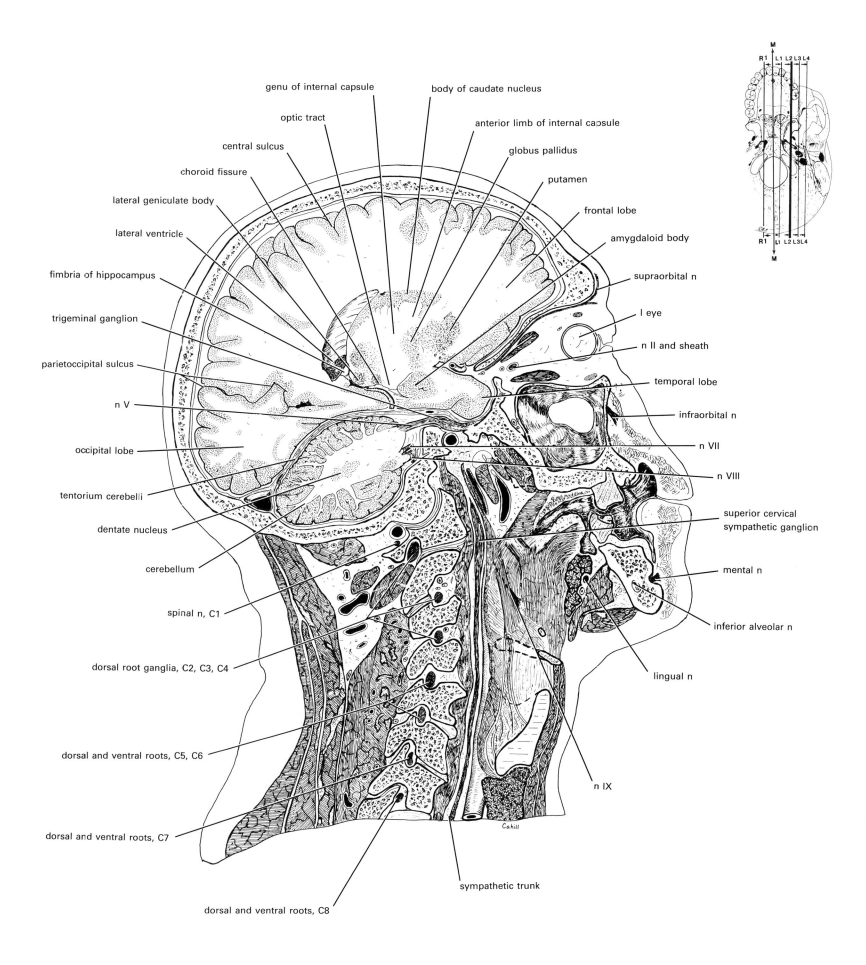

genu of internal capsule

body of caudate nucleus

optic tract

anterior limb of internal capsule

central sulcus

globus pallidus

choroid fissure

putamen

lateral geniculate body

frontal lobe

lateral ventricle

amygdaloid body

fimbria of hippocampus

supraorbital n

trigeminal ganglion

l eye

parietoccipital sulcus

n II and sheath

n V

temporal lobe

occipital lobe

infraorbital n

tentorium cerebelli

n VII

dentate nucleus

n VIII

cerebellum

superior cervical sympathetic ganglion

spinal n, C1

mental n

dorsal root ganglia, C2, C3, C4

inferior alveolar n

dorsal and ventral roots, C5, C6

lingual n

dorsal and ventral roots, C7

n IX

dorsal and ventral roots, C8

sympathetic trunk

Cahill

Section L2 from midline.

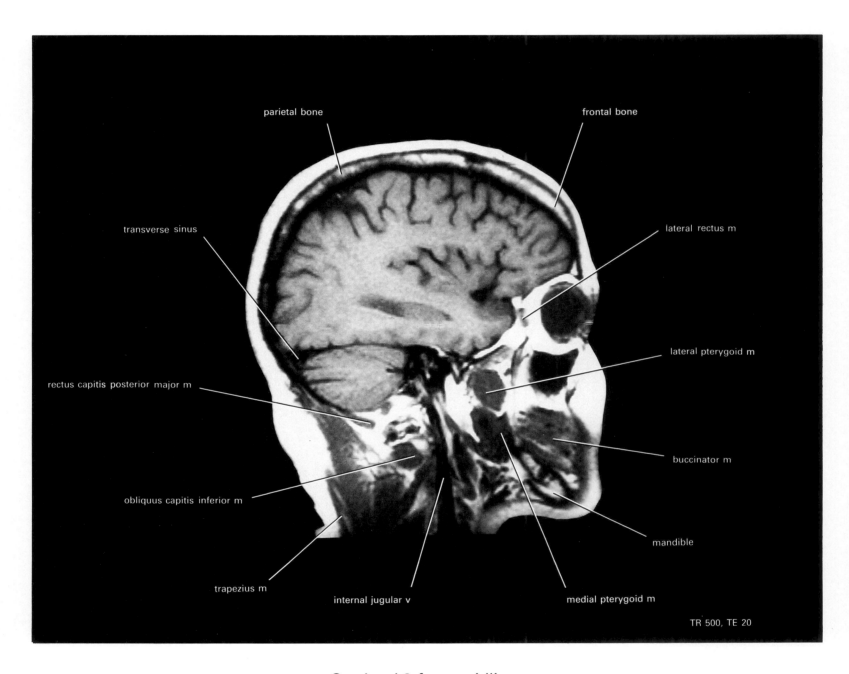

parietal bone

frontal bone

transverse sinus

lateral rectus m

lateral pterygoid m

rectus capitis posterior major m

buccinator m

obliquus capitis inferior m

mandible

trapezius m

internal jugular v

medial pterygoid m

TR 500, TE 20

Section L3 from midline.

BONES AND MUSCLES

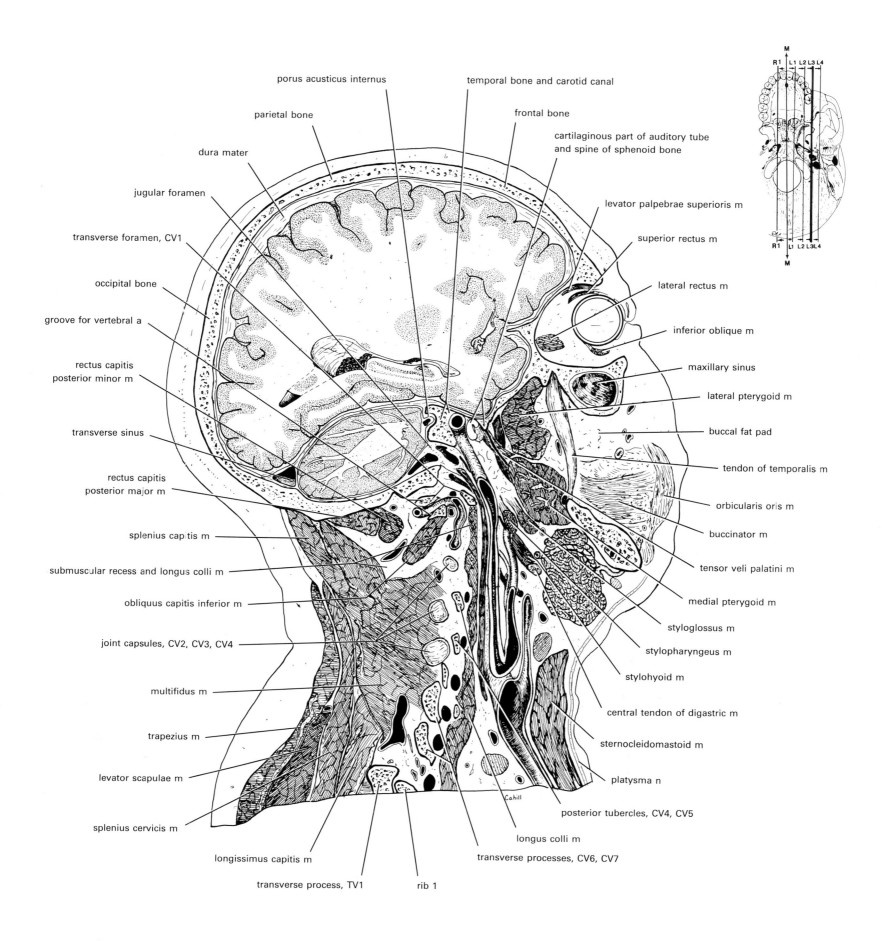

porus acusticus internus

parietal bone

dura mater

jugular foramen

transverse foramen, CV1

occipital bone

groove for vertebral a

rectus capitis
posterior minor m

transverse sinus

rectus capitis
posterior major m

splenius capitis m

submuscular recess and longus colli m

obliquus capitis inferior m

joint capsules, CV2, CV3, CV4

multifidus m

trapezius m

levator scapulae m

splenius cervicis m

longissimus capitis m

transverse process, TV1

rib 1

temporal bone and carotid canal

frontal bone

cartilaginous part of auditory tube
and spine of sphenoid bone

levator palpebrae superioris m

superior rectus m

lateral rectus m

inferior oblique m

maxillary sinus

lateral pterygoid m

buccal fat pad

tendon of temporalis m

orbicularis oris m

buccinator m

tensor veli palatini m

medial pterygoid m

styloglossus m

stylopharyngeus m

stylohyoid m

central tendon of digastric m

sternocleidomastoid m

platysma n

posterior tubercles, CV4, CV5

longus colli m

transverse processes, CV6, CV7

Section L3 from midline.

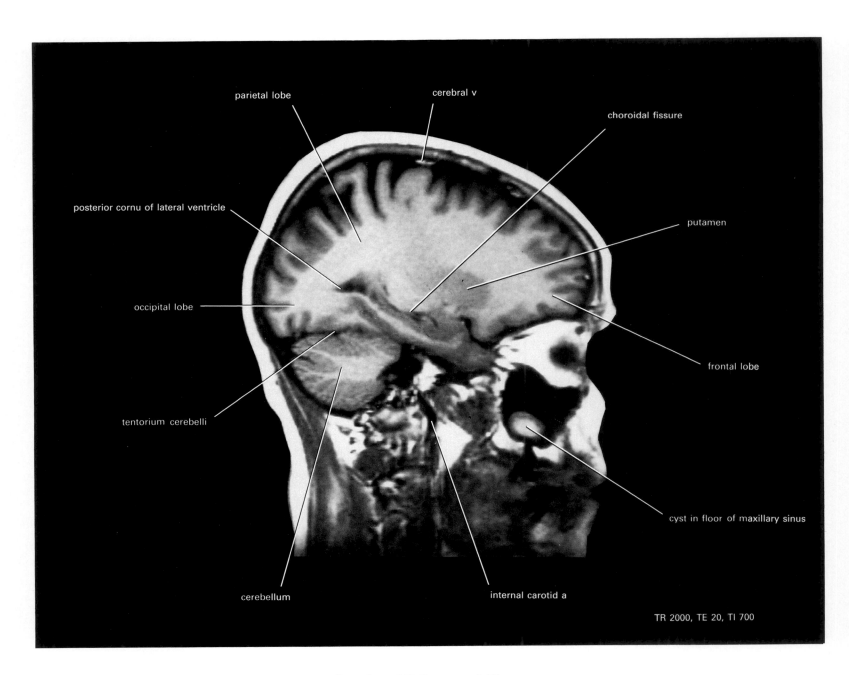

Section L3 from midline.

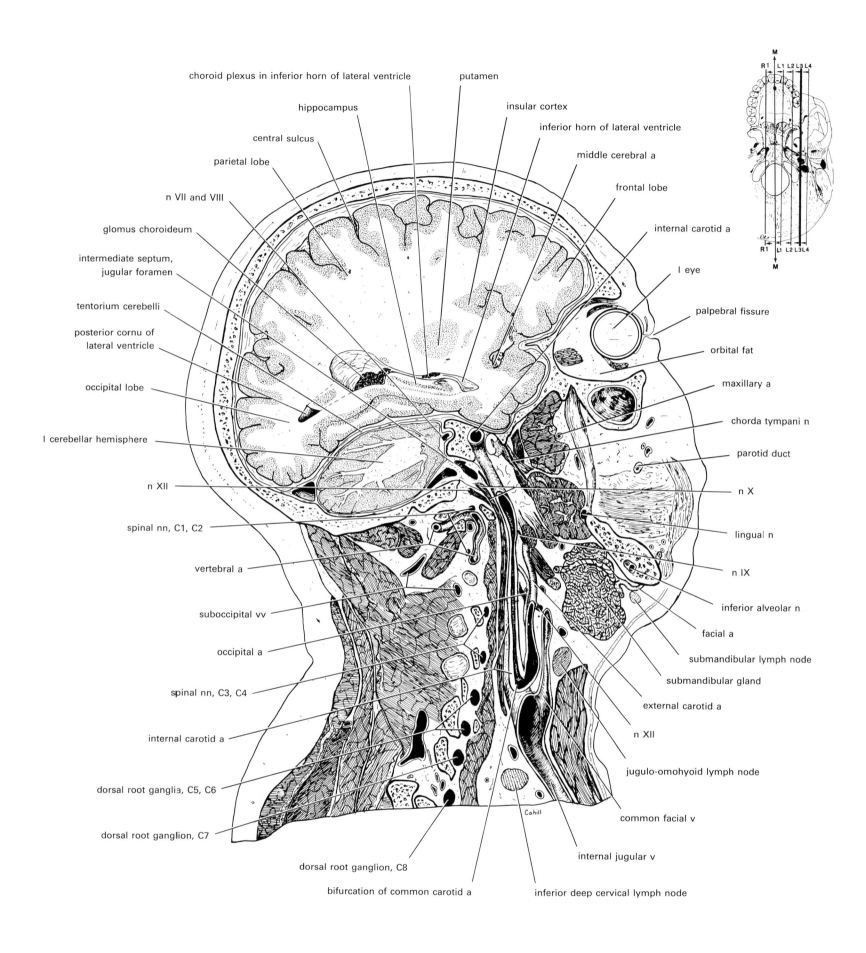

choroid plexus in inferior horn of lateral ventricle

hippocampus

central sulcus

parietal lobe

n VII and VIII

glomus choroideum

intermediate septum,
jugular foramen

tentorium cerebelli

posterior cornu of
lateral ventricle

occipital lobe

l cerebellar hemisphere

n XII

spinal nn, C1, C2

vertebral a

suboccipital vv

occipital a

spinal nn, C3, C4

internal carotid a

dorsal root ganglia, C5, C6

dorsal root ganglion, C7

dorsal root ganglion, C8

bifurcation of common carotid a

putamen

insular cortex

inferior horn of lateral ventricle

middle cerebral a

frontal lobe

internal carotid a

l eye

palpebral fissure

orbital fat

maxillary a

chorda tympani n

parotid duct

n X

lingual n

n IX

inferior alveolar n

facial a

submandibular lymph node

submandibular gland

external carotid a

n XII

jugulo-omohyoid lymph node

common facial v

internal jugular v

inferior deep cervical lymph node

Cahill

Section L3 from midline.

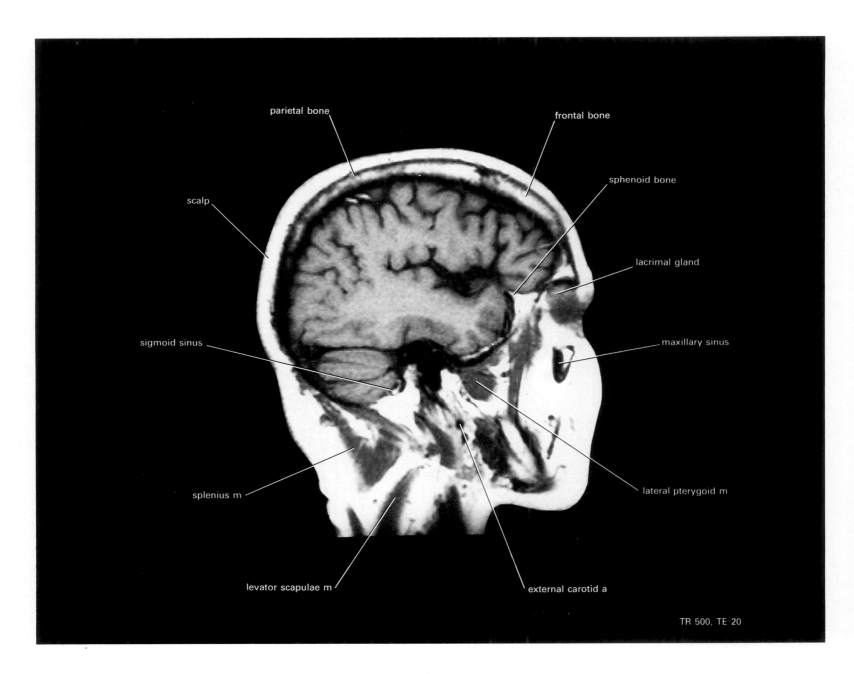

Section L4 from midline.

BONES AND MUSCLES

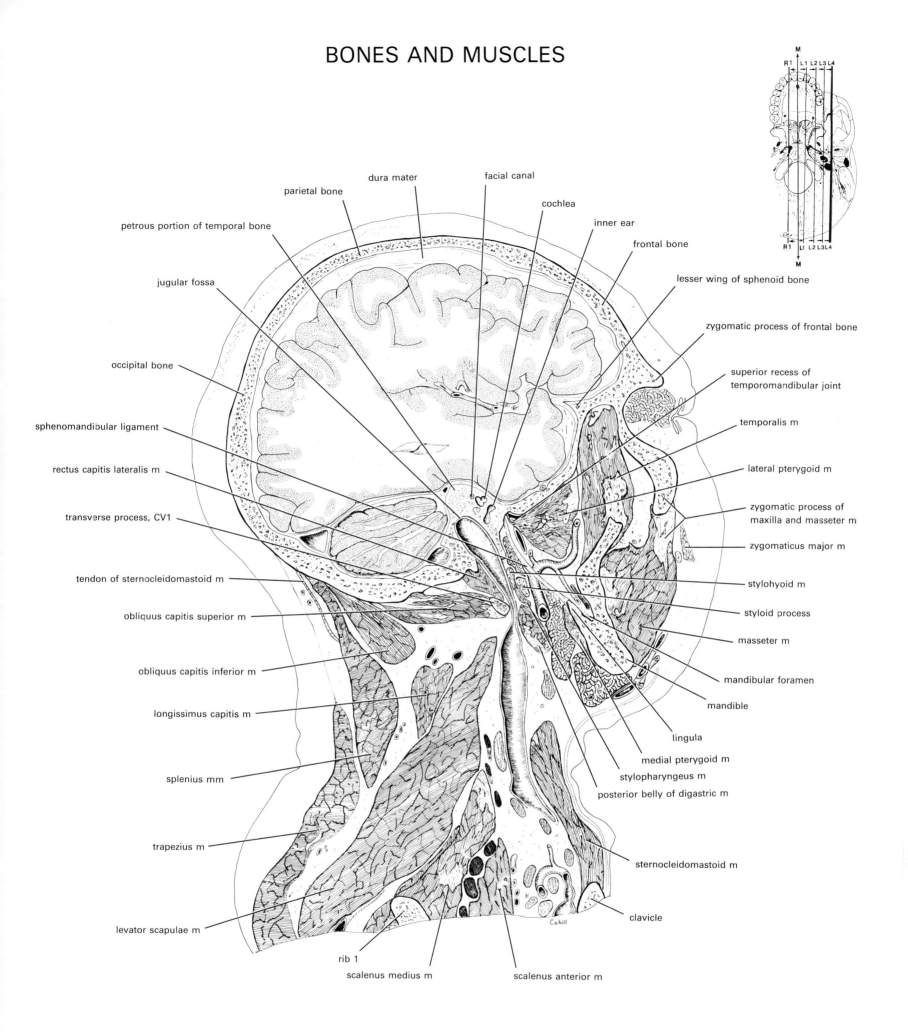

parietal bone

dura mater

facial canal

cochlea

inner ear

frontal bone

petrous portion of temporal bone

lesser wing of sphenoid bone

jugular fossa

zygomatic process of frontal bone

superior recess of temporomandibular joint

occipital bone

temporalis m

sphenomandibular ligament

lateral pterygoid m

rectus capitis lateralis m

zygomatic process of maxilla and masseter m

transverse process, CV1

zygomaticus major m

tendon of sternocleidomastoid m

stylohyoid m

obliquus capitis superior m

styloid process

masseter m

obliquus capitis inferior m

mandibular foramen

longissimus capitis m

mandible

splenius mm

lingula

medial pterygoid m

stylopharyngeus m

posterior belly of digastric m

trapezius m

sternocleidomastoid m

clavicle

levator scapulae m

rib 1

scalenus medius m

scalenus anterior m

Section L4 from midline.

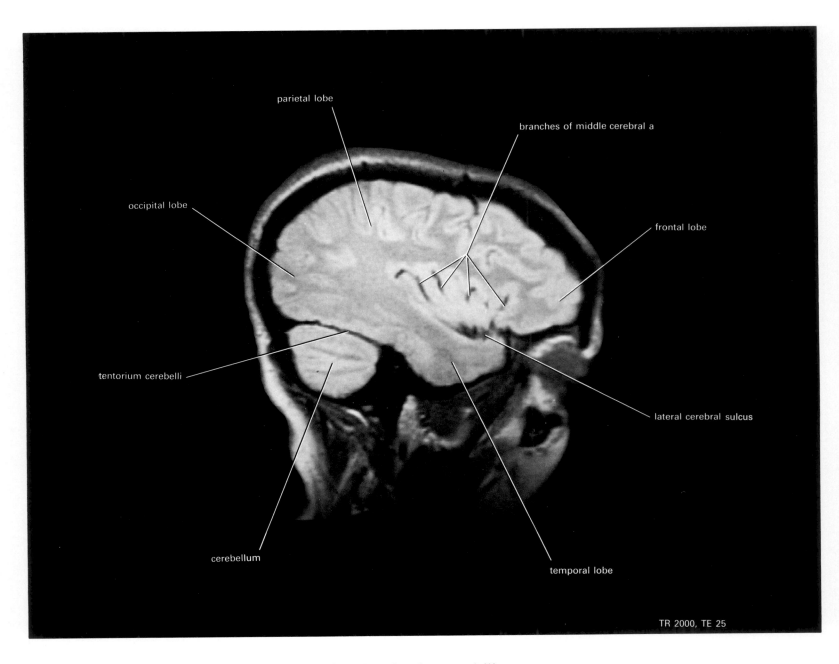

Section L4 from midline.

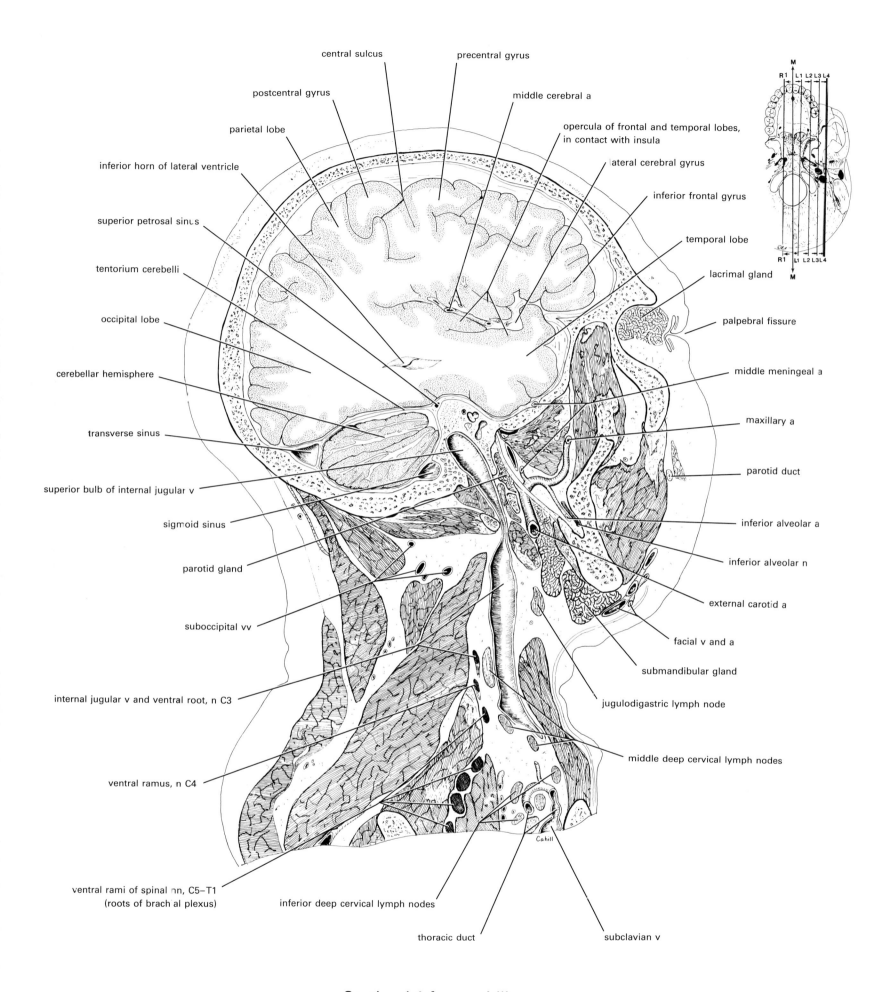

central sulcus

precentral gyrus

postcentral gyrus

middle cerebral a

parietal lobe

opercula of frontal and temporal lobes, in contact with insula

inferior horn of lateral ventricle

lateral cerebral gyrus

superior petrosal sinus

inferior frontal gyrus

tentorium cerebelli

temporal lobe

occipital lobe

lacrimal gland

cerebellar hemisphere

palpebral fissure

transverse sinus

middle meningeal a

superior bulb of internal jugular v

maxillary a

sigmoid sinus

parotid duct

parotid gland

inferior alveolar a

suboccipital vv

inferior alveolar n

internal jugular v and ventral root, n C3

external carotid a

ventral ramus, n C4

facial v and a

submandibular gland

jugulodigastric lymph node

middle deep cervical lymph nodes

ventral rami of spinal nn, C5–T1
(roots of brachial plexus)

inferior deep cervical lymph nodes

thoracic duct

subclavian v

Section L4 from midline.

The Head and Neck in Coronal Planes

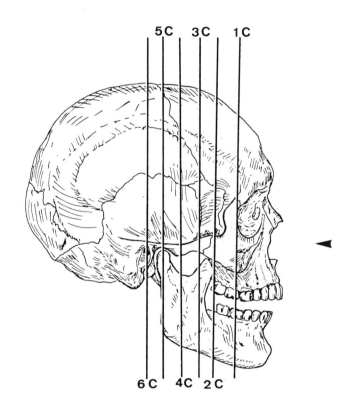

5C 3C 1C

6C 4C 2C

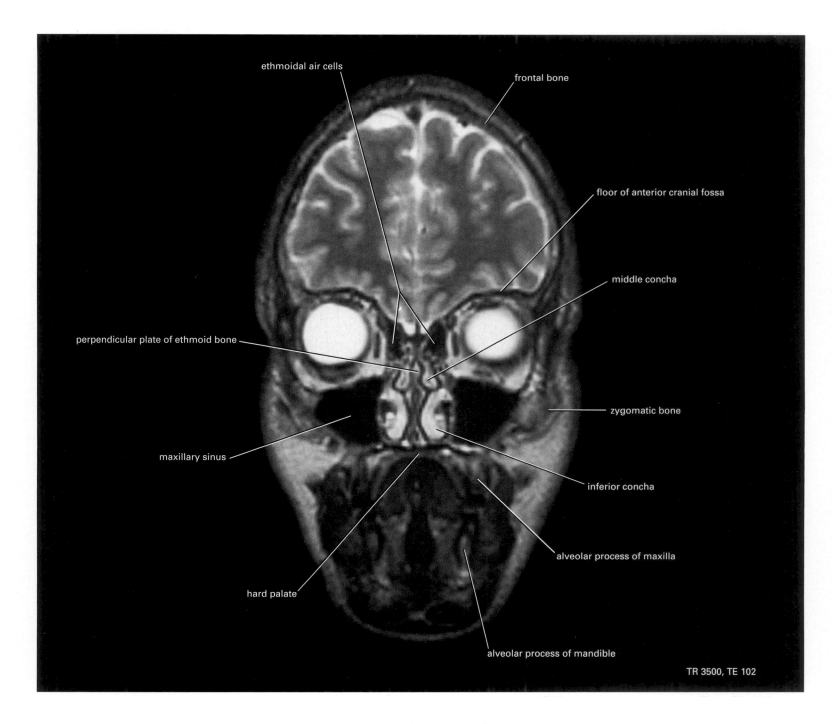

ethmoidal air cells

frontal bone

floor of anterior cranial fossa

middle concha

perpendicular plate of ethmoid bone

zygomatic bone

maxillary sinus

inferior concha

alveolar process of maxilla

hard palate

alveolar process of mandible

TR 3500, TE 102

Section 1C from the front.

BONES

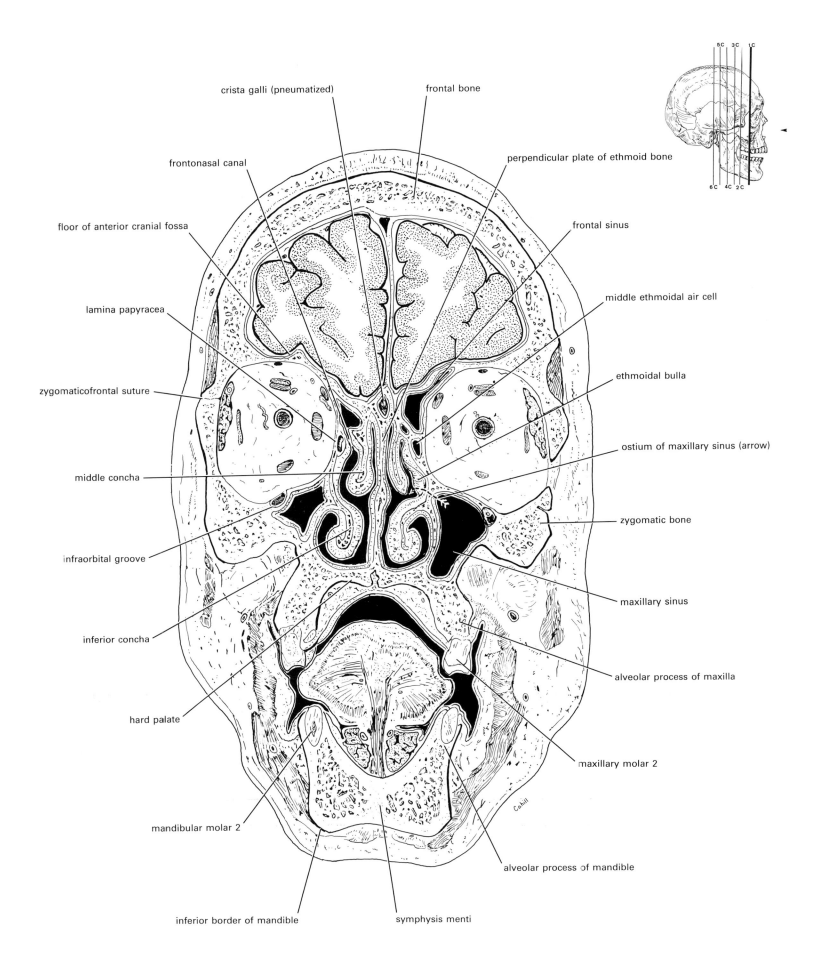

crista galli (pneumatized)

frontal bone

frontonasal canal

perpendicular plate of ethmoid bone

floor of anterior cranial fossa

frontal sinus

middle ethmoidal air cell

lamina papyracea

ethmoidal bulla

zygomaticofrontal suture

ostium of maxillary sinus (arrow)

middle concha

zygomatic bone

infraorbital groove

maxillary sinus

inferior concha

hard palate

alveolar process of maxilla

mandibular molar 2

maxillary molar 2

inferior border of mandible

symphysis menti

alveolar process of mandible

5C 3C 1C

6C 4C 2C

Cahill

Section 1C from the front.

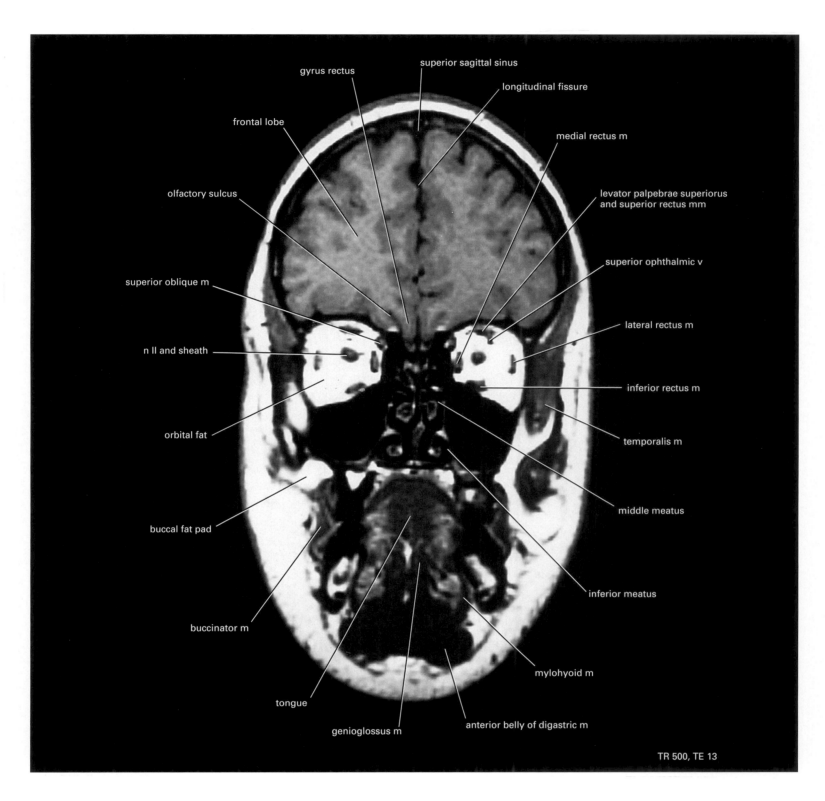

Section 1C from the front.

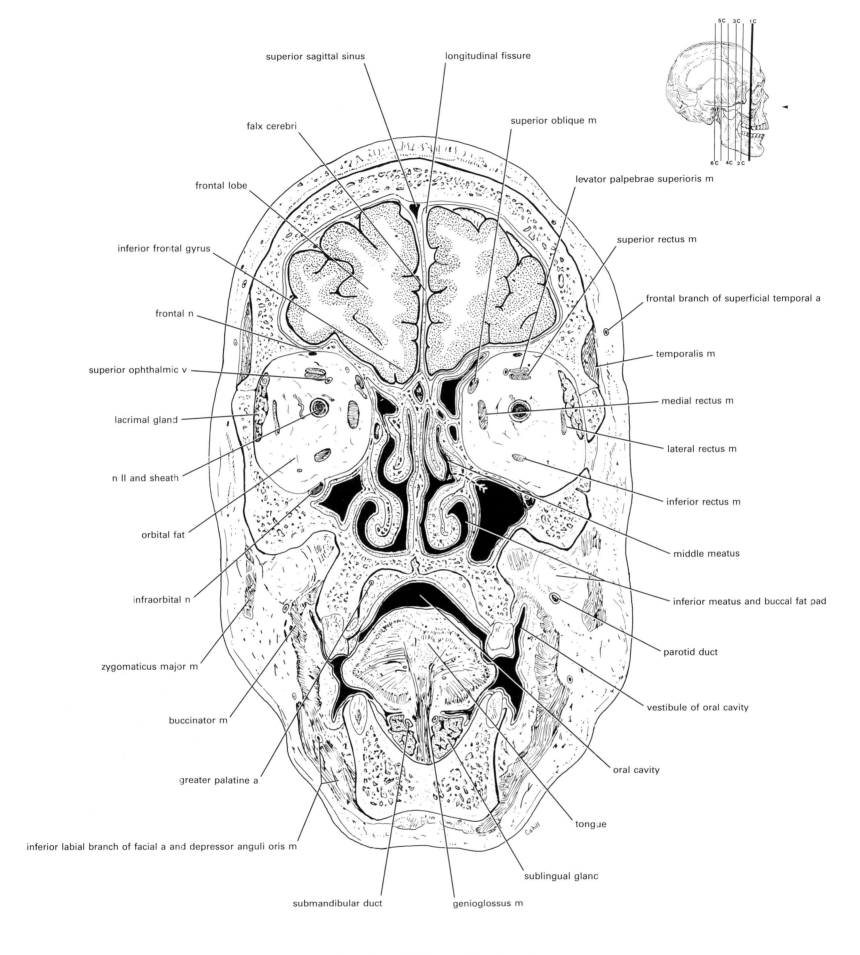

superior sagittal sinus

longitudinal fissure

falx cerebri

superior oblique m

frontal lobe

levator palpebrae superioris m

inferior frontal gyrus

superior rectus m

frontal n

frontal branch of superficial temporal a

superior ophthalmic v

temporalis m

lacrimal gland

medial rectus m

n II and sheath

lateral rectus m

orbital fat

inferior rectus m

infraorbital n

middle meatus

zygomaticus major m

inferior meatus and buccal fat pad

buccinator m

parotid duct

greater palatine a

vestibule of oral cavity

inferior labial branch of facial a and depressor anguli oris m

oral cavity

tongue

submandibular duct

sublingual gland

genioglossus m

Section 1C from the front.

BONES

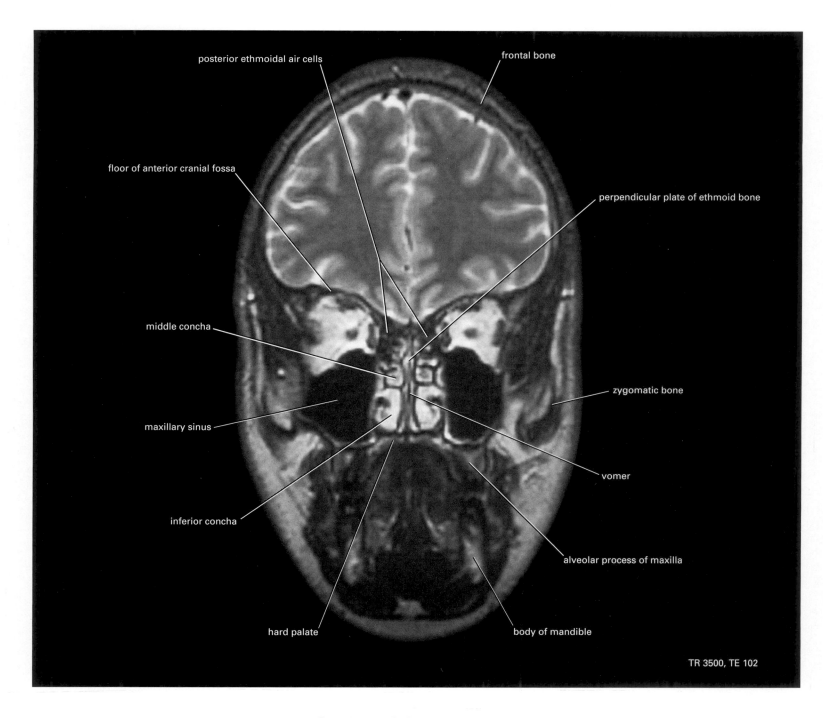

posterior ethmoidal air cells

frontal bone

floor of anterior cranial fossa

perpendicular plate of ethmoid bone

middle concha

zygomatic bone

maxillary sinus

vomer

inferior concha

alveolar process of maxilla

hard palate

body of mandible

TR 3500, TE 102

Section 2C from the front.

BONES

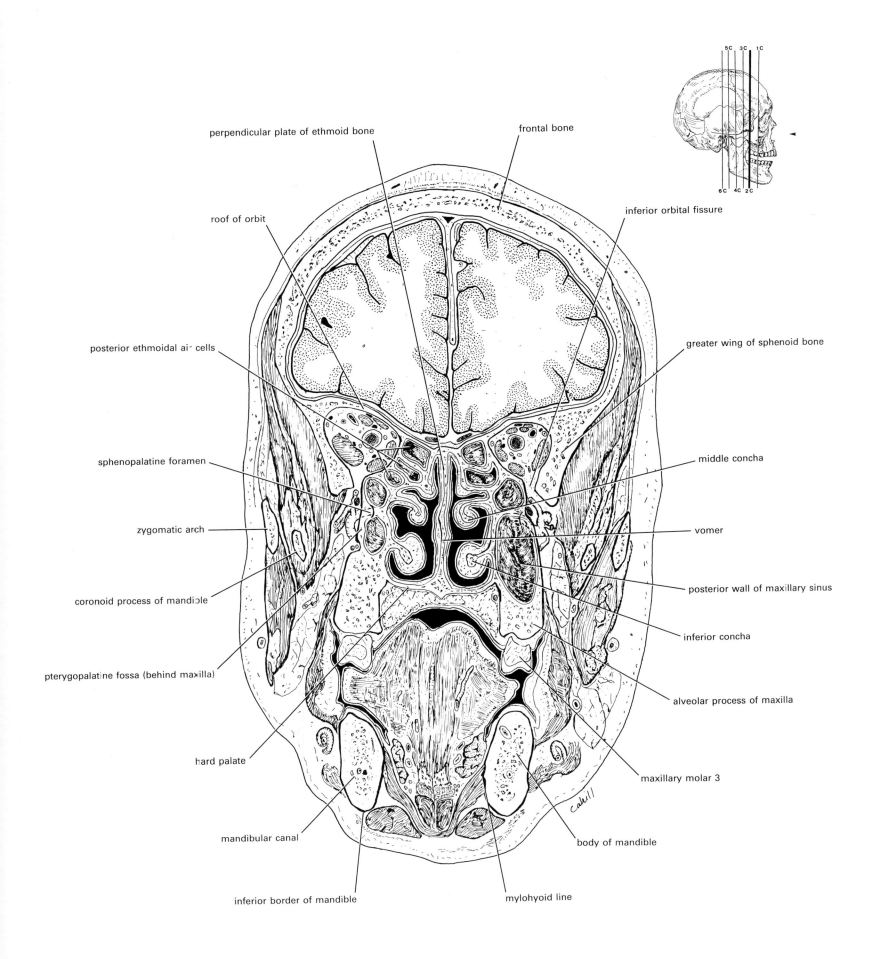

perpendicular plate of ethmoid bone

frontal bone

roof of orbit

inferior orbital fissure

posterior ethmoidal air cells

greater wing of sphenoid bone

sphenopalatine foramen

middle concha

zygomatic arch

vomer

coronoid process of mandible

posterior wall of maxillary sinus

pterygopalatine fossa (behind maxilla)

inferior concha

hard palate

alveolar process of maxilla

mandibular canal

maxillary molar 3

inferior border of mandible

body of mandible

mylohyoid line

Section 2C from the front.

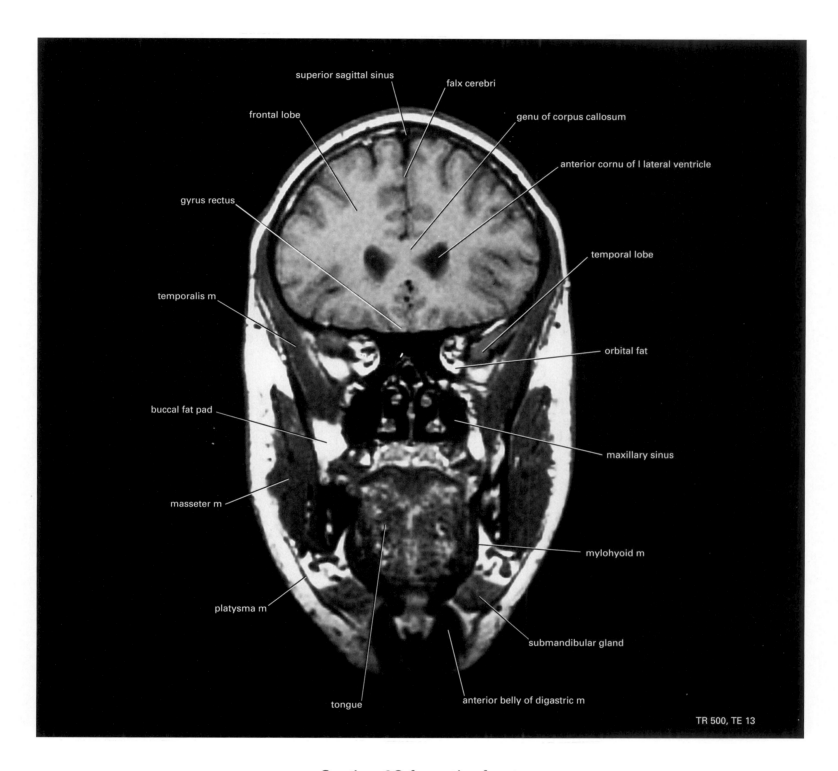

Section 2C from the front.

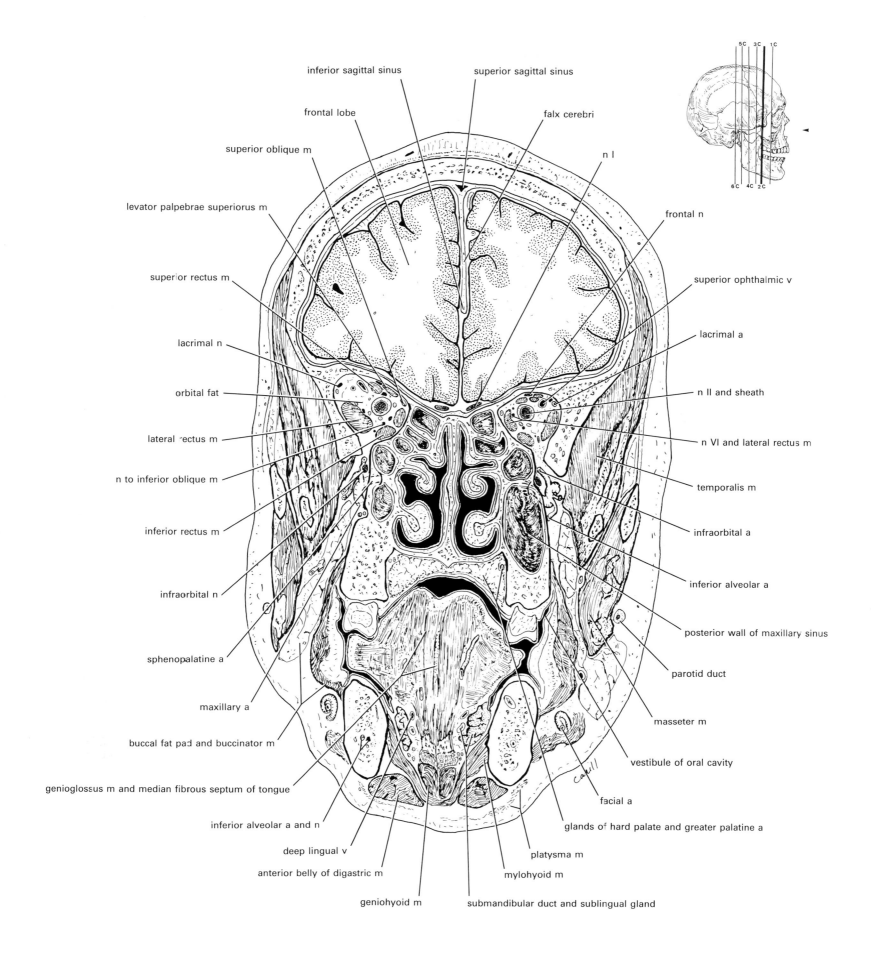

inferior sagittal sinus

superior sagittal sinus

frontal lobe

falx cerebri

superior oblique m

n I

levator palpebrae superiorus m

frontal n

superior rectus m

superior ophthalmic v

lacrimal n

lacrimal a

orbital fat

n II and sheath

lateral rectus m

n VI and lateral rectus m

n to inferior oblique m

temporalis m

inferior rectus m

infraorbital a

infraorbital n

inferior alveolar a

sphenopalatine a

posterior wall of maxillary sinus

parotid duct

maxillary a

masseter m

buccal fat pad and buccinator m

vestibule of oral cavity

genioglossus m and median fibrous septum of tongue

facial a

inferior alveolar a and n

glands of hard palate and greater palatine a

deep lingual v

platysma m

anterior belly of digastric m

mylohyoid m

geniohyoid m

submandibular duct and sublingual gland

Section 2C from the front.

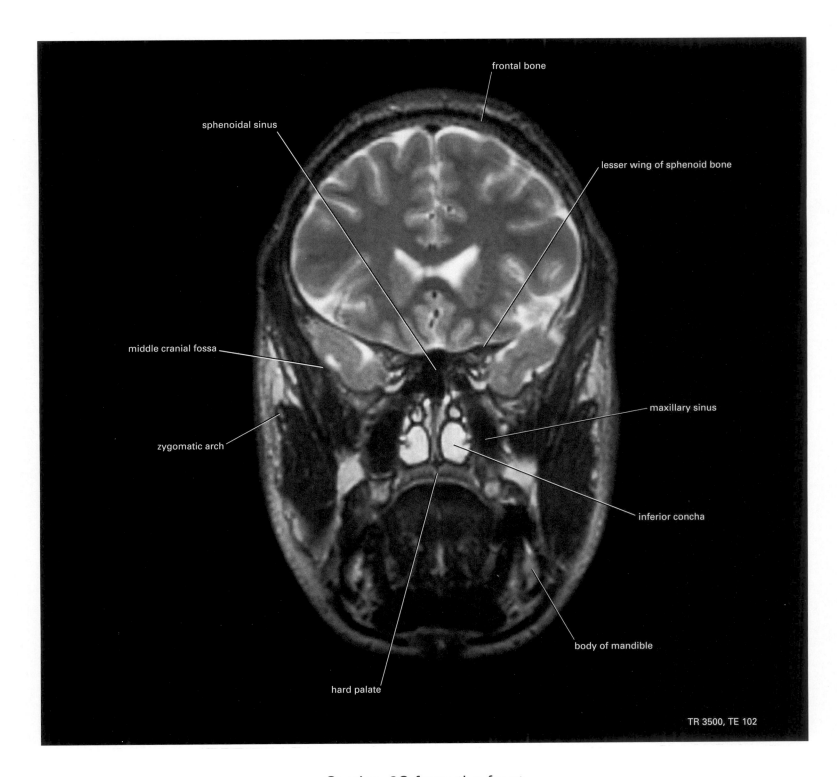

frontal bone

sphenoidal sinus

lesser wing of sphenoid bone

middle cranial fossa

maxillary sinus

zygomatic arch

inferior concha

body of mandible

hard palate

TR 3500, TE 102

Section 3C from the front.

BONES

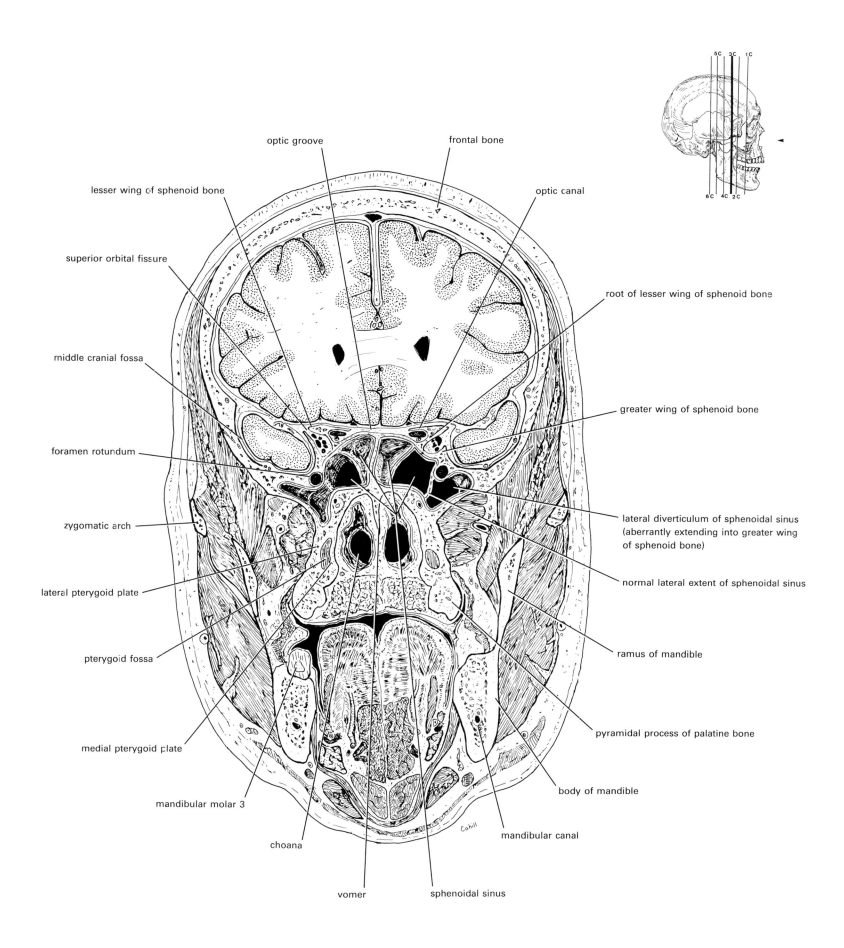

optic groove

frontal bone

lesser wing of sphenoid bone

optic canal

superior orbital fissure

root of lesser wing of sphenoid bone

middle cranial fossa

greater wing of sphenoid bone

foramen rotundum

lateral diverticulum of sphenoidal sinus
(aberrantly extending into greater wing
of sphenoid bone)

zygomatic arch

normal lateral extent of sphenoidal sinus

lateral pterygoid plate

ramus of mandible

pterygoid fossa

pyramidal process of palatine bone

medial pterygoid plate

body of mandible

mandibular molar 3

mandibular canal

choana

vomer

sphenoidal sinus

Section 3C from the front.

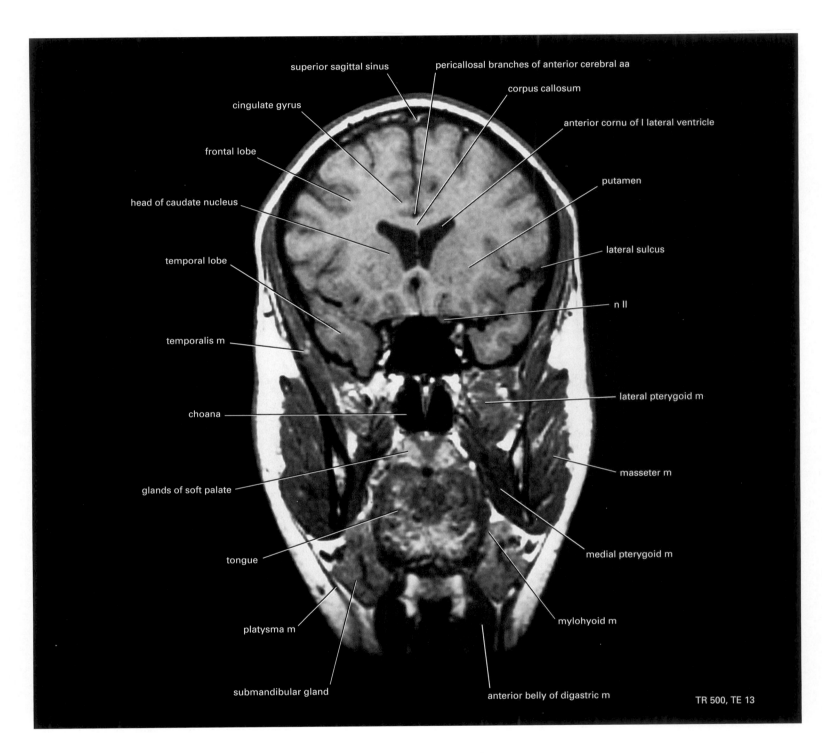

Section 3C from the front.

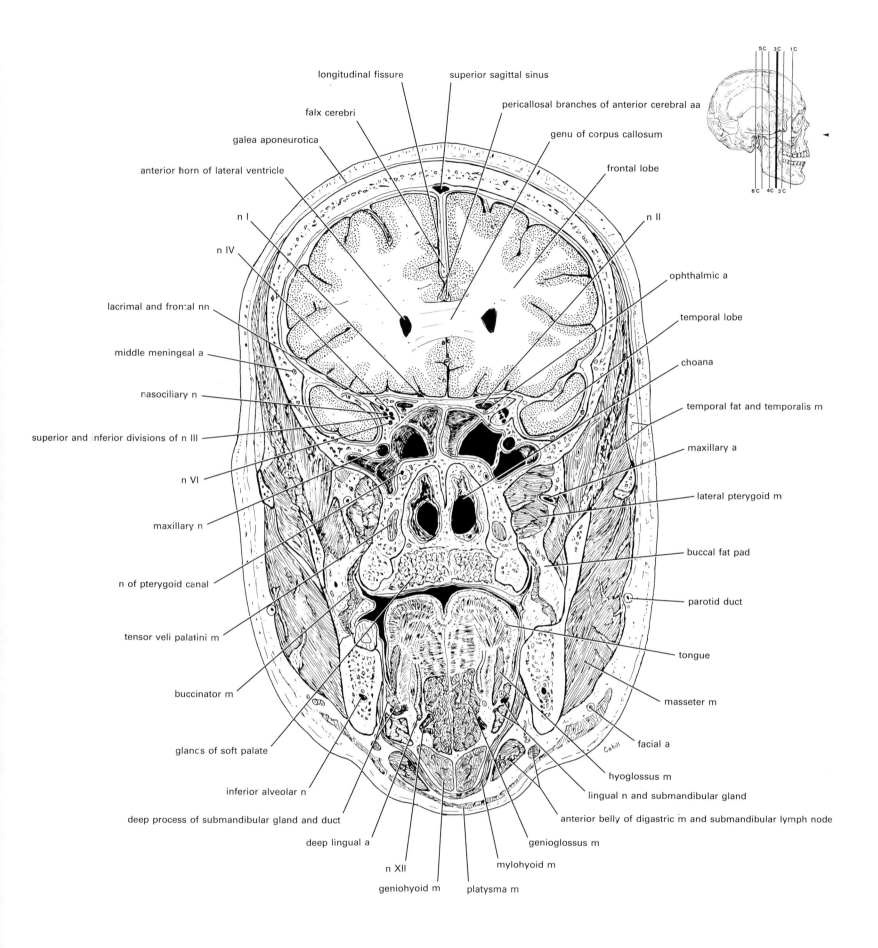

longitudinal fissure

superior sagittal sinus

falx cerebri

pericallosal branches of anterior cerebral aa

galea aponeurotica

genu of corpus callosum

anterior horn of lateral ventricle

frontal lobe

n I

n II

n IV

ophthalmic a

lacrimal and frontal nn

temporal lobe

middle meningeal a

choana

nasociliary n

temporal fat and temporalis m

superior and inferior divisions of n III

maxillary a

n VI

lateral pterygoid m

maxillary n

buccal fat pad

n of pterygoid canal

parotid duct

tensor veli palatini m

tongue

buccinator m

masseter m

glands of soft palate

facial a

inferior alveolar n

hyoglossus m

deep process of submandibular gland and duct

lingual n and submandibular gland

deep lingual a

anterior belly of digastric m and submandibular lymph node

n XII

genioglossus m

geniohyoid m

mylohyoid m

platysma m

Section 3C from the front.

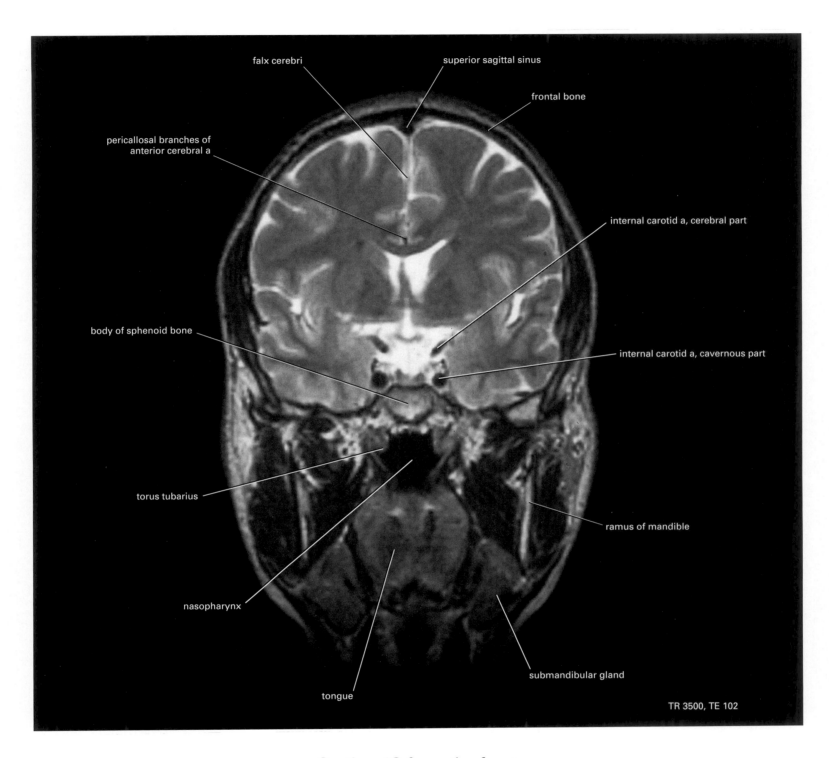

Section 4C from the front.

BONES, VESSELS, AND VISCERA

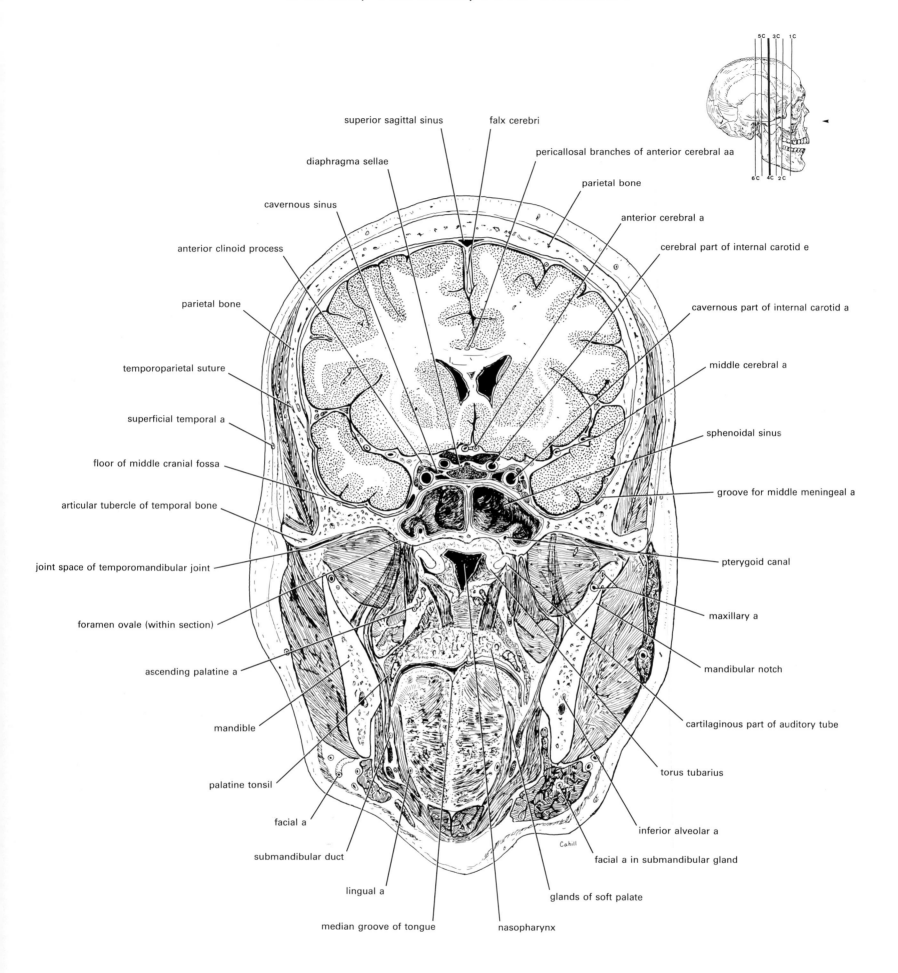

superior sagittal sinus

falx cerebri

diaphragma sellae

pericallosal branches of anterior cerebral aa

cavernous sinus

parietal bone

anterior clinoid process

anterior cerebral a

parietal bone

cerebral part of internal carotid e

temporoparietal suture

cavernous part of internal carotid a

superficial temporal a

middle cerebral a

floor of middle cranial fossa

sphenoidal sinus

articular tubercle of temporal bone

groove for middle meningeal a

joint space of temporomandibular joint

pterygoid canal

foramen ovale (within section)

maxillary a

ascending palatine a

mandibular notch

mandible

cartilaginous part of auditory tube

palatine tonsil

torus tubarius

facial a

inferior alveolar a

submandibular duct

facial a in submandibular gland

lingual a

glands of soft palate

median groove of tongue

nasopharynx

Cahill

Section 4C from the front.

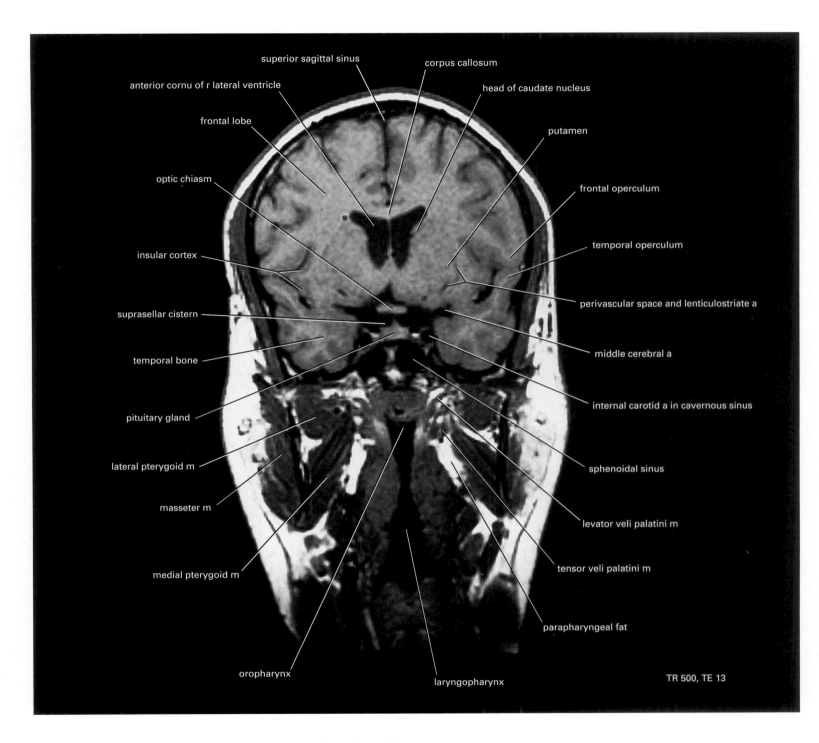

superior sagittal sinus

corpus callosum

anterior cornu of r lateral ventricle

head of caudate nucleus

frontal lobe

putamen

optic chiasm

frontal operculum

temporal operculum

insular cortex

suprasellar cistern

perivascular space and lenticulostriate a

temporal bone

middle cerebral a

pituitary gland

internal carotid a in cavernous sinus

lateral pterygoid m

sphenoidal sinus

masseter m

levator veli palatini m

medial pterygoid m

tensor veli palatini m

parapharyngeal fat

oropharynx

laryngopharynx

TR 500, TE 13

Section 4C from the front.

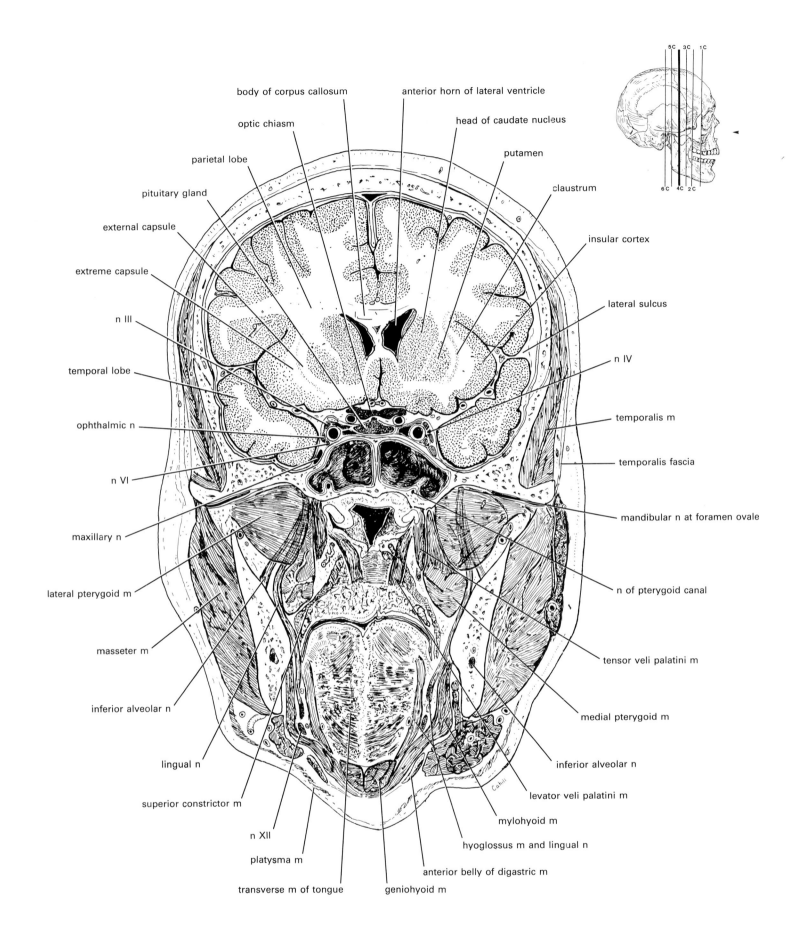

body of corpus callosum

anterior horn of lateral ventricle

optic chiasm

head of caudate nucleus

parietal lobe

putamen

pituitary gland

claustrum

external capsule

insular cortex

extreme capsule

lateral sulcus

n III

n IV

temporal lobe

temporalis m

ophthalmic n

temporalis fascia

n VI

mandibular n at foramen ovale

maxillary n

n of pterygoid canal

lateral pterygoid m

tensor veli palatini m

masseter m

medial pterygoid m

inferior alveolar n

inferior alveolar n

lingual n

levator veli palatini m

superior constrictor m

mylohyoid m

n XII

hyoglossus m and lingual n

platysma m

anterior belly of digastric m

transverse m of tongue

geniohyoid m

Section 4C from the front.

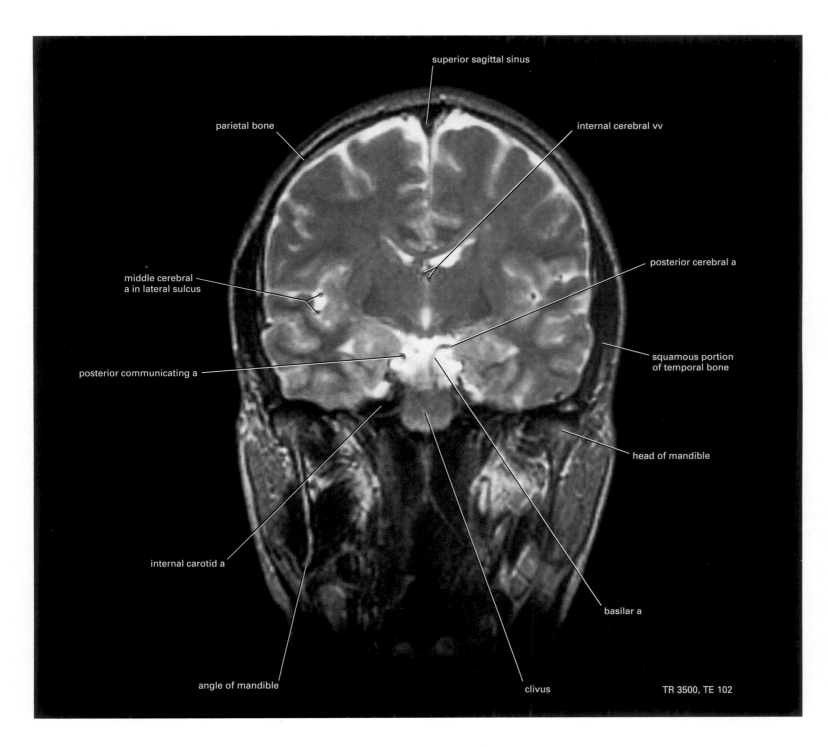

Section 5C from the front.

BONES, VESSELS, AND VISCERA

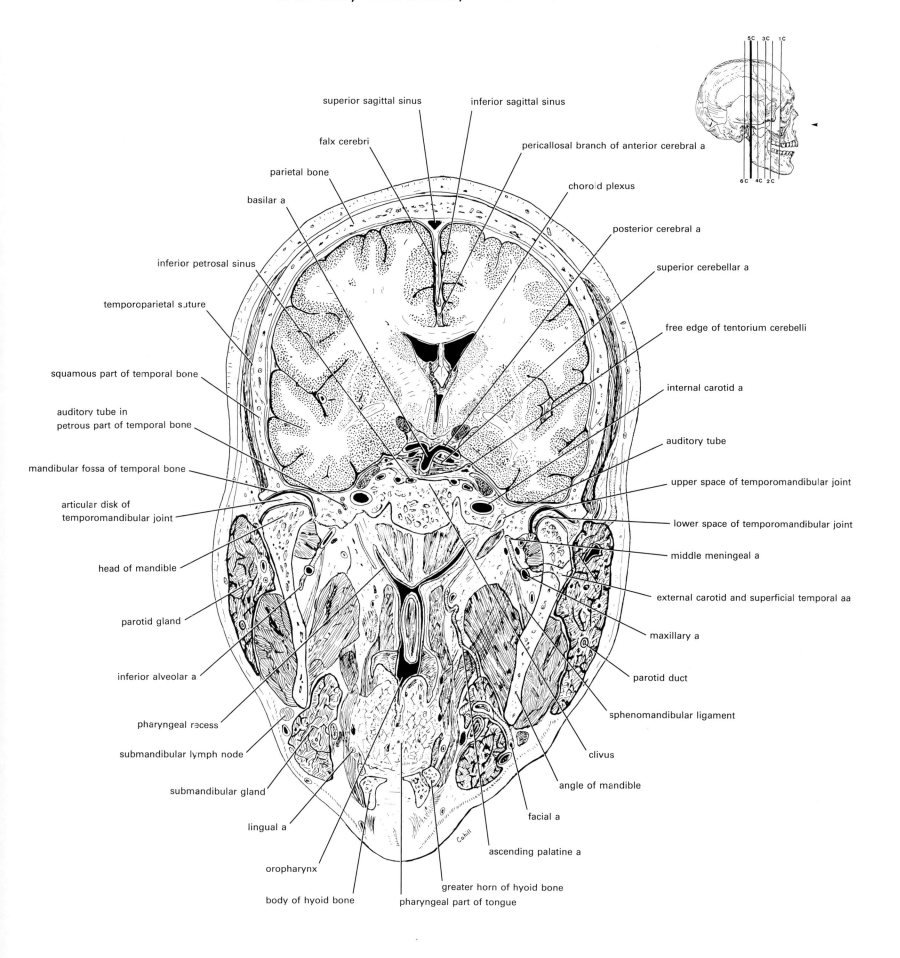

superior sagittal sinus

inferior sagittal sinus

falx cerebri

pericallosal branch of anterior cerebral a

parietal bone

choroid plexus

basilar a

posterior cerebral a

inferior petrosal sinus

superior cerebellar a

temporoparietal suture

free edge of tentorium cerebelli

squamous part of temporal bone

internal carotid a

auditory tube in
petrous part of temporal bone

auditory tube

mandibular fossa of temporal bone

upper space of temporomandibular joint

articular disk of
temporomandibular joint

lower space of temporomandibular joint

middle meningeal a

head of mandible

external carotid and superficial temporal aa

parotid gland

maxillary a

inferior alveolar a

parotid duct

pharyngeal recess

sphenomandibular ligament

submandibular lymph node

clivus

submandibular gland

angle of mandible

lingual a

facial a

oropharynx

ascending palatine a

body of hyoid bone

greater horn of hyoid bone

pharyngeal part of tongue

Section 5C from the front.

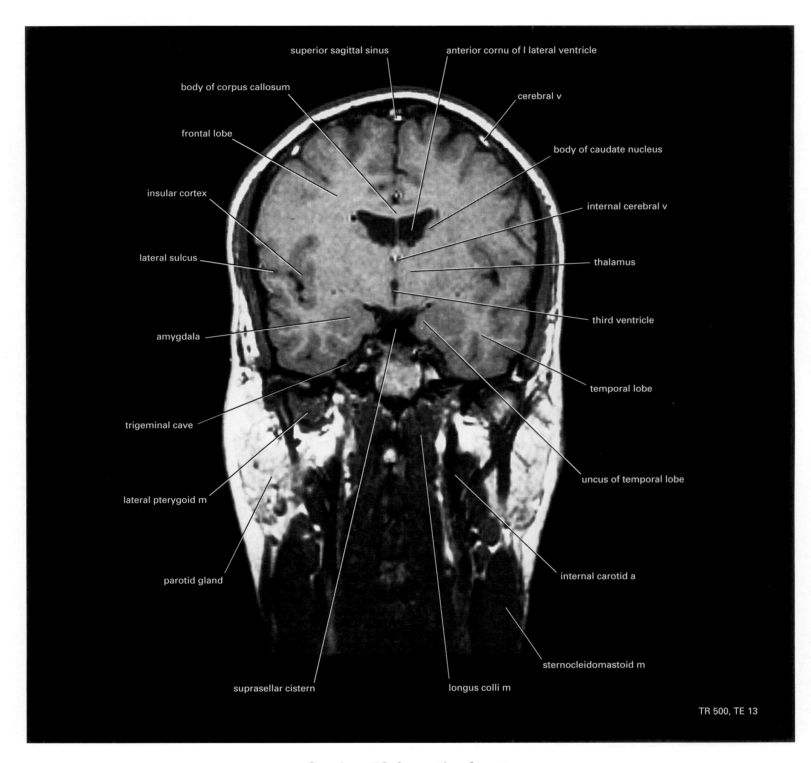

Section 5C from the front.

NERVOUS SYSTEM AND MUSCLES

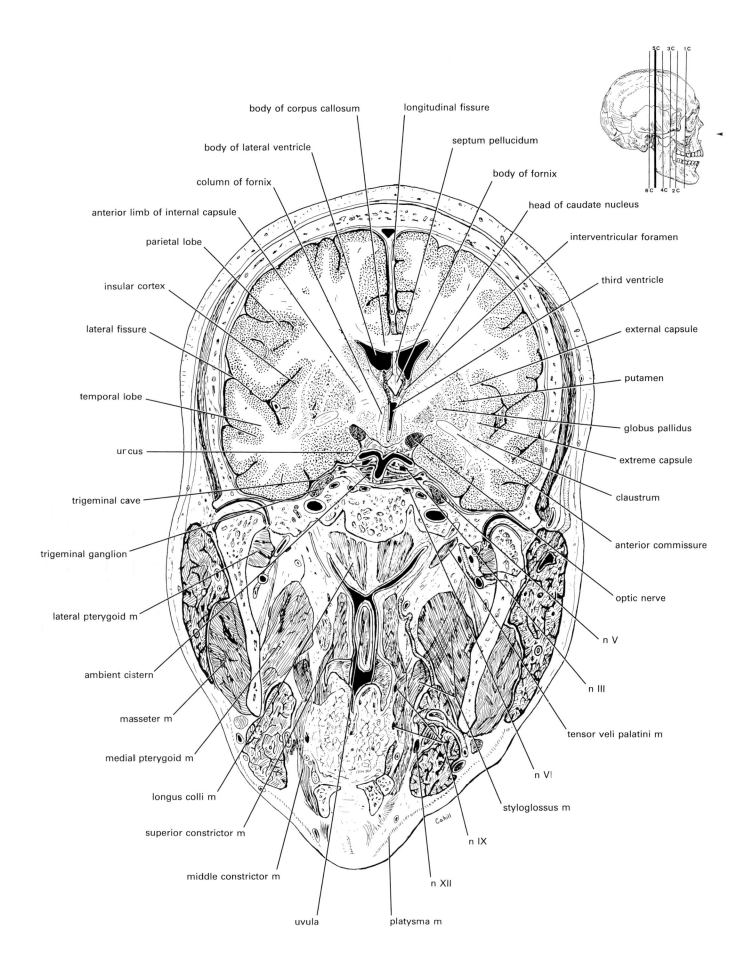

body of corpus callosum

longitudinal fissure

body of lateral ventricle

septum pellucidum

column of fornix

body of fornix

anterior limb of internal capsule

head of caudate nucleus

parietal lobe

interventricular foramen

insular cortex

third ventricle

lateral fissure

external capsule

temporal lobe

putamen

ur cus

globus pallidus

trigeminal cave

extreme capsule

claustrum

trigeminal ganglion

anterior commissure

lateral pterygoid m

optic nerve

ambient cistern

n V

masseter m

n III

medial pterygoid m

tensor veli palatini m

longus colli m

n VI

superior constrictor m

styloglossus m

middle constrictor m

n IX

uvula

n XII

platysma m

Cahill

Section 5C from the front.

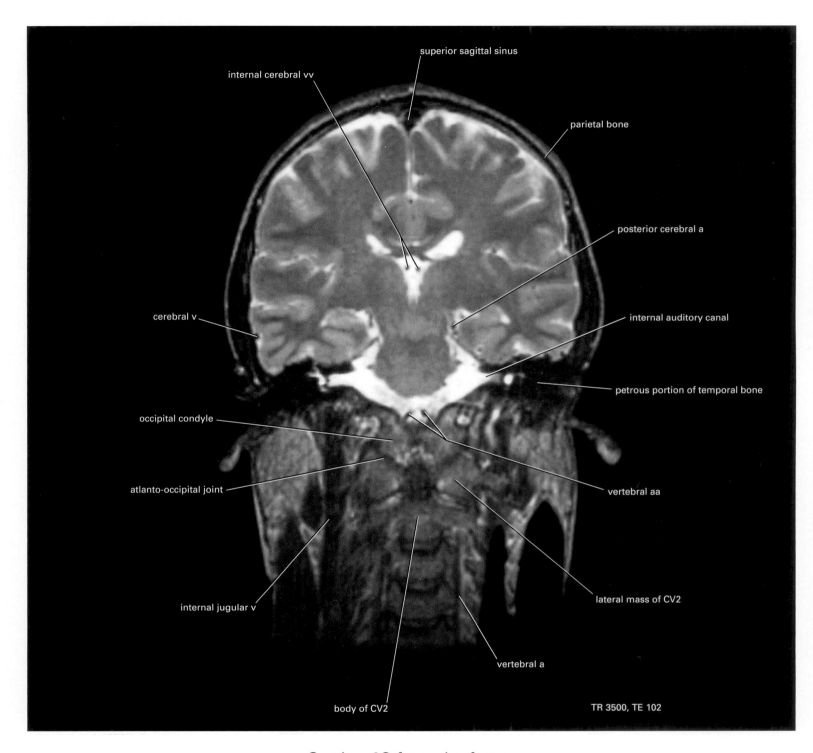

Section 6C from the front.

BONES, VESSELS, AND VISCERA

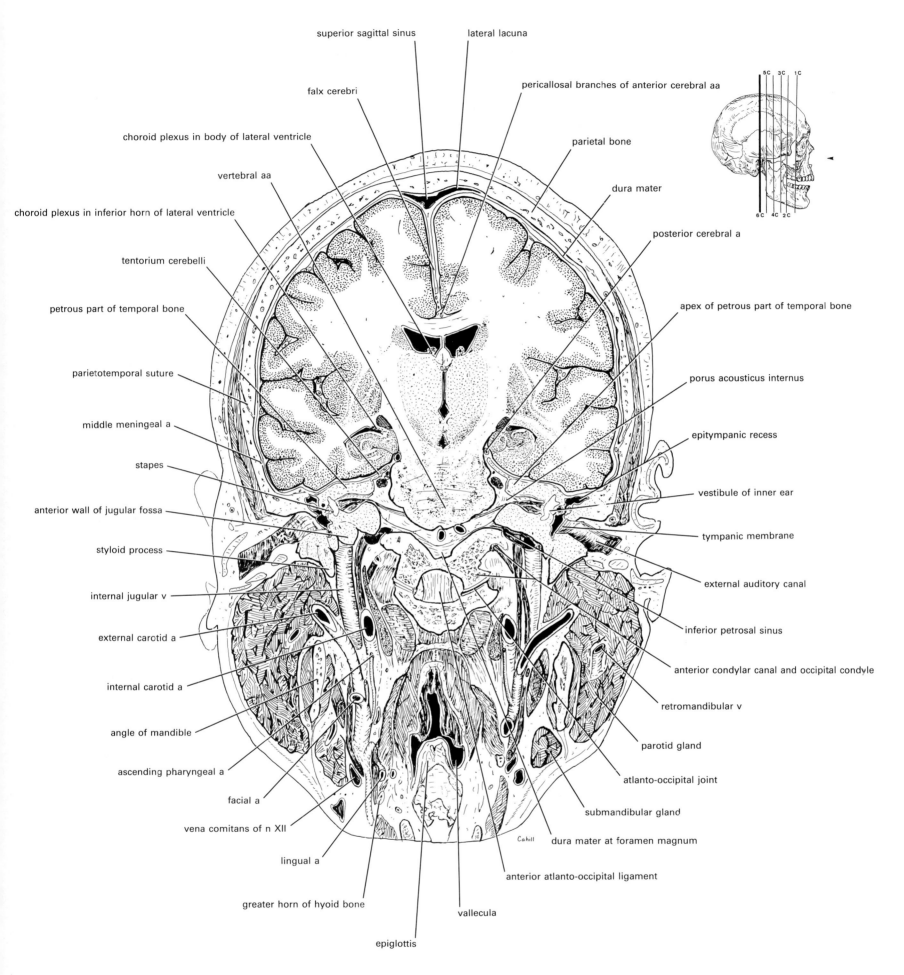

superior sagittal sinus

lateral lacuna

falx cerebri

pericallosal branches of anterior cerebral aa

choroid plexus in body of lateral ventricle

parietal bone

vertebral aa

dura mater

choroid plexus in inferior horn of lateral ventricle

posterior cerebral a

tentorium cerebelli

apex of petrous part of temporal bone

petrous part of temporal bone

parietotemporal suture

porus acousticus internus

middle meningeal a

epitympanic recess

stapes

vestibule of inner ear

anterior wall of jugular fossa

tympanic membrane

styloid process

external auditory canal

internal jugular v

inferior petrosal sinus

external carotid a

anterior condylar canal and occipital condyle

internal carotid a

retromandibular v

angle of mandible

parotid gland

ascending pharyngeal a

atlanto-occipital joint

facial a

submandibular gland

vena comitans of n XII

dura mater at foramen magnum

lingual a

anterior atlanto-occipital ligament

greater horn of hyoid bone

vallecula

epiglottis

Cahill

Section 6C from the front.

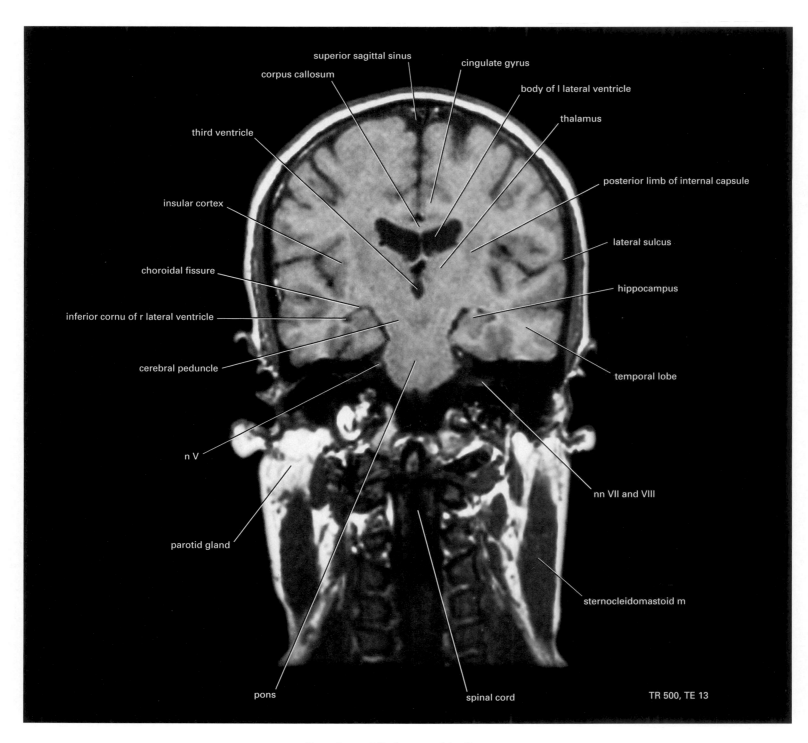

superior sagittal sinus

cingulate gyrus

corpus callosum

body of l lateral ventricle

third ventricle

thalamus

posterior limb of internal capsule

insular cortex

lateral sulcus

choroidal fissure

hippocampus

inferior cornu of r lateral ventricle

cerebral peduncle

temporal lobe

n V

nn VII and VIII

parotid gland

sternocleidomastoid m

pons

spinal cord

TR 500, TE 13

Section 6C from the front.

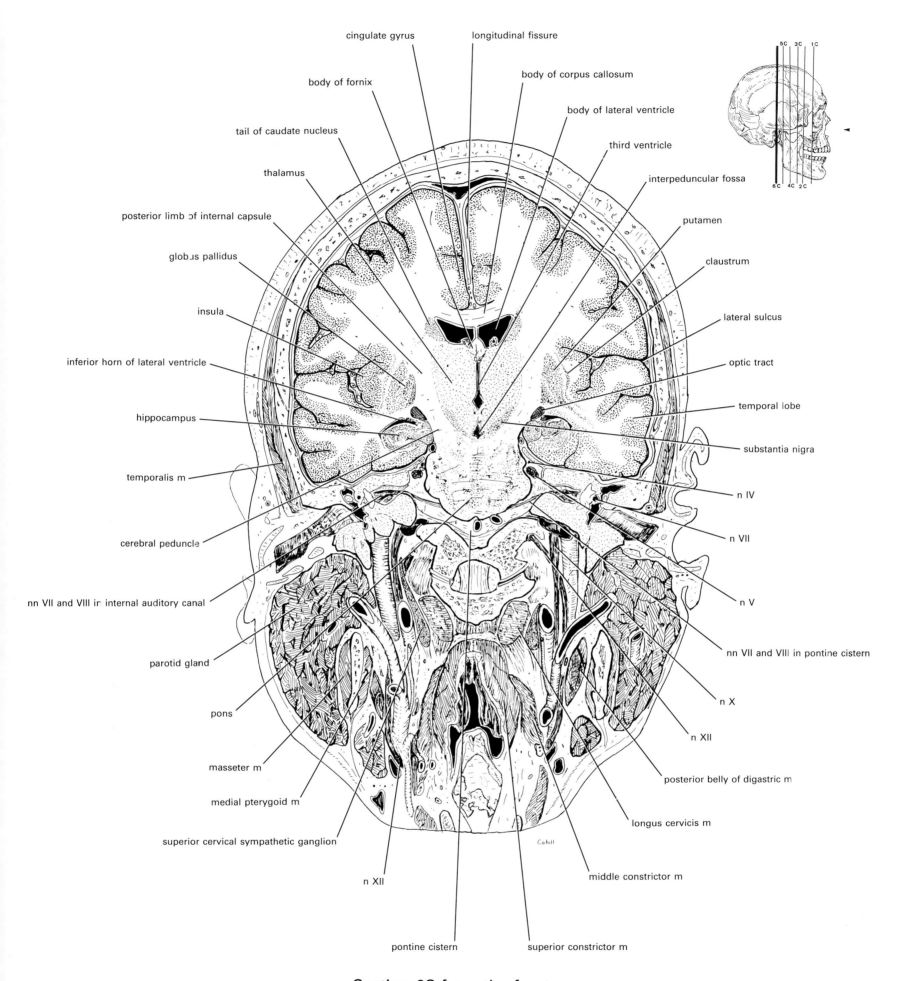

cingulate gyrus

longitudinal fissure

body of fornix

body of corpus callosum

tail of caudate nucleus

body of lateral ventricle

thalamus

third ventricle

posterior limb of internal capsule

interpeduncular fossa

globus pallidus

putamen

insula

claustrum

inferior horn of lateral ventricle

lateral sulcus

hippocampus

optic tract

temporalis m

temporal lobe

cerebral peduncle

substantia nigra

nn VII and VIII in internal auditory canal

n IV

parotid gland

n VII

pons

n V

masseter m

nn VII and VIII in pontine cistern

medial pterygoid m

n X

superior cervical sympathetic ganglion

n XII

n XII

posterior belly of digastric m

longus cervicis m

middle constrictor m

pontine cistern

superior constrictor m

Cahill

Section 6C from the front.

The Cervical Spine in Sagittal and Axial Planes

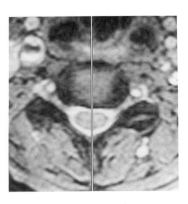

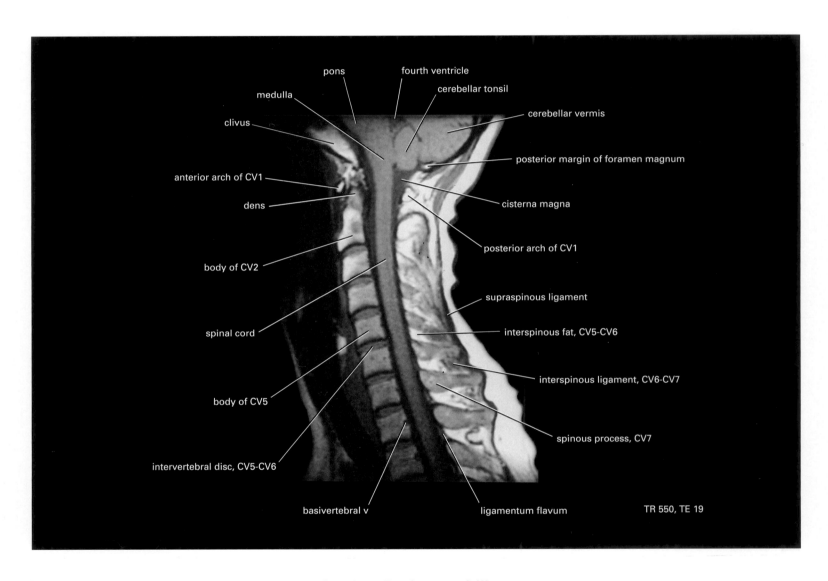

pons
fourth ventricle
cerebellar tonsil
medulla
cerebellar vermis
clivus
posterior margin of foramen magnum
anterior arch of CV1
dens
cisterna magna
posterior arch of CV1
body of CV2
supraspinous ligament
spinal cord
interspinous fat, CV5-CV6
interspinous ligament, CV6-CV7
body of CV5
spinous process, CV7
intervertebral disc, CV5-CV6
basivertebral v
ligamentum flavum
TR 550, TE 19

Section R1 from midline.

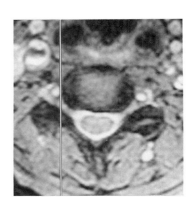

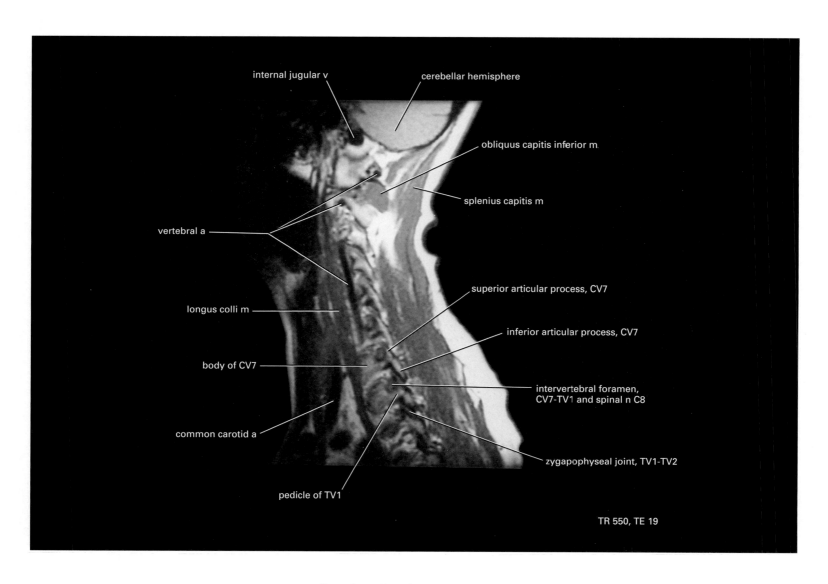

internal jugular v

cerebellar hemisphere

obliquus capitis inferior m

splenius capitis m

vertebral a

superior articular process, CV7

longus colli m

inferior articular process, CV7

body of CV7

intervertebral foramen, CV7-TV1 and spinal n C8

common carotid a

zygapophyseal joint, TV1-TV2

pedicle of TV1

TR 550, TE 19

Section R2 from midline.

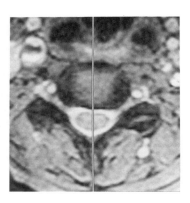

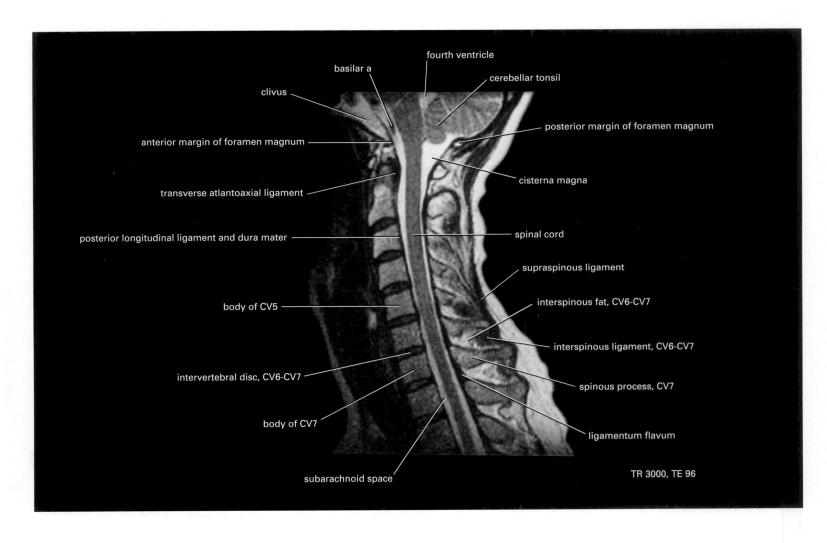

fourth ventricle

basilar a

clivus

cerebellar tonsil

posterior margin of foramen magnum

anterior margin of foramen magnum

cisterna magna

transverse atlantoaxial ligament

posterior longitudinal ligament and dura mater

spinal cord

supraspinous ligament

interspinous fat, CV6-CV7

body of CV5

interspinous ligament, CV6-CV7

intervertebral disc, CV6-CV7

spinous process, CV7

body of CV7

ligamentum flavum

subarachnoid space

TR 3000, TE 96

Section R3 from midline.

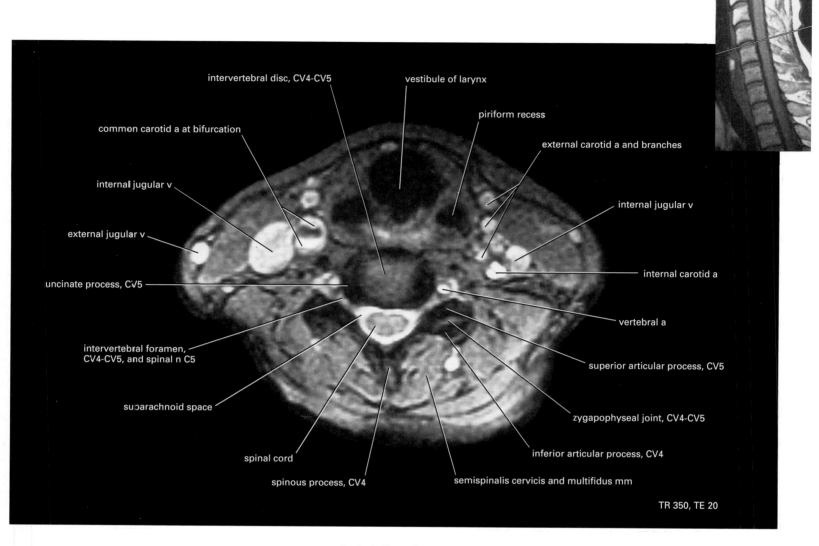

Axial Section 1.

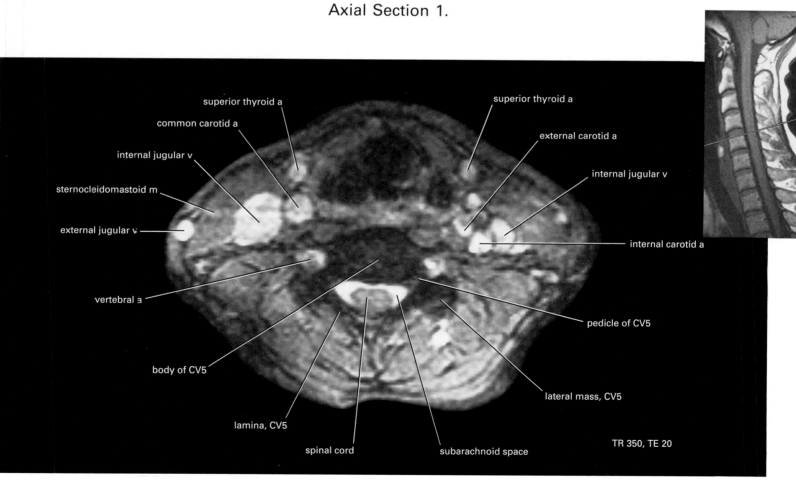

Axial Section 2.

The Thoracic Spine in Sagittal and Axial Planes

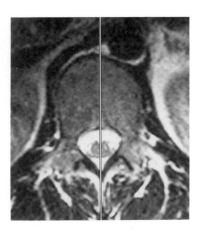

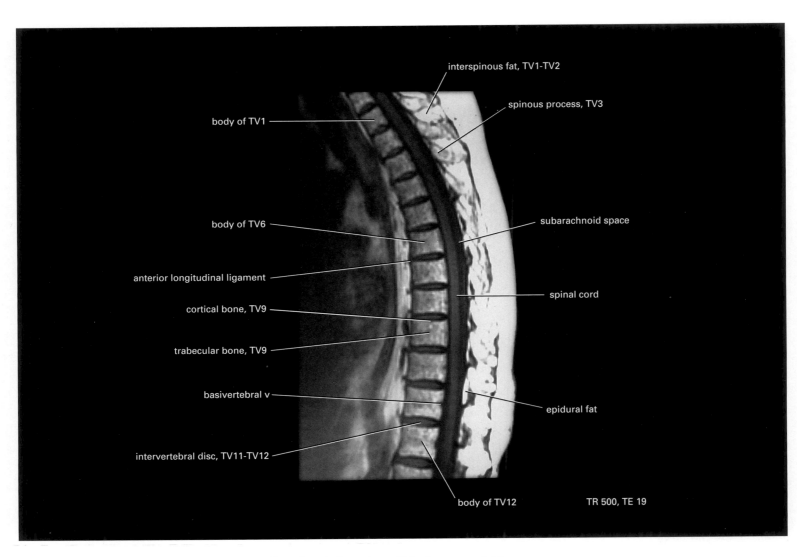

interspinous fat, TV1-TV2

spinous process, TV3

body of TV1

subarachnoid space

body of TV6

anterior longitudinal ligament

spinal cord

cortical bone, TV9

trabecular bone, TV9

basivertebral v

epidural fat

intervertebral disc, TV11-TV12

body of TV12

TR 500, TE 19

Sagittal Section R1 from midline.

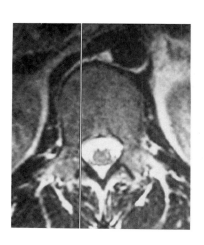

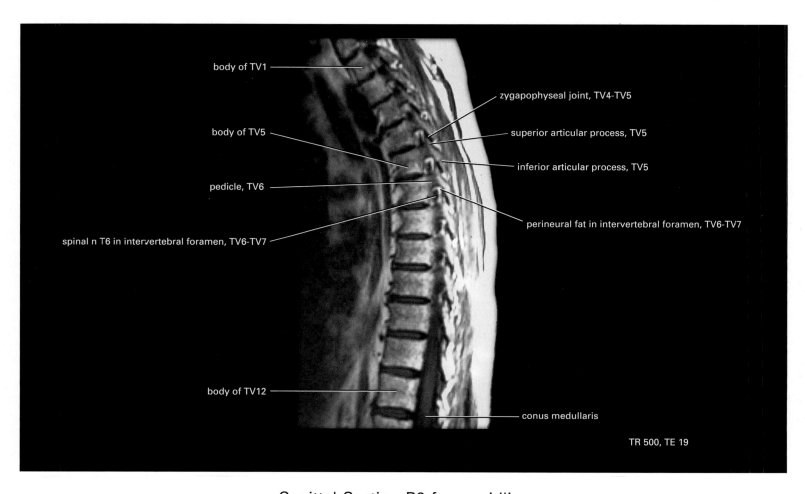

body of TV1 ———	
	zygapophyseal joint, TV4-TV5
body of TV5 ———	superior articular process, TV5
	inferior articular process, TV5
pedicle, TV6 ———	
	perineural fat in intervertebral foramen, TV6-TV7
spinal n T6 in intervertebral foramen, TV6-TV7 ———	
body of TV12 ———	
	conus medullaris

TR 500, TE 19

Sagittal Section R2 from midline.

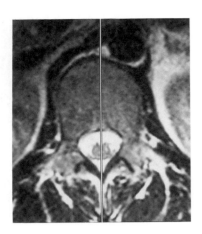

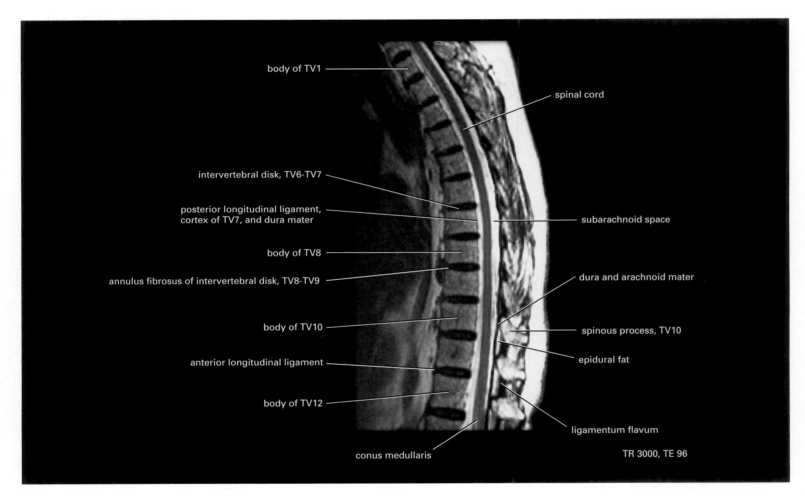

body of TV1

spinal cord

intervertebral disk, TV6-TV7

posterior longitudinal ligament,
cortex of TV7, and dura mater

subarachnoid space

body of TV8

annulus fibrosus of intervertebral disk, TV8-TV9

dura and arachnoid mater

body of TV10

spinous process, TV10

anterior longitudinal ligament

epidural fat

body of TV12

conus medullaris

ligamentum flavum

TR 3000, TE 96

Sagittal Section R3 from midline.

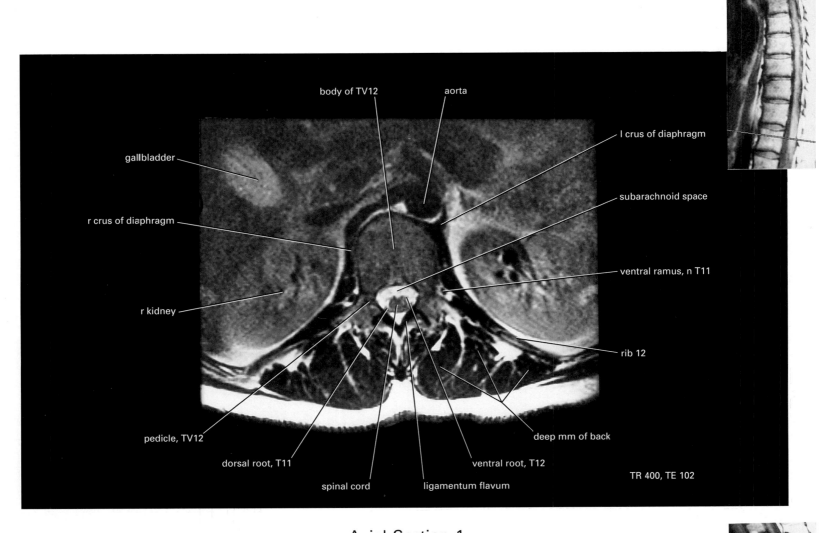

Axial Section 1.

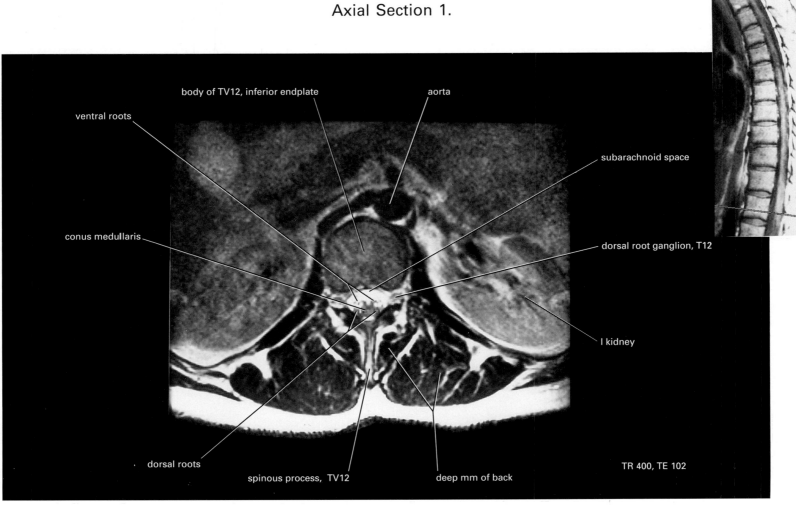

Axial Section 2.

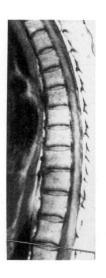

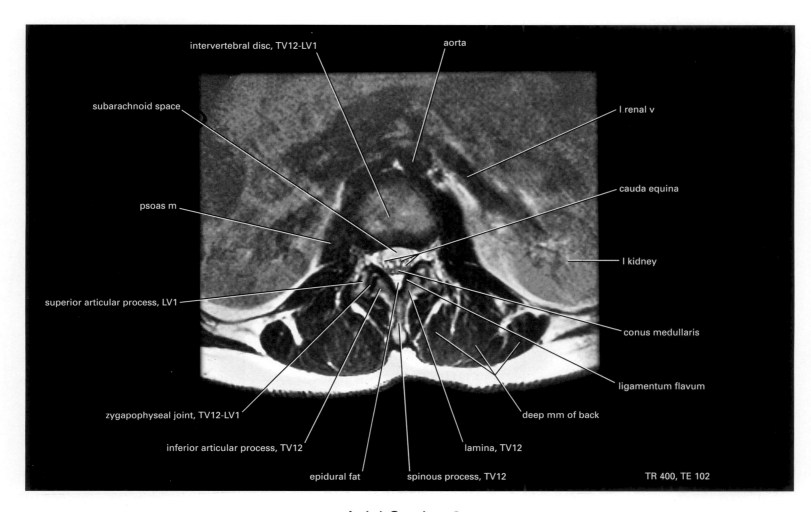

intervertebral disc, TV12-LV1

aorta

subarachnoid space

l renal v

cauda equina

psoas m

l kidney

superior articular process, LV1

conus medullaris

ligamentum flavum

zygapophyseal joint, TV12-LV1

deep mm of back

inferior articular process, TV12

lamina, TV12

epidural fat

spinous process, TV12

TR 400, TE 102

Axial Section 3.

The Lumbar Spine in Sagittal, Axial, and Coronal Planes

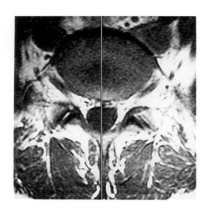

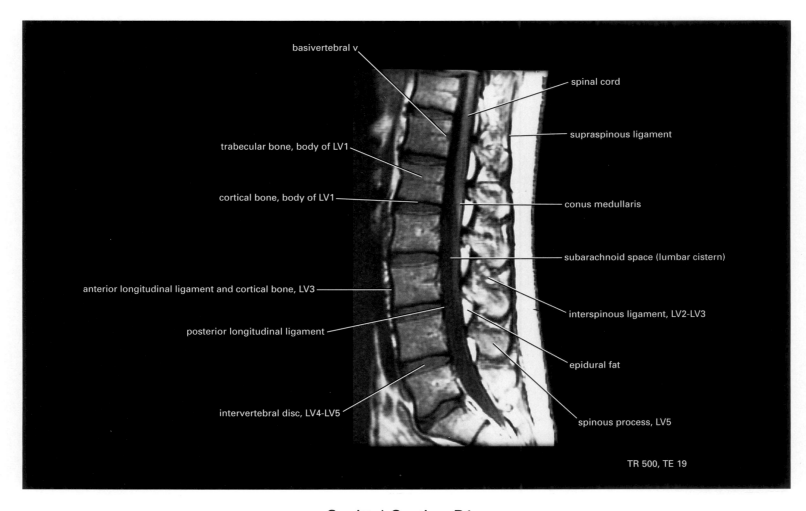

basivertebral v

spinal cord

trabecular bone, body of LV1

supraspinous ligament

cortical bone, body of LV1

conus medullaris

subarachnoid space (lumbar cistern)

anterior longitudinal ligament and cortical bone, LV3

posterior longitudinal ligament

interspinous ligament, LV2-LV3

epidural fat

intervertebral disc, LV4-LV5

spinous process, LV5

TR 500, TE 19

Sagittal Section R1.

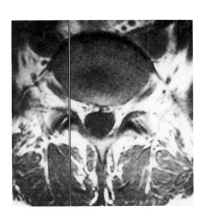

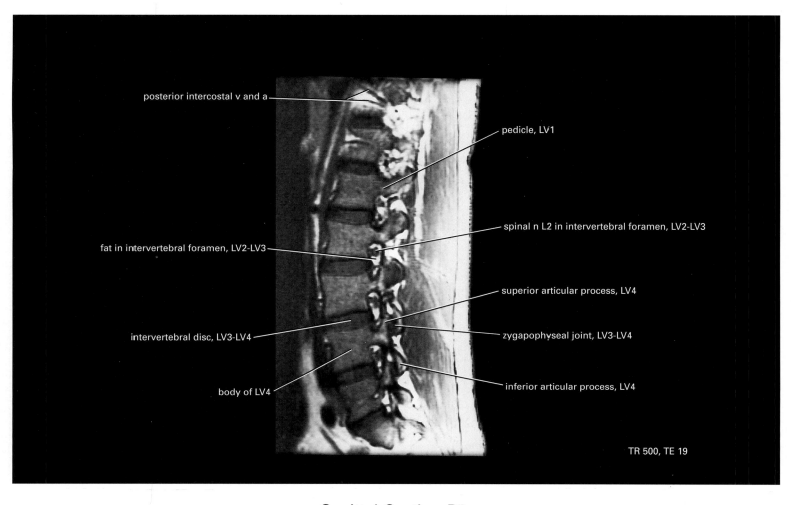

posterior intercostal v and a

pedicle, LV1

spinal n L2 in intervertebral foramen, LV2-LV3

fat in intervertebral foramen, LV2-LV3

superior articular process, LV4

intervertebral disc, LV3-LV4

zygapophyseal joint, LV3-LV4

body of LV4

inferior articular process, LV4

TR 500, TE 19

Sagittal Section R2.

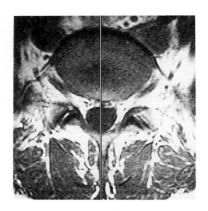

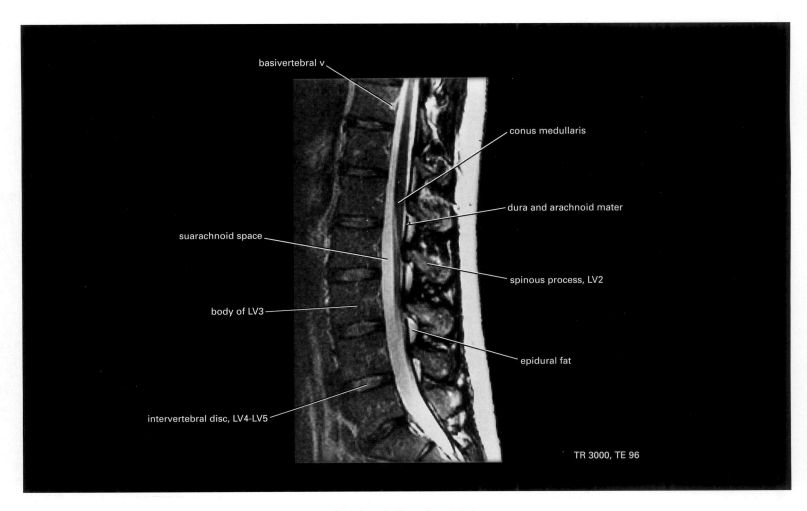

basivertebral v

conus medullaris

dura and arachnoid mater

suarachnoid space

spinous process, LV2

body of LV3

epidural fat

intervertebral disc, LV4-LV5

TR 3000, TE 96

Sagittal Section R3.

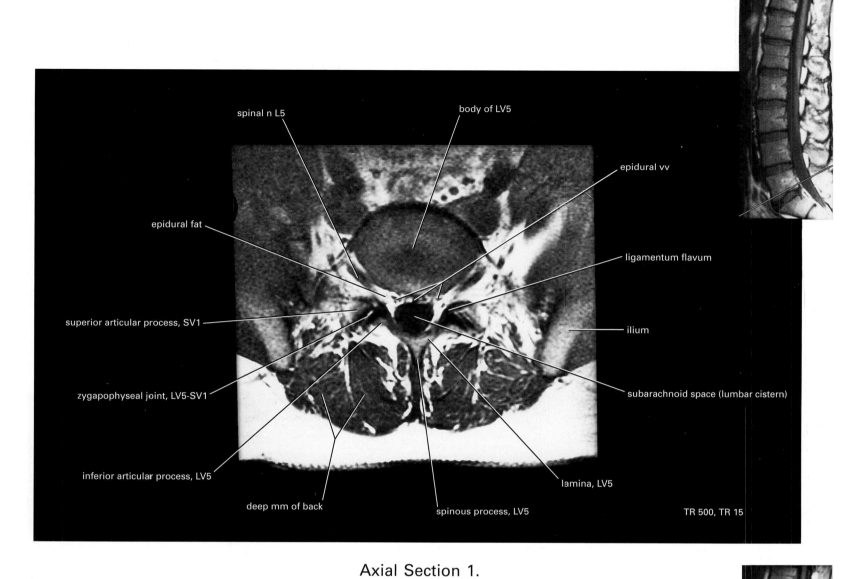

spinal n L5

body of LV5

epidural vv

epidural fat

ligamentum flavum

superior articular process, SV1

ilium

zygapophyseal joint, LV5-SV1

subarachnoid space (lumbar cistern)

inferior articular process, LV5

lamina, LV5

deep mm of back

spinous process, LV5

TR 500, TR 15

Axial Section 1.

intervertebral disc, LV5-SV1

epidural vv

superior articular process, SV1

spinal n L5

fat in intervertebral foramen, LV5-SV1

zygapophyseal joint, LV5-SV1

spinal n S1

inferior articular process, LV5

epidural fat

ligamentum flavum

lamina, LV5

subarachnoid space (lumbar cistern)

spinous process, LV5

TR 500, TE 15

Axial Section 2.

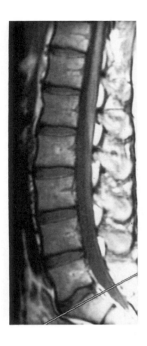

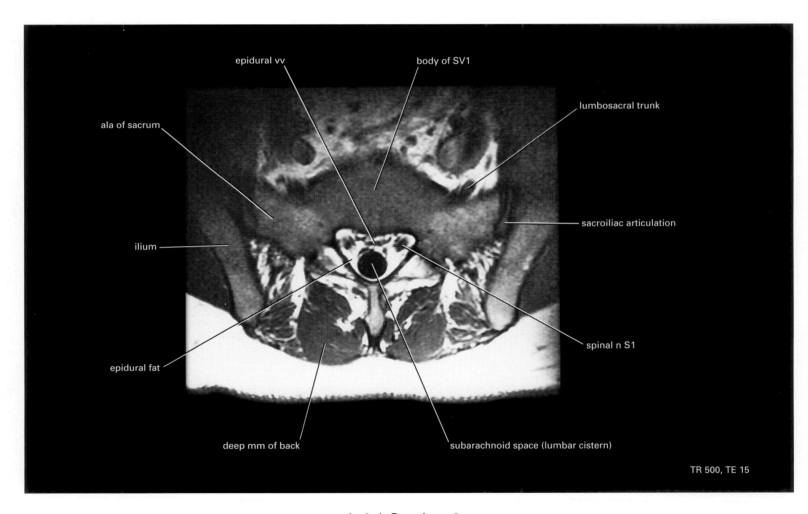

epidural vv   body of SV1

lumbosacral trunk

ala of sacrum

sacroiliac articulation

ilium

spinal n S1

epidural fat

deep mm of back   subarachnoid space (lumbar cistern)

TR 500, TE 15

Axial Section 3.

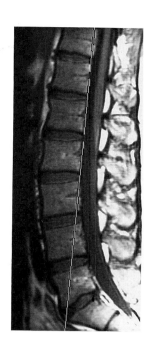

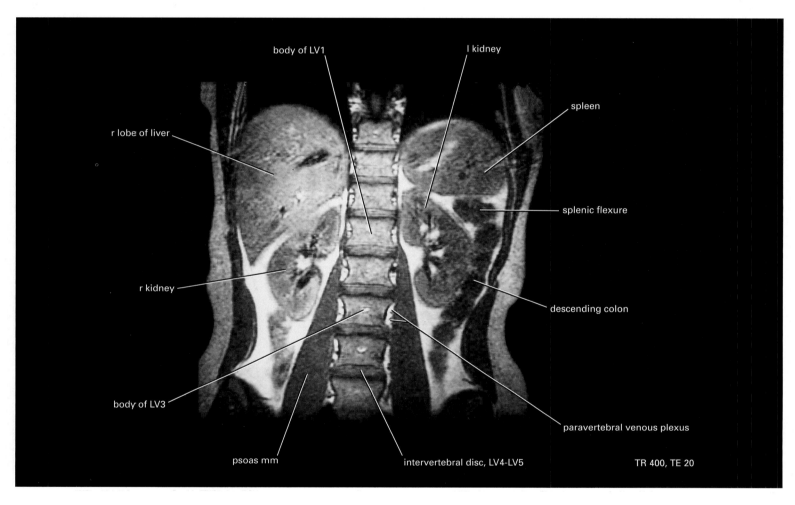

body of LV1

l kidney

spleen

r lobe of liver

splenic flexure

r kidney

descending colon

body of LV3

paravertebral venous plexus

psoas mm

intervertebral disc, LV4-LV5

TR 400, TE 20

Coronal Section 1.

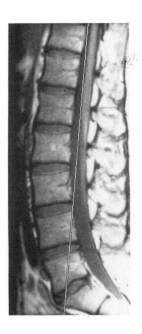

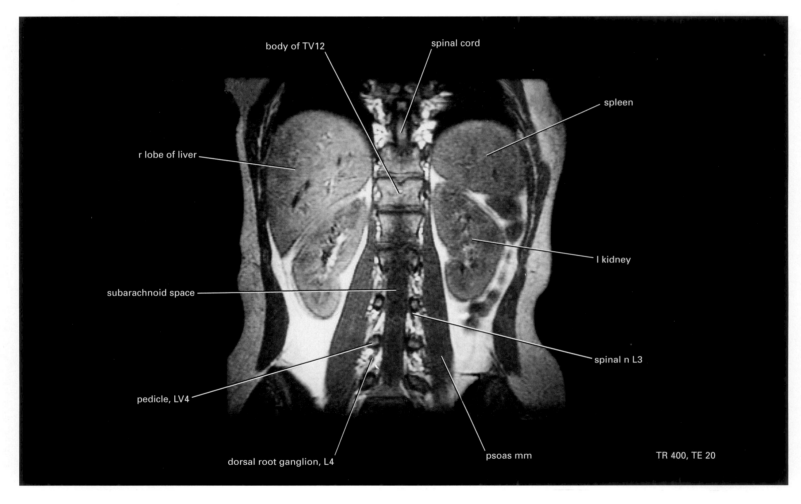

Coronal Section 2.

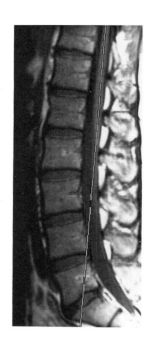

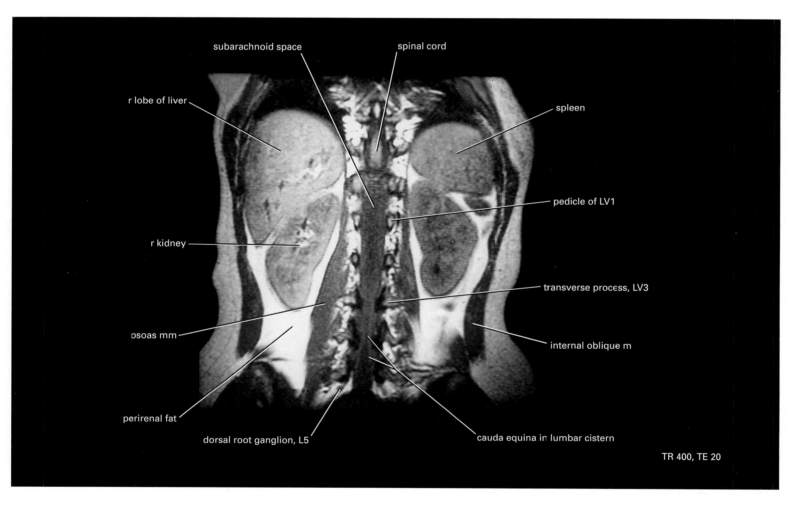

subarachnoid space

spinal cord

r lobe of liver

spleen

r kidney

pedicle of LV1

transverse process, LV3

psoas mm

internal oblique m

perirenal fat

dorsal root ganglion, L5

cauda equina in lumbar cistern

TR 400, TE 20

Coronal Section 3.

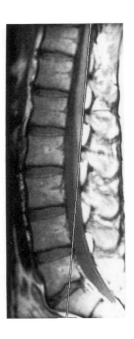

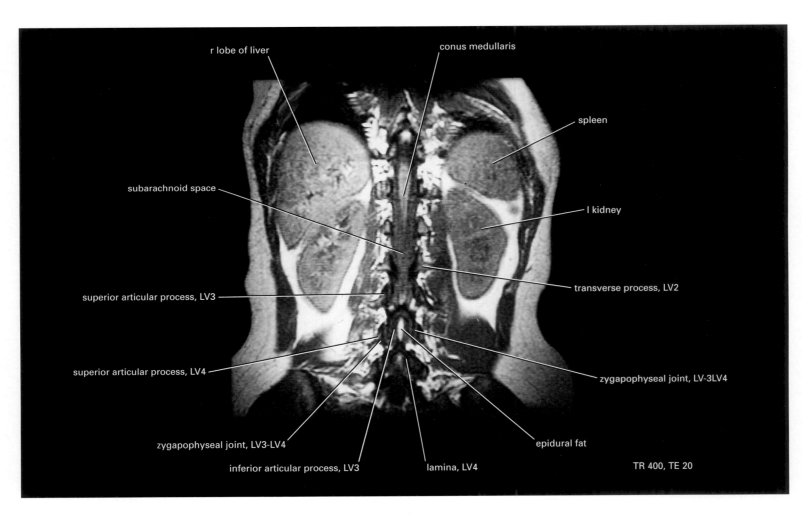

Coronal Section 4.

Index

Dura mater, 37, 42, 215, 231, 245, 249, 275, 282, 288, 294
    at foramen magnum, 275

Ear,
    inner, 249
        vestibule of, 275
    lobule of, 211
    tragus of, 204
Elbow, joint space of, 145
Epicondyle,
    of humerus,
        lateral, 144
        medial, 144
Epiglottis, 217, 219, 223, 227, 233, 275
    cut edge of, 220
Esophagus, 4–19, 22–23, 223, 233
Ethmoid bone,
    perpendicular plate of, 188, 190, 202–203, 254–255, 258–259
Eye, 190, 200–204, 241–243, 247
Eye lid, upper, 201

Falx cerebelli, 184–186
Falx cerebri, 177–186, 193–200, 204, 219, 227, 229, 257, 260–261, 266–267, 271, 275
Fascia,
    antebrachial, 146
    brachial, 140–143
    cervical investing, 190, 213, 219
    crural, 104–107
    gluteal, 53, 57–60, 70–81, 85
    inferior, of urogenital diaphragm, 66
    ischiorectal, 86
    lata, 90–91, 94, 96–99
    renal, 44
    superficial, 140–144, 146, 148, 151, 153–154
    temporalis, 186, 189, 205, 269
    thoracolumbar, 23, 25, 28, 33–37, 44
    transverse, deep, 108–109
Fasiculus, superior fronto–occipital, 196
Fat,
    epicardial, 13–14, 16–18, 23
    epidural, 286, 288, 292, 295–296, 300
        posterior, 290, 294
    extraperitoneal, 44
    in intercondylar notch of femur, 135
    interspinous,
        CV5-CV6, 280
        CV6-CV7, 282
        TV1-TV2, 286
    in intervertebral foramen, 287, 293, 295
    orbital, 198–202, 205, 247, 256–257, 260–261
    palatine, 241
    parapharyngeal, 207, 211–212
    pararenal, 26, 28–29, 42, 44
    perineural, 287
    periorbital, 203
    peripharyngeal, 268
    perirenal, 299
    popliteal, 123, 134–137
    retropubic, 62
    subcutaneous, of scalp, 193–194
    temporal, 265
Fat pad,
    buccal, 207, 208–210, 212, 245, 256–257, 260–261, 265
    of heel, 108–109
    infrapatellar, 124–128, 131
    intrapatellar, 101–102, 130–132
    midpalmar, 155
    suprapatellar, 124–127, 130
Femur, 60–66, 84–94, 98–99, 123–124
    articular cartilage of, 124–126
    distal epiphyseal line of, 122
    head of, 60–63, 78, 80–84
        ligament of, 62, 80, 82
    intercondylar notch of, fat in, 135
    lateral condyle of, 126–128, 130–134, 136
        facet for, 130
    medial condyle of, 120–123, 130–35
    neck of, 62–64, 84–86
    popliteal surface of, 126–127
    shaft of, 123, 125–127, 131–133

cortical bone of, 131
    trabecular bone of, 131
Fibula, 103–111
    head of, 103–104, 106, 109–110, 127–128, 134–136
    neck of, 127
Fimbria,
    of hippocampus, 180, 185, 243
    of uterine tube, 75–76
Fissure,
    choroid, 183, 199, 225, 242–243, 246, 276
    horizontal, 12–14
    labial (oral), 212, 241
    lateral, 273
    longitudinal, 177–180, 182, 184, 193–196, 240, 256–257, 265, 273, 277
    oblique, 8–19, 22–23, 158, 168–169
    orbital,
        inferior, 259
        superior, 188–190, 201–202, 237, 263
    palpebral, 247, 251
    pterygomaxillary, 205, 237
    sylvian, 199
Flexure,
    hepatic, 30, 37, 45, 49
    splenic, 22–24, 42, 297
Floculus, of cerebellum, 205
Fold(s),
    aryepiglottic, 233
    axillary, posterior, 10
    glossoepiglottic, median, 219
    rectal, transverse, 59
    sublingual, 215
Foramen(ina),
    epiploic, 28
    infraorbital, 237
    interventricular, 182, 198, 229, 273
    intervertebral,
        CV2-CV3, 214
        CV4-CV5, 220, 283
        CV5-CV6, 237
        CV7-CV8, 281
        LV1-LV2, 28–29
        LV2-LV3, 28, 32, 293
        LV5–S1, 295
        TV6-TV7, 287
    jugular, 189, 205–206, 245, 249
        intermediate septum of, 247
    lacerum, 190, 237, 267
    magnum, 190, 208, 226–227, 231, 275
        anterior margin of, 282
        posterior margin of, 280, 282
    mandibular, 249
    mental, 237
    obturator, 86
    ovale, 190, 204, 267, 269
    rotundum, 263
    sacral,
        pelvic,
            SV1, 54–55
            SV3, 57
    sciatic, greater, 73
    sphenopalatine, 204, 259
    spinosum, 190
    stylomastoid, 190, 207
    transverse, 3, 211, 217, 220, 223, 245
Fornix(ices), 197, 228–229
    of brain
        body of, 180–181, 197, 273, 277
        columns of, 181–184, 198–200, 273
        crus of, 181, 198–199
    vaginal,
        lateral, 84–85
        posterior, 82
Fossa,
    acetabular, 60, 80
    cranial,
        anterior, 187, 254–255, 258
        middle, 204, 262–263, 267
        posterior, 189, 206–207, 209
    incisive, 211, 227
    infracapsular, 172
    infratemporal, 204–205
        roof of, 190

interpeduncular, 185, 229, 277
ischiorectal, 62–66, 82, 84–85, 87–94
jugular, anterior wall of, 275
mandibular, 205, 271
    ovalis, 16
    popliteal, 98
    pterygoid, 208, 263
    pterygopalatine, 190, 204, 259
popliteal, 125–126, 134, 136
scapular,
    infraspinous, 158–159, 173
    supraspinous, 158–159
subscapular, 173
suprascapular, floor of, 170–171
Frontal bone, 177–184, 186, 188–189, 193–199, 222–223, 226–227, 236, 244–245, 248–249, 254–255, 258–259, 262–263, 266
    nasal process of, 200
    near coronal suture, 237
    orbital part of, 187
    zygomatic process of, 200–201
Frontal lobe, 198
Fundus,
    of gallbladder, 35
    of stomach, 23–24
    of uterus, 75

Galea aponeurotica, 265
Gallbladder, 30, 32, 33–35, 43–45, 48–49, 289
    neck of, 30–31
Ganglion(a),
    aorticorenal, 3, 44
    celiac, 26–27, 43
    dorsal root, 29
        C2, 225
        C3, 243
        C4, 243
        C5, 247
        C6, 247
        C7, 247
        C8, 225, 247
        L1, 29
        L3, 34–35
        L4, 36–37, 298
        L5, 299
        T1, 4
        T12, 43, 289
    geniculate, 205
    mesenteric,
        inferior, 33
        superior, 28
    sympathetic, 7–8
        superior cervical, 212, 214, 216, 243, 277
    trigeminal, 188–189, 202, 225, 243, 273
Genu,
    of corpus callosum, 180–183, 197–198, 229, 234–235, 260, 265
    of internal capsule, 182, 224–225, 243
Gland(s)
    lacrimal, 188–189, 201, 248, 251, 257
    of palate (palatine),
        hard, 241, 261
        soft, 264–265, 267
    parotid, 190, 207–217, 251, 271–272, 276–277
    pineal, 199, 229
    pituitary, 202, 228, 268–269; see also Stalk, hypophysial
        anterior, 227
        posterior, 229
    prostate, 62–64
    sublingual, 216–218, 223, 261
    submandibular, 215–220, 247, 251, 260, 264–266, 271, 275
        deep process of, 241, 265, 267
    suprarenal (adrenal),
        left, 26–28, 42–43
        right, 24–27, 42–43
    thyroid, 4–7, 241
    vestibular, greater, 92–93
Globus pallidus, 182–184, 198–199, 224–225, 243, 273, 277
Glomus choroideum, 181, 199, 225, 247
Gray matter, periaqueductal, 184, 201